Superficial Bladder Cancer

Edited by

Francesco Pagano
*Department of Urology, University of Padova,
Padova, Italy*

William R. Fair
*Urology Service, Department of Surgery,
Memorial Sloan-Kettering Cancer Center,
New York, USA*

Editorial Co-ordinator

Pierfrancesco Bassi
*Department of Urology, University of Padova,
Padova, Italy*

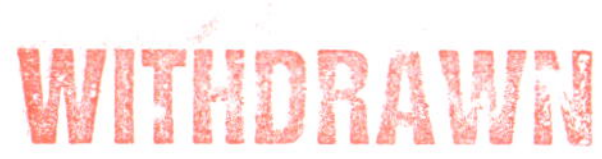

I S I S
MEDICAL
M E D I A

—

Oxford

Typeset by
Creative Associates, Oxford, UK

Printed and bound by
GZ Printek S.A.L., Bilbao, Spain

Distributed by
Oxford University Press, Saxon Way West,
Corby, Northamptonshire NN18 9ES, UK

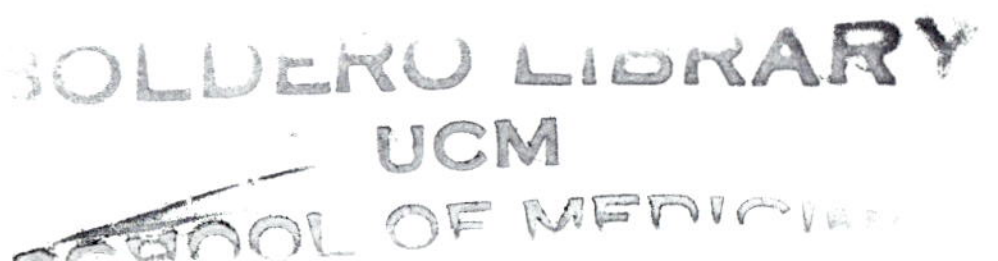

Contents

List of contributors

Giuseppe Abatangelo
Department of Urology, University of Padova, Via Giustiniani 2, Padova, Italy

Paul D. Abel
*Reader and Honorary Consultant Urologist, Department of Surgery, Royal
Postgraduate Medical School, Hammersmith Hospitals and Ealing Hospital Trust,
Du Cane Road, London, UK*

Friedrich Balck
*Professor of Psychosomatic Medicine, Department of Psychosomatic Medicine and
Psychotherapy, Medical University of Lübeck, Germany*

Pierfrancesco Bassi
Department of Urology, University of Padova, Via Giustiniani 2, Padova, Italy

Andreas Böhle
Assistant Professor of Urology, Department of Urology, University of Lübeck, Germany

Christian R. A. G. Bouffioux
*Professor, Medical Director, University Hospital of Liege, Medical Direction, CHU Sart
Tilman, Liege, Belgium*

Peter Boyle
*Professor and Director, Division of Epidemiology and Biostatistics, European Institute
of Oncology, Via Ripamonti 435, Milan, Italy*

Peter A. Cybulski
*Division of Urology, The University of Toronto and The Toronto Hospital, 200 Elizabeth
Street, EN14-205, Toronto, Ontario, Canada*

Guido Dalbagni
*Assistant Attending Surgeon, Memorial Sloan-Kettering Cancer Center, New York,
NY, USA*

Frans M. J. Debruyne
*Professor and Chairman, Department of Urology, University Hospital Nijmegen,
Geert Grooteplein 16, P.O. Box 9101, Nijmegen, The Netherlands*

Theo M. de Reijke
*Department of Urology, Academic Medical Center, University of Amsterdam,
Meibergdreef 9, Amsterdam, The Netherlands*

William R. Fair
Chief, Urologic Surgery, Memorial Sloan-Kettering Cancer Center, 1275 York Avenue, New York; Professor of Urology, Cornell University Medical Center, New York, USA

Yves Fradet
Professor of Urology, Laval University Cancer Research Center, L'Hotel-Dieu de Quebec, 11 cote du Palais, Quebec, Canada

Dieter Jocham
Professor and Chairman, Department of Urology, University of Lübeck, Germany

Michael A. S. Jewett
Professor and Chairman, Division of Urology, The University of Toronto and The Toronto Hospital, 200 Elizabeth Street, EN14-205, Toronto, Ontario, Canada

Gholam R. Khakpour
Division of Urology, The University of Toronto and The Toronto Hospital, 200 Elizabeth Street, EN14-205, Toronto, Ontario, Canada

Karlheinz Kurth
Professor and Chairman, Department of Urology, Academic Medical Center, University of Amsterdam, Meibergdreef 9, Amsterdam, The Netherlands

Donald L. Lamm
Professor and Chairman, Department of Urology, Robert C. Byrd Health Sciences Center of West Virginia University, P.O. Box 9651, Morgantown, West Virginia, USA

Patrick Maisonneuve
Deputy Director, Division of Epidemiology and Biostatistics, European Institute of Oncology, Via Ripamonti 435, Milan, Italy

J. Mansel Harris
Assistant Professor of Surgery, Division of Urology, University of Texas Health Science Center, 7703 Floyd Curl Drive, San Antonio, Texas, USA

William M. Murphy
Professor of Pathology, Department of Pathology, Immunology and Laboratory Medicine, University of Florida, College of Medicine, P.O. Box 100275, Gainesville, Florida, USA

Pavel Napalkov
Head, Urological Carcinogenesis Programme, Division of Epidemiology and Biostatistics, European Institute of Oncology, Via Ripamonti 435, Milan, Italy

Francesco Pagano
Department of Urology, University of Padova, Via Giustiniani 2, Padova, Italy

Gianluigi Pappagallo
Division of Medical Oncology, Clinical Trials Office, Noale, Italy

Nicola Piazza
Department of Urology, University of Padova, Via Giustiniani 2, Padova, Italy

Michael F. Sarosdy
Professor of Surgery; Chief, Division of Urology, University of Texas Health Science Center, 7703 Floyd Curl Drive, San Antonio, Texas, USA

Jack A. Schalken
Professor and Research Director, Department of Urology, University Hospital Nijmegen, Geert Grooteplein 16, P.O. Box 9101, Nijmegen, The Netherlands

R. Sylvester
EORTC Data Center, Avenue E. Mounier, 1200, Brussels, Belgium

Adrian P.M. van der Meijden
Department of Urology, Ziekengasthuis, Bosch Medicentrum, P.O. Box 90153, Den Bosch, The Netherlands

H. G. van der Poel
Department of Urology, University Hospital Nijmegen, Geert Grooteplein 16, P.O. Box 9101, Nijmegen, The Netherlands

Jorn von Wietersheim
Department of Psychosomatic Medicine and Psychotherapy, Medical University of Lübeck, Germany

J. A. Witjes
Department of Urology, University Hospital Nijmegen, Geert Grooteplein 16, P.O. Box 9101, Nijmegen, The Netherlands

Preface

Intravesical therapy of superficial bladder cancer represents one of the most successful achievements in the treatment of solid tumours in humans before the end of the century.

During the last decade, the urological community has witnessed a steady accumulation of knowledge related to endocavitary therapy together with an improvement in the results obtained, in both short- and long-term tumour control, and in the control of disease progression. Progress in the field of topical therapy has rendered superficial bladder cancer one of the major fast-developing areas in oncology, while also providing better clarification and more thorough exploration of many other aspects.

Some of the changing concepts urologists have been faced with recently include: a critical reassessment of intravesical chemotherapy; the more extensive use of immunotherapy; the onset of new BRMs (also active by oral route); new modalities (laser, PDT) and new approaches (combination chemo-immunotherapy). The fall-out of these new therapeutic strategies is heralding substantial innovations in the management of bladder cancer by opening new pathways and promoting new approaches. Some of these innovative treatment modalities may also be adopted in many other oncological diseases.

As a consequence of this endless achievement, both from a clinical point of view and from the researcher's perspective, urologists feel the need for periodical and comprehensive evaluation in order to understand where all these developments are taking us. The main purpose of this book is to offer the reader an up-date of the major advances achieved over the last few years as well as possible future developments. The book reports the most significant improvements in almost every field of the current knowledge on superficial bladder cancer, spanning from molecular biology to the most sophisticated forms of disease management.

For this reason, we hope that this book will provide both the experienced urologist in clinical practice and the resident in training with the most up-to-date criteria which may be incorporated into the clinical management of superficial bladder cancer. Hopefully, it will also act as a catalyst for further research innovation in a field which has proven to be more fertile than many others in the realm of solid tumours.

Francesco Pagano
William R. Fair

CHAPTER 1

Epidemiology of bladder cancer

P. Napalkov, P. Maisonneuve and P. Boyle

Introduction

There are few epidemiological studies on the topic of superficial bladder cancer and little is known about the epidemiology of this independent entity; hence this chapter will focus on what is known about bladder cancer.

Cancer of the urinary bladder is, overall, the eleventh most common form of cancer world-wide. Bladder cancer exhibits moderate international variation in incidence, although, to some extent, the differences may be dependent on whether so-called 'benign papillomas' of the bladder are included with the overtly malignant neoplasms. It was estimated that in 1985 there was a total of 243,000 incident cases, of which the estimated 182,000 in men and 51,000 in women represented 4.7% and 1.3% of their total cancer burden, respectively [1]. If the prevalence of bladder cancer is defined to include cancer patients who are alive between up to 5 years after diagnosis there are an estimated 781,000 patients throughout the world with bladder cancer who require medical care [2]. Transitional-cell carcinomas comprise more than 90% of bladder cancers in western countries, and most of the remainder are squamous-cell carcinomas [3,4]. In contrast, the prevalence of squamous-cell carcinoma is considerably higher in Egypt and the Middle East where infection by *Schistosoma Haematobium* is endemic.

Descriptive epidemiology of bladder cancer

Geographical differences in incidence rates

The five highest rates of bladder cancer in men are found in regions of Italy: Trieste (34.0 per 100,000), Florence (33.5), Torino (32.6), Varese (31.0) and Romagna (30.3) (Table 1.1). Other high rates are recorded from white population groups of the United States, the Basque country of Spain and Denmark. Low incidence rates are recorded from populations of the developing world. In women, the incidence rates are much lower than in men; the highest in women (7.4) would rank 138th out of 166 in men. Of potential interest are the high rates in women in Scotland where three of the regions (west, south-east and north-east) have rates among the ten highest recorded. Rates are elevated in several industrialized countries particularly Italy and

Table 1.1 Ten highest and lowest incidence rates of bladder cancer internationally c1983 to c1990.

	Bladder, male ICD9 188 registry	Cases	Rate*	Bladder, female ICD9 188 registry	Cases	Rate
Highest	Italy, Trieste	181	34.0	US, New Orleans: White	208	7.4
	Italy, Florence	1036	33.5	UK, West Scotland	1029	7.3
	Italy, Torino	765	32.6	US, Detroit: White	940	7.3
	Italy, Varese	823	31.0	US, S.E. Scotland	439	7.0
	Italy, Romagna	242	30.3	US, Connecticut: White	973	6.9
	US, Detroit: White	2512	27.1	Kuwait: Non-Kuwaitis	29	6.8
	US, Hawaii: White	209	27.1	Denmark	1719	6.7
	US, New Orleans: White	539	26.8	Italy, Trieste	64	6.7
	Spain, Basque Country	688	26.4	UK, N.E. Scotland	179	6.7
	Denmark	5327	26.3	Canada, Quebec	1596	6.6
Lowest	Peru, Trujillo	16	3.7	India, Ahmedabad	35	0.8
	Philippines, Rizal	115	3.7	Paraguay, Asuncion	13	0.8
	Thailand, Khon Kaen	33	3.7	Israel: Non-Jews	6	0.7
	India, Bombay	412	3.6	The Gambia	2	0.7
	India, Ahmedabad	145	3.5	Kyrgyzstan	26	0.6
	India, Bangladore	150	3.3	India, Madras	33	0.6
	Algeria, Setif	24	2.2	India, Bangalore	21	0.5
	US, Los Angeles: Filipino	10	1.8	US, Los Angeles: Korean	1	0.4
	The Gambia	9	1.8	Thailand, Khon Kaen	4	0.3
	India, Madras	97	1.8	Algeria, Setif	2	0.2

Source: Parkin DM, Muir CS, Whelan S, Gao YT, Ferlay J and Powell J (eds) Cancer Incidence in Five Continents, Vol VI (IARC Scientific Publication No.120). Lyon: International Agency for Research on Cancer, 1992.
*Annual average, age-adjusted incidence rate per 100,000 people (years).

Switzerland. For a large number of registries in the remainder of Europe and North America, rates are a little lower. The lowest rates occur in Asia, notably in India. Rates in Japan are slightly higher. Other populations with high levels in women include white populations of the United States (Table 1.1).

Bladder cancer is also frequent in countries of the Middle East and Africa where *schistosomiasis* is endemic. For example, it accounts for some 29% of all cancer in males and 11% of those in females reported to the Cairo Metropolitan Cancer Registry. In Baghdad, bladder cancer accounts for 13% of all malignant neoplasms in males [5]. A predominance of squamous-cell carcinomas is observed in areas where bladder cancer is related to schistosomiasis in contrast to the overwhelming preponderance of transitional-cell tumours seen elsewhere [6,7]. In the Bulawayo region of Zimbabwe 71% of all bladder cancer cases were squamous-cell carcinomas and 28% of bladder cancers were attributable to schistosomiasis [8]. A study from Egypt demonstrated recent changes in the *Schistosoma*-associated bladder cancer.

There is a shift in pathological findings from predominantly squamous-cell types towards transitional-cell types which is paralleled by an increased incidence of low-degree schistosomal infestation [6]. Nonetheless, the urothelial/squamous ratio varies greatly, being 3 in Cali, Colombia; 7 in Birmingham, England; 30 in Alameda County; and 70 in Sweden, possibly due in part to differences in pathological interpretation [9]. Recent analysis of the SEER (Surveillance Epidemiology and End Results Programme) data from the United States demonstrated that transitional-cell carcinoma accounts for 93.6% of all urinary bladder cancers. The ratio of transitional-cell carcinomas to squamous-cell carcinomas was 45 to 1 and to adenocarcinomas 67 to 1. The proportion of squamous-cell carcinoma increase among both sexes with age, reaching 2.1% among males and 4.4% among females in patients of 85 years and older [4].

Race

Rates for Afro-Americans are uniformly about half those in white Americans, apparently due in part to an under-reporting of early-stage tumours [10]. Incidence data for a sufficiently long period of time for different races are available only from the few cancer registries in North America. For example, in Alameda County (California) between 1963 and 1988, age-adjusted incidence rates from bladder cancer increased among both white (Caucasian) men and black (African–American) men with the incidence rate almost two times higher in white men throughout the period of observation (Fig. 1.1). Although the incidence rates for white women remained fairly stable throughout the whole period of observation they were higher than in Afro-American women. Differences in incidence rates around a factor of 1.5–2 between Afro-Americans and whites were also reported from the other cancer registries with a relatively long period of observation.

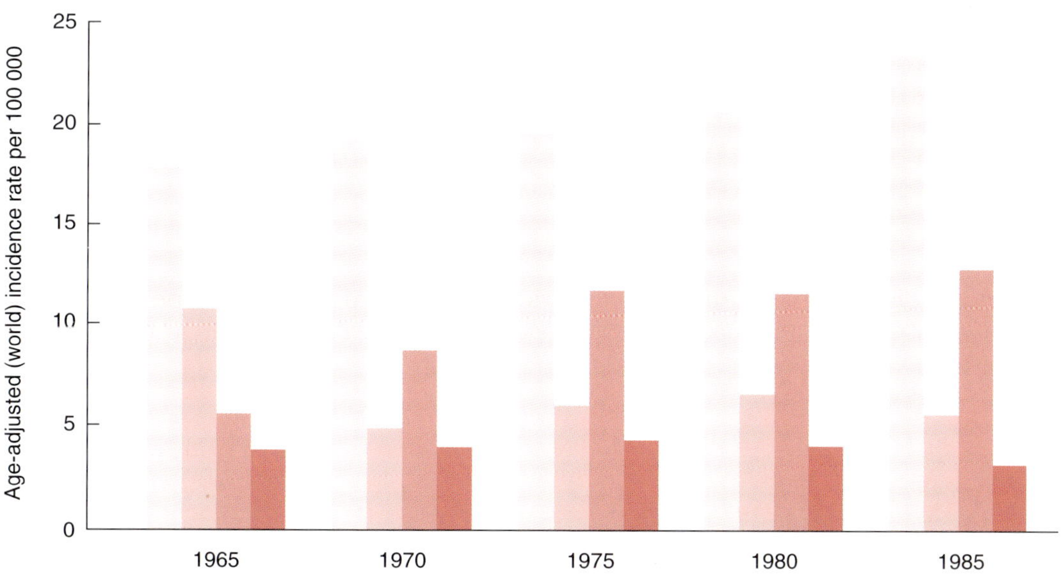

Figure 1.1. Trends in incidence rates of bladder cancer: USA, California, Alameda County (incidence rates age-adjusted, world-standardized, per 100 000). White, males; white, females; black, males; black, females. Data abstracted from: Parkin DM, Muir CS, Whelan S et al. (eds) Cancer Incidence in Five Continents, Vol VI (IARC Scientific Publication No.120). Lyon, International Agency for Research on Cancer, 1992.

While the incidence rate of bladder cancer in whites is considerably greater than in blacks, 72% of whites have localized disease at diagnosis as compared to 50% among blacks [11]. A study of the 1,860 bladder cancer cases and 3,934 population-based controls from the National Bladder Cancer Study showed that while non-whites were at a lower risk of non-invasive bladder cancer than whites (RR = 0.4), risk for invasive bladder cancer is similar among whites and non-whites (RR = 1.1), which may indicate racial differences in health practices related to bladder cancer detection [12]. Rates in Chinese and Japanese in the United States are comparable to those in African–Americans [1,13–16]. Rates among Hispanics residing in several regions of the United States are approximately half of those observed for non-Hispanic whites [17]. A study of 593 bladder cancer patients of known smoking status, and of randomly selected controls, demonstrated that ethnic differences in bladder cancer between Hispanics, Asians and non-Hispanic whites may be related to smoking and occupational exposures [18]. In a study from Hawaii the stage and histological grades of bladder cancer were compared among white and Japanese patients. It was found that grade-I papillary tumours comprised 43% of all bladder cancers in men of both races, and 37.5% in white and 31% in Japanese women [19]. These findings indicate that racial differences in the incidence of bladder cancer may not be accounted for only by increased numbers of superficial tumours diagnosed in whites. In a population of European origin living in Southern Africa for over 30 years the incidence rate of bladder cancer was unusually higher than normally seen in white populations in Europe and Northern America [20].

Age and incidence rates

There were about 1000 cases of bladder cancer before the age of 30 reported from 166 cancer registries around the world [1]. The average incidence rates (per 100,000) were less than one per 100 000 for men younger than 30 years of age and for women younger than 40 years. Similar to prostate and kidney cancer, bladder cancer exhibits an increasing incidence over the age of 50 [21]. The age-specific incidence rates increase dramatically after 40 years of age for both sexes and reach 107.9 for men and 25.6 for women in their late 60s, which is generally the median age for diagnosis of bladder cancer (Fig. 1.2). It appears that tumour behaviour may vary with age at presentation. However, bladder cancer potency for multifocal disease, recurrence and progression is more likely linked to the stage and grade at presentation rather than to age [22]. Several studies suggest that older patients are at increased risk for high-grade tumours which carry more aggressive tumour behaviour [23]. Bladder cancer progression rates in younger and older patients with similar tumour grades appears to be the same [24].

Gender differences in incidence rates

Women are much less affected by the disease than men [21]. In different populations the male to female ratio varies between 2 and 4, and the geographic variation is smaller among women than in men. In Egypt the male-female ratio changed from 7.8:1 in 1962–1967 to 4.9:1 in 1987–1992, which may be explained by more exposure of women to schistosomal infestation in the recent period [6]. In the National Bladder Cancer Study (National Cancer Institute, USA). which involved 2,806 white individuals

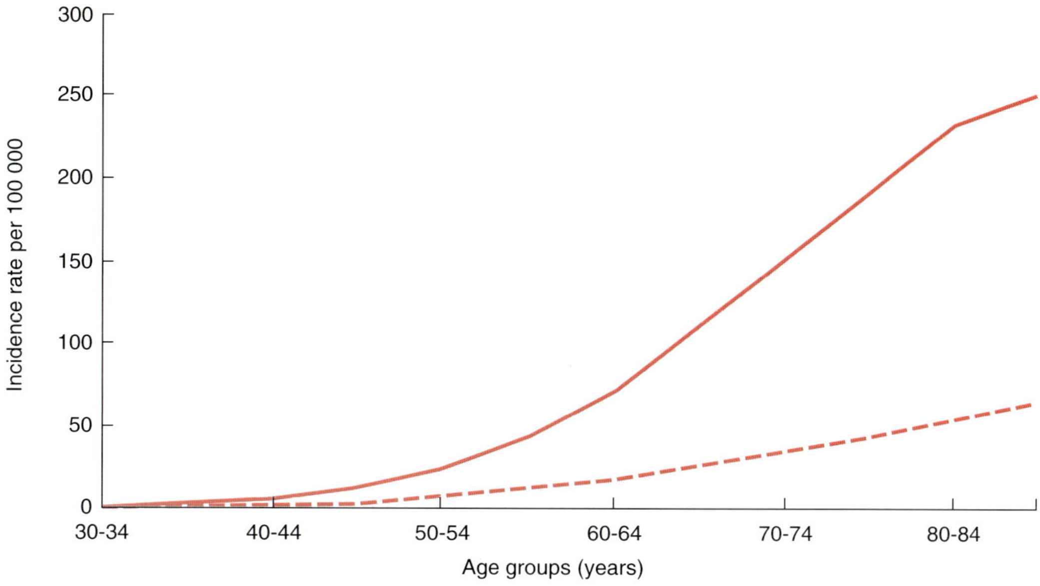

Figure 1.2. Age-specific incidence rates of bladder cancer from 166 cancer registries around the world (C83–C87). ——— males; - - - - females. Data abstracted from: Parkin DM, Muir CS, Whelan S et al (eds) Cancer Incidence in Five Continents, Vol VI (IARC Scientific Publication No. 120). Lyon, International Agency for Research on Cancer, 1992.

with bladder cancer and 5,258 controls, it was estimated that even in the absence of exposure to known carcinogenic factors (i.e. cigarettes and occupational factors) the risk of bladder cancer for men was almost three times higher than in women [25]. Anton-Culver *et al* [18] reported an even higher risk for bladder cancer associated with gender which reached 5.95 (95% CI 4.36–8.12) for males relative to females after adjustment for ethnicity, smoking status, occupation, and age. A study from Denmark showed significantly smaller increases in cohort-specific risk for bladder cancer in women than in men (3.7 vs. 6.1 times, respectively). Because the difference could not be explained by trends in tobacco consumption or occupational exposures, it was suggested, rather proactively, that women may be less susceptible than men to developing tobacco related bladder cancer [26]. There may be some previously unidentified environmental exposures, anatomic differences, or hormonal factors that can account for an apparent difference in bladder cancer incidence rates between men and women. Some laboratory studies suggest an influence of androgen and oestrogen hormones on oncogenesis in bladder tissue. It was demonstrated that parous women were at decreased risk relative to nulliparous women (OR = 0.67, 95% CI = 0.44–1.00), after adjustment for age, tobacco use, and previous bladder infection. This may indicate that oncogenesis in transitional cell tissue of the human bladder is influenced by sex hormones, and that hormonal changes related to pregnancy may decrease risk for developing bladder cancer [27].

Temporal trends in bladder cancer

Temporal trends in incidence of bladder cancer may be artefactually influenced by coding practices with regard to registration of 'bladder papilloma' changing with time. In The Netherlands the increase in incidence rates from 25.9 to 40.7 in males and from 3.1 to 8.5 in females observed between 1975 and 1989 has largely been caused by changed classification systems and reporting of non-invasive pTa tumours which were previously classified as papillomas [28].

The analysis of cohort-specific risks for both men and women from 1943 to 1987 in Denmark showed that risks increased in the beginning of the period, but then levelled off. There was no increase in risk for bladder cancer in the cohorts born after 1930. Another finding was the smaller increase in risk for women than for men which could not be explained by difference in smoking status or occupational exposures. The authors suggested that women may be less susceptible than men to developing bladder cancer attributable to smoking [26].

In the United States between 1973–1977 and 1983–1987 there has been a 17% increase in age-adjusted incidence rates among black males followed by a 16% increase in white males, and an 11% increase among white females. During the same period of observation there were no significant changes in incidence rates for black females. While there was a 14% increase in age-adjusted incidence rates for transitional-cell carcinoma in males a 10% increase for females, the rates for squamous-cell carcinoma and adenocarcinoma have not changed. There was an estimated 1% annual change in incidence for cancers of the urinary bladder among males and females of all races between 1973 and 1987 [4]. In Ontario (Canada) the comparison of age-adjusted incidence rates of bladder cancer between 1979 and 1983 and 1984–1988 showed a 2% increase for males, while the rate remained stable for females [29].

During a 15-year period between 1968 and 1982 there was a 2.3% increase in incidence among the Chinese male population of Singapore without any significant increase for females [30]. A similar increase of 2.3% for bladder cancer was reported during a 10-year period of observation between 1981 and 1990 for the male population in Bulgaria [31].

Notwithstanding, there are substantial increases reported in the incidence rates of bladder cancer in males with rates doubling over the two decades covered by incidence statistics in several regions (Table 1.2). The exception to this general rule may be the more interesting to investigate; in non-Maoris in New Zealand the incidence rate has remained fairly constant (Table 1.2). Incidence rates of bladder cancer for females increased slowly but steadily in different populations around the world (Table 1.3).

Mortality data from bladder cancer are freer from the possible confounding effects of international variation in coding practice *vis-à-vis* papilloma influencing comparisons of rates between countries. Improved detection rates of bladder cancer may significantly contribute to the difference between incidence and mortality trends [32]. Investigators from the Netherlands performed statistical modelling of bladder cancer mortality data from 1955 to 1988. They found that the risk of dying from bladder cancer increased from the 1885 birth cohort to the 1910 cohort and decreased thereafter, which may be explained by changes in smoking behaviour [33].

In the United States in 1995 there have been 7500 deaths from bladder cancer in men and 3700 in women, which makes bladder cancer the fourth most common cause of cancer deaths in men [34]. Mortality from bladder cancer constitutes about 20% of the incidence rates in whites, but 32% in black males and 36% in black females (Fig. 1.3). During a period of approximately 30 years 5-year survival rates increased both for whites and blacks from 53 and 24 to 81 and 60, respectively

Table 1.2 Incidence of bladder cancer in selected cancer registries, c1960–c1990.

Cancer incidence in five continents	Males					
	Volume I[1]	Volume II[2]	Volume III[3]	Volume IV[4]	Volume V[5]	Volume VI[6]
Canada, Manitoba	12.61	14.07	15.29	15.22	17.87	18.58
Canada, Saskatchewan	13.29	11.84	14.91	16.05	17.88	19.17
US, Alameda: White		17.85	19.16	19.65	20.83	23.60
US, Alameda: Black		10.88	8.64	11.95	11.62	12.95
US, Connecticut	16.80	19.93	21.30	22.29		
US, Connecticut: White					25.21	26.12
US, Connecticut: Black					10.13	11.24
India, Bombay		2.28	2.85	3.50	4.33	3.63
Japan, Miyagi	4.14	4.72	3.72	5.27	6.39	7.83
Denmark	10.78	12.37	16.06	20.55	24.75	26.33
				22.00		
Finland	6.74	7.38	8.66	9.93	12.74	12.99
Norway	4.89	6.21	9.69	14.61	16.99	19.74
Sweden	8.42	9.83	11.86	13.75	15.47	16.93
UK, Birmingham	10.22	11.52	16.92	17.09	16.88	18.59
New Zealand: Non-maori		12.12	10.78	12.80	13.55	12.71

(1) From Doll R, Payne P, Waterhouse J, eds. Cancer Incidence in Five Continents, Vol I, Lyon, International Agency for Research on Cancer, 1966 [13].
(2) From Doll R, Muir CS, Waterhouse J, eds. Cancer Incidence in Five Continents, Vol II, Lyon, International Agency for Research on Cancer, 1970 [14].
(3) From Waterhouse J, Muir CS, Correa P and Powell J, eds. Cancer Incidence in Five Continents, Vol III (IARC Scientific Publication No.15). Lyon, International Agency for Research on Cancer, 1976 [15].
(4) From Waterhouse J, Muir CS, Shanmugaratnam K and Powell J, eds. Cancer Incidence in Five Continents, Vol IV (IARC Scientific Publication No.42). Lyon, International Agency for Research on Cancer, 1982 [16].
(5) From Muir CS, Waterhouse JAH, Mack T, Powell J, Whelan S, eds. Cancer Incidence in Five Continents, Vol V (IARC Scientific Publication No.88). Lyon, International Agency for Research on Cancer, 1987 [125].
(6) From Parkin DM, Muir CS, Whelan S, Gao YT, Ferlay J and Powell J, eds. Cancer Incidence in Five Continents, Vol VI (IARC Scientific Publication No.120). Lyon, International Agency for Research on Cancer, 1992 [124].

(Fig. 1.4). However, blacks had significantly lower survival rates than whites throughout all periods of observation from circa 1960 to circa 1990. The stage-to-stage comparison of 5-year survival rates between whites and Afro-Americans showed constantly lower survival rates for Afro-Americans for localized, regional and distant tumours (Fig. 1.5). Overall, both age-adjusted and truncated (35–64 years) mortality rates slowly decreased for both sexes between 1965 and 1989.

In Canada, both the truncated and overall age-adjusted mortality rates have been decreasing slowly but steadily in both males and females. Birth cohort examination shows that, in males, the rates are quite stable for cohorts born before 1910. For

Table 1.3 Incidence of bladder cancer in selected cancer registries, c1960–c1990

	Females					
Cancer incidence in five continents	Volume I[1]	Volume II[2]	Volume III[3]	Volume IV[4]	Volume V[5]	Volume VI[6]
Canada, Manitoba	2.27	3.54	4.44	4.66	4.74	5.18
Canada, Saskatchewan	2.44	3.34	2.94	4.06	4.40	5.66
US, Alameda: White		5.59	5.13	6.12	6.70	5.82
US, Alameda: Black		3.94	3.94	4.55	4.14	3.23
US, Connecticut	4.98	5.89	5.70	6.02		
US, Connecticut: White					7.35	6.93
US, Connecticut: Black					4.34	4.24
India, Bombay		0.77	1.08	0.88	0.97	0.94
Japan, Miyagi	1.79	1.55	1.35	1.62	1.95	2.31
Denmark	3.42	3.76	4.24	5.44	6.17	6.74
				5.64		
Finland	1.34	1.62	1.80	2.26	2.53	2.40
Norway	1.99	2.18	3.03	3.97	4.82	5.00
Sweden	2.90	3.50	3.77	4.15	4.21	4.60
UK, Birmingham	2.33	2.75	3.95	4.48	4.38	5.14
New Zealand: Non-maori		2.38	2.58	3.42	3.35	3.20

(1) From Doll R, Payne P, Waterhouse J, eds. Cancer Incidence in Five Continents, Vol I, Lyon, International Agency for Research on Cancer, 1966.
(2) From Doll R, Muir CS, Waterhouse J, eds. Cancer Incidence in Five Continents, Vol II, Lyon, International Agency for Research on Cancer, 1970.
(3) From Waterhouse J, Muir CS, Correa P and Powell J, eds. Cancer Incidence in Five Continents, Vol III (IARC Scientific Publication No.15). Lyon, International Agency for Research on Cancer, 1976.
(4) From Waterhouse J, Muir CS, Shanmugaratnam K and Powell J, eds. Cancer Incidence in Five Continents, Vol IV (IARC Scientific Publication No.42). Lyon, International Agency for Research on Cancer, 1982.
(5) From Muir CS, Waterhouse JAH, Mack T, Powell J, Whelan S, eds. Cancer Incidence in Five Continents, Vol V (IARC Scientific Publication No.88). Lyon, International Agency for Research on Cancer, 1987.
(6) From Parkin DM, Muir CS, Whelan S, Gao YT, Ferlay J and Powell J, eds. Cancer Incidence in Five Continents, Vol VI (IARC Scientific Publication No.120). Lyon, International Agency for Research on Cancer, 1992.

cohorts born after than, a slight decrease in rates in successive birth cohorts was observed. For females, the rates have been decreasing in successive birth cohorts for all age groups examined.

In Japan, the overall age-adjusted mortality rates in males showed a slightly increasing trend between 1958 and 1975, and has been relatively stable or even slightly decreasing ever since. The truncated rates in males remained stable until 1975, and was then followed by a slow but steady decrease. In females, both the truncated and overall age-adjusted mortality rates have been decreasing continuously since 1958. Birth-cohort examination indicates that in males the rates increased in

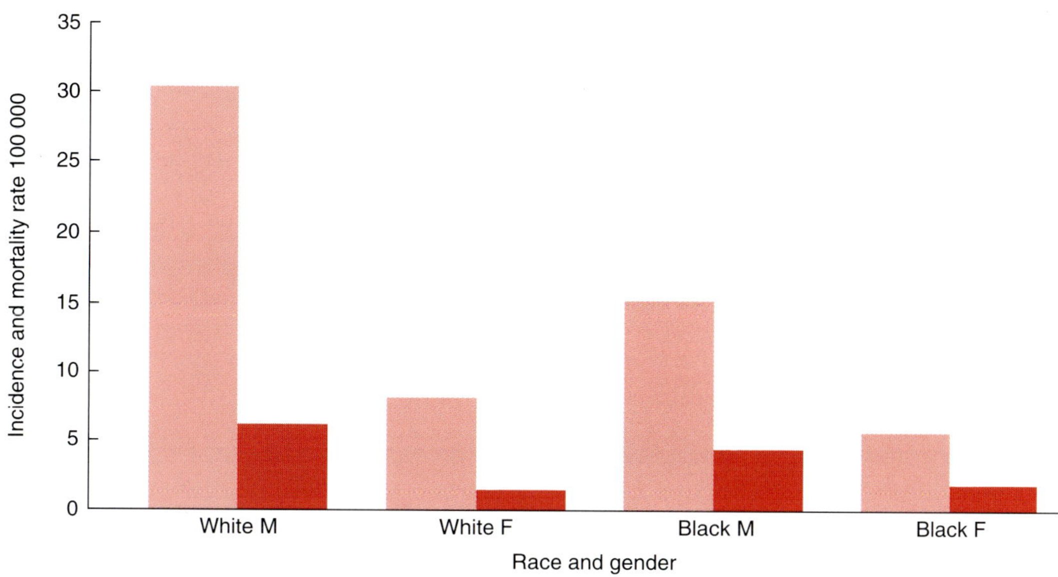

Figure 1.3 Incidence and mortality age-standardized rates for bladder cancer (per 100 000) among whites and blacks (SEER program, 1985). ■ *Incidence;* ■ *mortality. Data abstracted from: Annual Cancer Statistics Review, Publication No. 88-2789. Bethesda, Maryland, US Department of Health and Human Services, National Institute of Health, 1987.*

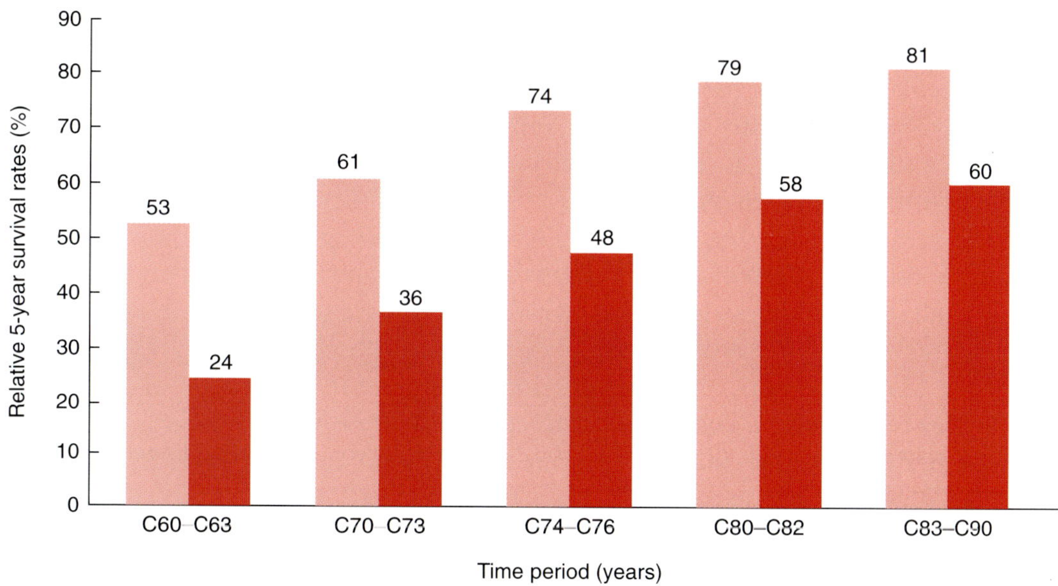

Figure 1.4 Trends in cancer relative 5-year survival rate (%) by race and years of diagnosis in the USA (C60–C90). ■ *White;* ■ *black. Data abstracted from: Wingo PA, Tong T, Bolden S. Cancer statistics 1995. Ca-A Cancer Journal for Clinicians 45: 8–30, 1995.*

successive birth cohorts for those born before 1900 in both males and females. For cohorts born after that, the rates have stabilized or even slightly decreased in males. In females, the rates have been decreasing rapidly in successive birth cohorts.

In Czechoslovakia, both the truncated and overall age-adjusted mortality rates have been increasing in both males and females since 1968, although the increase in

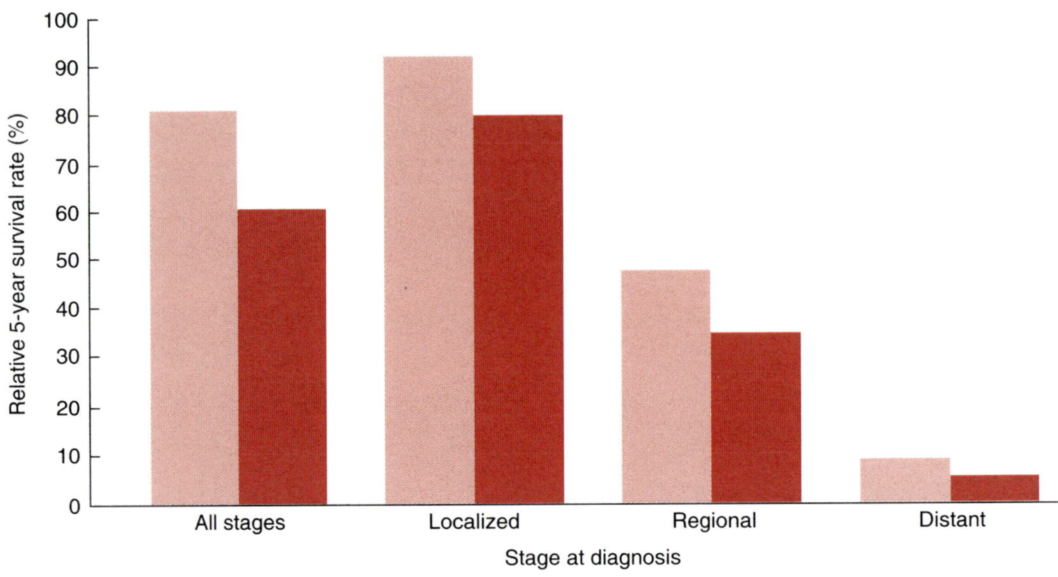

Figure 1.5. Five-year relative survival rates (%) by race and stage at diagnosis in the USA (C83–C90). White; black. *Data abstracted from: Wingo PA, Tong T, Bolden S. Cancer statistics 1995. Ca-A Cancer Journal for Clinicians 45: 8–30, 1995.*

females is slow. Birth-cohort examination shows an increase in rates in successive birth cohorts for most of the age groups in both sexes.

In Germany, the truncated rate has been decreasing since 1968 in males and since 1978 in females. The overall age-adjusted mortality rates, however, remained relatively stable for the entire study period. Birth-cohort examination shows that rates have either stabilized or decreased in successive birth cohorts for those born after 1905 in both males and females.

In Denmark, there has been a slight increase in overall age-adjusted mortality rates in males since 1967. However, no systematic change has taken place in truncated rates in both males and females and in overall age-adjusted mortality rates in females. Examination of rates by birth cohorts suggests than in both males and females the rates have been increasing in successive birth cohorts for those aged over 55. For those under 55, rates have been decreasing in successive birth cohorts.

In the United Kingdom, both the truncated and overall age-adjusted mortality rates showed a slight increase in males between 1958 and 1967. The rates, however, have been decreasing ever since. In females, there is no clear time-trend in both truncated and overall age-adjusted mortality rates during the entire study period. Birth cohort examination shows quite similar rates in successive birth cohorts for those born after 1905 in both males and females, except for the age group 30–34 which experienced an increase in rates in successive birth cohorts.

In Italy, the overall age-adjusted mortality rates showed a linear increasing trend between 1957 and 1987 in males. The truncated rates also showed an increase between 1957 and 1983, however, there was a decrease thereafter. In females, although there was no systematic change in the overall age-adjusted mortality rates, the truncated rates underwent a slight decrease from 1981. Birth-cohort examination indicates an increase in successive birth cohorts in males for those aged over 55. For those aged below 55, the rates have stabilized. In females, and increase in rates in successive birth cohorts was observed only for those aged over 70. The rates have been decreasing or stable for all other age groups.

Overall incidence of bladder cancer increases at a rate of around 1% per year. During the same period of time there has also been a slow, but steady decrease in mortality from bladder cancer in men (Table 1.4) and the rates decreased or remained fairly stable for women (Table 1.5). It appears that improvement of diagnostic techniques and their availability are the major factors contributing to the difference in incidence and mortality trends. Changes in classification of bladder cancer (i.e. papillomas to Ta tumours) may also help count towards a temporal increase in incidence rates.

Analytical epidemiology

Tobacco smoking

Bladder cancer is a neoplasm for which the evidence of an association with cigarette smoking is overwhelming [35]; the only remaining question surrounds the strength of the association. In different regions of the world, smoking accounts for one-third to half of bladder cancers diagnosed among men and about one-quarter of that among women [36,37]. One slight difficulty is that cases in several studies have been recruited with 'cancer of the lower urinary tract' which comprises the renal pelvis, ureter, bladder and urethra.

For all cigarette smokers, estimated relative risks for smokers (relative to non-smokers) have been generally around 2.0 [38–42] although some higher estimates have been reported [37,43–46]. The large majority of studies find relationships between bladder-cancer risk and 'dose' of cigarettes smoked [44,47–49]. Furthermore, smokers of black tobacco appear to have a higher risk than smokers of blond cigarettes [50,51]. D'Avanzo *et al* [47] reported that black tobacco smokers had a 40% increased risk over those who smoked blond tobacco only. However, some studies suggest that this difference may be confounded by the depth of inhalation [48]. The predominant role of cigarette smoking is reflected in the geographical distribution of the disease, with high rates in predominantly urban areas of Europe and North America, although areas with extensive chemical industry and endemic schistosomiasis also tend to have high rates.

Several studies have looked at the association between smoking, type of the tumour, and disease progression. A case-control study, conducted in the Boston Metropolitan Area, demonstrated different risk for superficial and invasive bladder cancers. The tobacco-associated risk was 2.6 for superficial bladder cancer and 1.7 for invasive tumours. Only for patients younger than 60 years of age was the risk greater for invasive tumours [46]. Another study found higher risk (5.2) for invasive than for superficial tumours (3.0). After adjustment for stage, cigarette smoking was associated with higher risk of low-grade than high-grade tumours [12]. There is also some evidence that smoking may influence the natural history of bladder cancer [52]. In a follow-up study of 252 consecutive patients with histologically verified transitional-cell carcinoma (TCC) of the bladder 27% of the non-smokers and 40% of the smokers had died during the first 10 years after diagnosis, suggesting that smoking may be associated with higher mortality from the disease in the longer term [53].

Table 1.4 Bladder cancer age-adjusted mortality rates (all ages and truncated: 35–64 years) per 100 000. Period of observation from c1955 to c1989.

Country	Males													
	C55–C59		C60–C64		C65–C69		C70–C74		C75–C79		C80–C84		C85–C89	
	All	35–64	All	35–64	All	35–64	All	35–64	All	35–64	All	35–64	All	35–64
USA					5.05	4.71	5.08	4.36	4.85	3.89	4.37	3.30	3.87	2.95
Canada	5.39	4.77	5.36	4.54	5.44	4.41	5.50	4.39	5.12	3.95	4.92	3.65	4.72	3.25
Japan	2.01	1.93	2.19	1.96	2.29	2.00	2.39	2.07	2.40	1.97	2.42	1.80	2.27	1.61
Czechoslovakia	4.93	6.52	6.10	6.75	6.55	6.22	5.92	5.55	6.62	6.22	7.12	7.20	7.36	7.20
Germany					7.02	6.44	7.03	6.04	7.18	6.02	7.31	5.77	7.00	4.92
Denmark	6.00	7.00	7.24	8.26	7.46	9.03	8.03	8.32	8.88	8.17	9.32	8.60	9.52	8.33
UK	6.87	7.68	7.36	7.59	7.80	7.67	8.00	7.39	7.84	6.69	7.56	6.18	7.42	5.84
Italy	1.62	2.73	1.80	2.87	2.01	3.28	2.44	3.91	2.85	4.81	3.54	5.69	4.08	6.15

Data abstracted from WHO mortality database and La Vecchia *et al.*, 1992.

Table 1.5 Bladder cancer age-adjusted mortality rates (all ages and truncated: 35–64 years) per 100 000. Period of observation from c1955 to c1989.

Country	Females													
	55–59		60–64		65–69		70–74		75–79		80–84		85–89	
	All	35–64	All	35–64	All	35–64	All	35–64	All	35–64	All	35–64	All	35–64
USA					1.67	1.55	1.54	1.43	1.41	1.25	1.29	1.09	1.18	0.97
Canada	1.87	1.63	1.81	1.37	1.72	1.36	1.58	1.28	1.50	1.28	1.39	1.09	1.28	0.93
Japan	0.93	1.20	0.95	1.02	0.98	1.08	0.94	0.84	0.83	0.65	0.78	0.52	0.69	0.42
Czechoslovakia	1.18	1.59	1.53	1.73	1.21	1.20	1.16	1.15	1.11	1.02	1.30	1.34	1.38	1.39
Germany					1.54	1.39	1.58	1.40	1.69	1.51	1.70	1.34	1.66	1.17
Denmark	2.28	2.15	2.27	2.24	2.28	2.53	2.29	2.44	2.66	3.08	2.52	2.73	2.45	2.66
UK	2.04	2.08	2.02	2.18	2.08	2.12	2.12	2.18	2.19	2.25	2.12	2.04	2.18	2.01
Italy	1.18	1.37	1.15	1.24	1.19	1.19	1.23	1.13	1.35	1.18	1.40	1.09	1.33	0.89

Data abstracted from WHO mortality database and La Vecchia *et al.*, 1992.

For males smoking over 20 cigarettes per day relative risk varies from around five in three studies conducted in North America [54–56] and one in Denmark [57] to between two and three in a number of other studies from the United States [58,59], France [60] and from Japan [61]. While a clear dose–response relationship was observed in many studies [43,45,49,55,56,61–63], several large studies report a levelling-off of the dose–response curve [57,58,64,65]. Hayes *et al* [46] found a dose–response trend for invasive bladder cancers, but not for superficial tumours. Such wide variations in the reported dose–response relationship could possibly be related to a number of factors including different study designs, different ways of smoking or different types of tobacco smoked; the apparent levelling-off could also reflect differences in data collection with underestimation of the levels of consumption by the subjects [35]. Several recent studies have found significant impact of smoking on the mutation of the *p17* and *p53* genes in bladder cancer leading to the suggestion of a hypothesis that certain carcinogens in tobacco may cause DNA damage and may produce specific mutations [66–68]. One of these studies demonstrated a significant association between the number of cigarettes smoked per day and *p53* nuclear overexpression with 2.3 higher risk for those smoking 1–2 packs per day and 8.4 for smoking more than two packs per day [67].

Duration of cigarette smoking shows a direct relationship with relative risks of bladder cancer with the risk rising to between 3 and 5 for 40 years of cigarette smoking [56,59,69]. In a small number of studies, cancers of the renal pelvis and ureter have been considered separately and these have all demonstrated a dose–response relationship with daily or cumulative consumption of tobacco and with relative risks generally higher than those reported for the bladder. For example, in the population-based study of McLaughlin *et al* [70] the overall relative risk for cancer of the renal pelvis and ureter among men who had ever smoked was 7.6.

The use of filter cigarettes has been examined in several studies with conflicting results, some studies reporting weaker effects, some reporting similar effects and yet others reporting greater effects than non-filter cigarettes [35]. A slight effect has been reported for inhaling [48,56,58,61] although not by every study [43]. Relative risks of bladder cancer associated with smoking cigarettes made from black (air-cured) tobacco have been reported to be twice the risks associated with the use of blond tobacco after all available information on potential confounders had been taken into account [44,62].

Many studies of bladder cancer report a lowering of risk in men after stopping cigarette smoking with the risk in ex-smokers falling to that compatible with non-smokers 15 years after quitting [35,71,72]. There also appears to be a increased risk of bladder cancer when smoking began at an earlier age [44]. Conflicting evidence is available on the role of pipe smoking in the aetiology of bladder cancer [35,45]. Although one study suggests that racial differences in risk for bladder cancer may be attributable to smoking [73] another did not find a statistically significant difference in the association between smoking and bladder cancer in blacks and whites [74].

It has even been suggested that women may be less susceptible than men to developing bladder cancer from cigarette smoking [26,73]. However, there is some evidence that smoking causes increased risk for smoking-related secondary cancers in female bladder cancer patients and this association is stronger than in males [75,76]. These observations deserve close attention and further research.

Alcohol consumption

Cohort studies on mortality according to level of alcohol consumption find no excess of bladder cancer [77–80]. A large number of case-control studies have investigated the association between alcohol intake and bladder cancer-risk and have found no association [54,55,63,64,81–85]. Only a few studies conducted in Germany, France and Turkey reported some increased risk and an element of dose–response [44,45,86,87]. Generally the risk estimates in these studies were significant only for the heaviest drinkers. Taken together, the available data show no association between risk of bladder cancer and alcohol consumption [36,88,89].

Coffee consumption

There have been two prospective studies of bladder-cancer risk and coffee consumption; one reported a non-significant positive association [90] while the other [91] showed no association. More than two dozen case-control studies have addressed the issue of coffee consumption and bladder cancer risk [92]. In the majority of studies (16/22) a weak positive association was seen with consumption of coffee as compared to non-drinkers; in seven of these the association was significant with a dose–response relationship present in three. No association was seen in the six remaining studies. The association persisted, but was less clear, when reported non-smokers were considered in 7 of the 16 studies suggesting that confounding by tobacco smoking is unlikely to be the sole explanation for this finding. The association was found in men and women suggesting that occupational factors could not fully explain this finding. Of four available case-control studies, three indicated a slightly increased risk for transitional-cell cancers of the renal pelvis and ureter but none of the results were significant. Viscoli *et al* [93] reviewed 35 case-control studies of the association between coffee consumption and bladder cancer published between 1971 and 1992. None of the eight studies that had met the criteria for design of analysis showed any evidence of an increase in risk of bladder cancer with coffee drinking in men or women after adjustment for the effects of cigarette smoking. Furthermore, inclusion of the data from the remaining 27 studies in an overall summarized estimate did not substantially change the findings. The authors concluded that there are no data suggesting a clinically significant association between coffee consumption and development of bladder cancer. Several recent case-control studies indicate a dose-dependent increase in risk of bladder cancer for consumption of coffee but these data are not consistent [12,45,94–96]. Taken as a whole the data are consistent with a weak positive relationship between coffee consumption and the occurrence of bladder cancers, but the possibility that this is due to bias or confounding cannot be excluded [92,97]. However, there is a lack of internal consistency within most of the positive studies which should keep the question of a causal association open; in some studies the association is present in women but not in men and in others vice versa and there is a lack of consistent dose–response.

Occupational, nutritional and other factors

Several other factors have been related to cancer of the urinary bladder, including occupational exposure to aromatic amines, coal tar and, possibly, other chemicals,

S. Haematobium and other infectious agents, and exposure to some drugs such as phenacetin, chlornaphazine and cyclophosphamide [32,36,98–100].

Occupational exposure has generally been considered to be the second most important risk for bladder cancer after smoking [99,101]. The proportion of bladder cancers attributable to occupation ranges between 16 and 24% in several investigations conducted in different countries [71]. Among occupations most frequently reported to be associated with an increased risk of bladder cancer are printing, plastics and synthetics, rubber, mining, metal, and dyestuff industries, and those professions which involve exposure to dyes, spray paints, zinc, oils, petroleum, stone dust, metal dust/fumes and herbicides [18,45,102–105]. Relative risks for bladder cancer in men and women who are engaged in these occupations are generally around a factor of 2 with higher risk for chemical and metal workers, press operators, and those who are exposed to dyes, paints and herbicides. A study of 2,893 white males employed in high-risk occupations diagnosed with primary bladder cancer in Missouri showed that when occupations were examined individually, motor vehicle operators, truck drivers, vehicle mechanics, other mechanics, and janitors were more likely to have high-grade or late-stage tumours [101]. The most common occupational carcinogens for bladder cancer are benziadine, 4-aminobiphenyl, 2-naphthylamine, aminobiphenyl, dichlorobenzidine, orthodianisidine and orthotoluidine [36,100,103]. Most of these exposures are regulated in many countries and occupational bladder cancer may be shrinking in importance in many western countries through a combination of legislation against carcinogens and a cleaner workplace. Some of the practices responsible for bladder cancer in the west may, however, be in the process of being exported to the developing world where occupational hygiene standards may not be so rigorously enforced as in the developed countries.

S. Haematobium infection is strongly related to the development of squamous cell bladder cancer, although the nature of this relationship is not completely resolved [106]. Several *in vivo* and *in vitro* studies demonstrated that inflammatory cells in patients which chronic cystitis may induce gene mutations on chromosomes 11 and 17p [66,107]. In Zimbabwe the proportion of bladder cancer attributable to schistosomiasis was estimated to be 28% [8], and about 80% of squamous cell carcinomas in Egypt are associated with chronic urinary bilharziasis [108]. A recent study from Egypt showed a considerable shift towards non-schistosomal bladder cancers and an increased average age at diagnosis of bladder cancer which may be attributed to the increased incidence of low infestation in recent years [6].

Although there were many observations on the occurrence of bladder cancer in patients who received treatment with the anticarcinogenic immunosuppressive drug, cyclophosphamide [100,109–113] there are only a few cohort and case-control studies that investigated this relationship. In a case-control study of 63 cases of bladder tumours and 188 controls among women who received cyclophosphamide therapy for ovarian cancer there was an approximately fourfold increase in risk for bladder cancer [114]. When 119 patients (76 women and 43 men) with refractory rheumatoid arthritis who were treated with oral cyclophosphamide were compared in a longitudinal cohort study with 119 control patients with rheumatoid arthritis, investigators found nine bladder tumours in the cyclophosphamide group compared with no bladder cancers in the control group [115]. The largest cohort study which also evaluated the dose–response relationship between cyclophosphamide and bladder cancer included a cohort of 6171 2-year survivors of non-Hodgkin's lymphoma. Of these patients, 48 developed secondary cancer of the bladder and were matched to 136 control subjects with non-Hodgkin's lymphoma who did not develop a second malignancy. There was 4.5-fold dose-dependent risk of bladder cancer (95% CI = 1.5–13.6) following therapy with cyclophosphamide. Risk was not significant among patients who received a total amount of cyclophosphamide of less than 20 g. However, in patients who received cumulative doses of 20–49 g and over 50 g there was 6-fold and 14.5-fold statistically significant risk, respectively, with a statistically test for linear trend [116].

It appears that consumption of large doses of phenacetin may cause $p53$ gene mutations and cause transitional-cell carcinomas of renal pelvis and bladder [36,117]. However, while some studies suggest that phenacetin may cause bladder urothelial cancers [118,119] the most recent findings are inconclusive and the latent period may range for more than 25 years.

Another widely used potential risk factor is saccharin; however, the results of extensive investigation are largely reassuring [98,120]. A review of the most recent epidemiological data revealed that there is no significant association between the use of artificial sweeteners and the risk of bladder cancer. A meta-analysis of all case-control studies demonstrated a relative risk of 0.97 and, in combination with laboratory studies of saccharin carcinogenicity, suggested that there is no association between saccharin and bladder cancer [121].

Additionally, the role of diet in bladder carcinogenesis has recently been considered, and there is some evidence that a diet rich in fresh fruit and vegetables and, possibly, vitamin A is protective [49,122]. In a cohort study of 11,580 residents of a retirement community, followed for 9 years, the only protective effect was found for vitamin C supplement use [123]. In a review of approximately 200 studies that examined the relationship between fruit and vegetable intake and 11 cancer sites strong evidence of a protective effect of fruit and vegetable consumption was seen in 23 of 38 studies. A number of studies have reported increased risks of bladder cancer associated with coffee consumption and an IARC Working Group considered that there was some evidence that coffee may be carcinogenic for the human bladder [92].

The observation that a number of heterogeneous factors have been related to bladder cancer is not surprising, since most substances or metabolites are excreted through the urinary tract and are consequently in direct contact with the mucosa of the bladder. For instance, there are several mutagenic substances in tobacco smoke, and the urine of smokers is mutagenic according to the Ames test. Quantitative assessment of the role of various factors is therefore important; qualitative assessment is not adequate. In developed countries, cigarette smoking is by far the most important single determinant of the disease; the relative risk is of the order of 3 to 5, and the population attributable risk has been estimated to be from around 50% to as high as 85% in British males. Occupational exposure to aromatic amines has been an important cause of bladder cancer in the past [98], and could still be responsible for an appreciable proportion of cases occurring nowadays in certain areas of the world with a large chemical industry but perhaps lacking the advanced standards of industrial hygiene present in advanced countries.

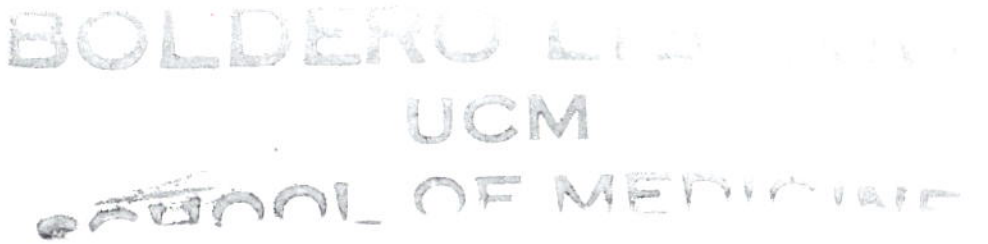

Acknowledgments

This work was conducted within the framework of support from the *Associazione Italiana per la Ricerca sul Cancro* (Italian Association for Cancer Research).

Summary

Cancer of the urinary bladder is the eighth most common form of cancer in males world-wide whose incidence rate exhibits moderate international variation. Incidence rates are two to four times higher in males than in females and there is generally a two-fold increased risk among whites when compared with non-whites. Incidence rates are also higher in the developed countries with the exception of some countries in Africa and Middle Asia where schistosomiasis is endemic. The large majority of bladder cancers occur in patients 60 years of age and older, and it appears that the progression rate is the same in younger and older patients with similar tumour grades. Mortality rates usually constitute about 20% of the incidence rates and there has been a slow but steady decline in mortality during the last 25–30 years in the countries from which mortality data for this period are available. It appears that a substantial increase in incidence rates in males, which has doubled over the last two decades, may be explained in large part by the improvement of diagnostic techniques and availability. Changes in classification and registration of low-stage 'papillomas' may also influence temporal trends in incidence of bladder cancer. There are few epidemiological studies on the topic of superficial bladder cancer, and hence this chapter will focus on what is known about bladder cancer. Tobacco smoking and some environmental factors associated with industrial exposure contribute to increasing the incidence of bladder cancer. Smoking is a major, well-established and avoidable risk factor for bladder cancer which accounts for up to half of bladder cancers among men and about one-quarter among women. There is evidence that smoking may influence the natural history of bladder cancers increasing the progression rate and mortality from this disease in the long term. It appears that females may be less susceptible than men to the bladder-specific carcinogenic effect of tobacco; however, this alone cannot explain gender differences in the incidence rates. Many studies demonstrated a dose–response effect of smoking as well as effect of duration, time from cessation, and age of starting on the risk of bladder cancer. Furthermore, the risk of bladder cancer declines considerably in men after stopping cigarette smoking and generally reaches the risk among non-smokers about 15 years after quitting. Among several other factors related to the developing of bladder cancer in certain areas of the world are occupational exposures to dyes, paints, aromatic amines, herbicides, and petroleum. Several occupations including textile, chemical, metal workers, truck drivers, and other mechanics are also associated with an excessive risk of bladder cancer. Chronic cystitis in the patients with bladder calculi, indwelling catheters, and among those infected with *Schistosoma Haematobium* is strongly related to the developing of bladder cancer, although the nature of this relationship is not clearly understood. Further epidemiological studies are needed to investigate the nature of the causal relationship between administration of cyclophosphamide, and the protective effects of fruit, vegetables and certain vitamin supplements in the diet. It appears that with increasing numbers of patients diagnosed with early-stage bladder cancer, due to the improvements in early diagnosis and increasing availability of diagnostic techniques, there will be relative increase in incidence and, hopefully, a further decrease in mortality from bladder cancer. Preventive regulatory measures directed to the decrease of smoking and some occupational exposures may considerably contribute to the reduction of bladder cancer.

References

1   Parkin DM, Pisani P, Ferlay J. Estimates of the worldwide incidence of eighteen major cancers in 1985. *Int J Cancer* 1993; **54**: 594–606.

2   Parkin DM, Pisani P, Ferlay J. *Worldwide burden of cancer*. In: Biennial Report 1994–1995 Lyon: IARC, 1995; 14–15.

3   Young RH, Eble JN. Unusual forms of carcinoma of the urinary bladder. *Hum Pathol* 1991; **22**(10): 948–65.

4   Lynch CF and Cohen MB. Urinary system. *Cancer* 1995; **75** (1 Suppl): 316–29.

5   Al-Fouadi A, Parkin DM. Cancer in Iraq. Seven years data from the Baghdad Tumour Registry. *Int J Cancer* 1984; **34**: 207–13.

6   Koraitim MM, Metwalli NE, Atta MA, ed-Sadr AA. Changing age incidence and pathological types of schistosoma-associated bladder carcinoma. *J Urol* 1995; **154**(5): 1714–16.

7   Burin GJ, Gibb HJ, Hill RN. Human bladder cancer: evidence for a potential irritation-induced mechanism. *Food Chem Toxicol* 1995; **33**(9): 785–95.

8   Vizcaino AP, Parkin DM, Boffetta P, Skinner ME. Bladder cancer: epidemiology and risk factors in Bulawayo, Zimbabwe. *Cancer Causes Control* 1994; **5**(6): 517–22.

9   Tulinius H. Frequency of some morphological types of neoplasm of five sites. In: Doll R, Muir C, Waterhouse J (eds) *Cancer Incidence in Five Continents*, Vol. III. Berlin: Springer-Verlag, 1970; 23–83.

10 Schairer C, Hartge P, Hoover RN, Silverman DT. Racial differences in bladder cancer risk: a case-control study. *Am J Epidemiol* 1988; **128**(5): 1027–37.

11 Smart CR. Bladder cancer survival statistics. *J Occup Med* 1990; **32**(9): 926–8.

12 Sturgeon SR, Hartge P, Silverman DT *et al.* Associations between bladder cancer risk factors and tumor stage and grade at diagnosis. *Epidemiology* 1994; **5**(2): 218–25.

13 Doll R, Payne P, Waterhouse J (eds) *Cancer Incidence in Five Continents*, Vol I. Lyon: International Agency for Research on Cancer, 1966.

14 Doll R, Muir CS, Waterhouse J (eds) *Cancer Incidence in Five Continents*, Vol II. Lyon: International Agency for Research on Cancer, 1970.

15 Waterhouse J, Muir CS, Correa P, Powell J. (eds) *Cancer Incidence in Five Continents*, Vol III (IARC Scientific Publication No. 15). Lyon: International Agency for Research on Cancer, 1976.

16 Waterhouse J, Muir CS, Shanmugaratnam K, Powell J. (eds) *Cancer Incidence in Five Continents*, Vol IV (IARC Scientific Publication No.42). Lyon: International Agency for Research on Cancer, 1982.

17 Davis FG, Persky VW, Ferre CD *et al.* Cancer incidence of Hispanics and non-Hispanic whites in Cook County, Illinois. *Cancer* 1995; **75**(12): 2939–45.

18 Anton Culver H, Lee Feldstein A, Taylor TH. Occupation and bladder cancer risk. *Am J Epidemiol* 1992; **136**: 89–94.

19 Stemmermann GN, Yoshizawa CN, Nomura *et al.* Urothelial cancer in white and Japanese patients in Hawaii: pathology. *J Urol* 1990; **144**(1): 44–6.

20 Bassett MT, Levy L, Chokunonga *et al.* Cancer in the European population of Harare, Zimbabwe, 1990–1992. *Int J Cancer* 1995; **63**(1): 24–8.

21 Mulholland SG, Stefanelli JL. Genitourinary cancer in the elderly. *Am J Kidney Dis* 1990; **16**(4): 324–8.

22 Kutarski PW, Padwell A. Transitional cell carcinoma of the bladder in young adults. *Br J Urol* 1993; **72**(5): 749–55.

23 Briggs NC, Young TB, Gilchrist KW, Vaillancourt AM, Messing EM. Age as a predictor of an aggressive clinical course for superficial bladder cancer in men. *Cancer* 1992; **69**(6): 1445–51.

24 Wan J, Grosman HB. Bladder carcinoma in patients 40 years and younger. *Cancer* 1989; **64**: 178–81.

25 Hartge P, Harvey EB, Linehan *et al.* Unexplained excess risk of bladder cancer in men. *J Natl Cancer Inst* 1990; **82**(20): 1636–40.

26 Skov T, Sprogel P, Engholm G, Frolund C. Cancer of the lung and urinary bladder in Denmark, 1943–87: a cohort analysis. *Cancer Causes Control* 1991; **2**(6): 365–9.

27 Cantor KP, Lynch CF, Johnson D. Bladder cancer, parity, and age at first birth. *Cancer Causes Control* 1992; **3**(1): 57–62.

28 Kiemeney LA, Coebergh JW, Koper NP *et al.* Bladder cancer incidence and survival in the south-eastern part of The Netherlands, 1975–1989. *Eur J Cancer* 1994; **30A**(8): 1134–7.

29 McLaughlin JR, Kreiger N, Marrett LD, Holowaty EJ. Cancer incidence registration and trends in Ontario. *Eur J Cancer* 1991; **27**(11): 1520–4.

30 Lee HP. Monitoring cancer incidence and risk factors in Singapore. *Ann Acad Med Singapore* 1990; **19**(2): 133–8.

31 Valerianova Z, Gill C, Duffy SW, Danon SE. Trends in incidence of various cancers in Bulgaria, 1981–1990. *Int J Epidemiol* 1994; **23**(6): 1117–26.

32 McCredie M. Bladder and kidney cancers. *Cancer Surv* 1994; **19–20**: 343–68.

33 Kiemeney LA, Verbeek AL, Nelemans PJ, Witjes JA, Straatman H. Bladder cancer mortality in The Netherlands, 1955–1988. *Br J Urol* 1992; **70**(1) 46–52.

34 Wingo PA, Tong T, Bolden S. Cancer statistics 1995. *Ca-A Cancer J Clinicians* 1995; **45**: 8–30.

35 IARC (International Agency for Research on Cancer). Tobacco smoking. *Monogr Eval Carcinog Risk Hum* **38**: Lyon: IARC, 1986.

36 Silverman DT, Hartge P, Morrison AS, Devesa SS. Epidemiology of bladder cancer. *Hematol Oncol Clin North Am* 1992; **6**(1): 1–30.

37 Parkin DM, Pisani P, Lopez AD, Masuyer E. At least one in seven cases of cancer is caused by smoking. Global estimates for 1985. *Int J Cancer* 1994; **59**: 494–504.

38 Mommsen S, Aagaard J. Tobacco as a risk factor in bladder cancer. *Carcinogenesis* 1983; **4**: 335–8.

39 Najem RG, Lourier DB, Seebode JJ *et al.* Life time occupation, smoking, caffeine, saccharin, hair dyes and bladder carcinogenesis. *Int J Epidemiol* 1982; **11**: 212–17.

40 Staszewski J. Smoking and cancer of the urinary bladder in males in Poland. *Br J Cancer* 1966; **20**: 32–5.

41 Tola S, Tenho M, Korkala ML, Järvinen E. Cancer of the urinary bladder in Finland. Association with occupation. *Int Arch Occup Environ Health* 1980; **46**: 43–51.

42 Siemiatycki J, Krewski D, Franco E, Kaiserman M. Associations between cigarette smoking and each of 21 types of cancer: a multi-site case-control study. *Int J Epidemiol* 1995; **24**(3): 504–14.

43 Lockwood K. On the etiology of bladder tumors in Kobenhavn-Frederiksberg. An inquiry of 369 patients and 369 controls. *Acta Pathol Microbiol Scand* 1961; **51** (Suppl.145).

44 Momas I, Daures JP, Festy B *et al.* Bladder cancer and black tobacco cigarette smoking. Some results from a French case-control study. *Eur J Epidemiol* 1994; **10**(5): 599–604.

45 Kunze E, Chang Claude J, Frentzel Beyme R. Lifestyle and occupational risk factors for bladder cancer in Germany. A case-control study. *Cancer* 1992; **69**(7): 1776–90.

46 Hayes RB, Friedell GH, Zahm SH, Cole P. Are the known bladder cancer risk-factors associated with more advanced bladder cancer? *Cancer Causes Control* 1993; **4**(2): 157–62.

47 D'Avanzo B, Negri E, La Vecchia C *et al.* Cigarette smoking and bladder cancer. *Eur J Cancer* 1990; **26**(6): 714–18.

48 Lopez-Abente G, Gonzalez CA, Errezola M *et al.* Tobacco smoke inhalation pattern, tobacco type, and bladder cancer in Spain. *Am J Epidemiol* 1991; **134**(8): 830–9.

49 Chyou PH, Nomura AM, Stemmermann GN. A prospective study of diet, smoking, and lower urinary tract cancer. *Ann Epidemiol* 1993; **3**(3): 211–16.

50 De Stefani E, Correa P, Fierro L *et al.* Black tobacco, mate, and bladder cancer. A case-control study from Uruguay. *Cancer* 1991; **67**(2): 536–40.

51 Vineis P. Black (air-cured) and blond (flue-cured) tobacco and cancer risk. I: Bladder cancer. *Eur J Cancer* 1991; **27**(11): 1491–3.

52 Fitzpatrick JM. Superficial bladder carcinoma. Factors affecting the natural history. *World J Urol* 1993; **11**(3): 142–7.

53 Raitanen MP, Nieminen P, Tammela TL. Impact of tumour grade, stage, number and size, and smoking and sex, on survival in patients with transitional cell carcinoma of the bladder. *Br J Urol* 1995; **76**(4): 470–4.

54 Wynder EL, Hoffmann D. Experimental contribution to tobacco smoke carcinogenicity. *Dtsch Med Wochenschr* 1963; **88**: 623–8.

55 Morgan RW, Jain MG. Bladder cancer: Smoking, beverages and artificial sweeteners. *Can Med Assoc J* 1974; **111**: 1067–70.

56 Howe GR, Burch JD, Miller AB *et al.* Tobacco use, occupation, coffee, various nutrients, and bladder cancer. *J Natl Cancer Inst* 1980; **64**: 701–13.

57 Jensen OM, Wahrendorf J, Blettner M, Knudsen JB, Sorensen BL. The Copenhagen case-control study of bladder cancer: role of smoking in invasive and non-invasive bladder tumours. *J Epidemiol Community Health* 1987; **41**(1): 30–6.

58 Cole P, Monson RR, Haning H, Friedell GH. Smoking and cancer of the lower urinary tract. *New Engl J Med* 1971; **284**: 129–34.

59 Wynder EL, Goldsmith R. The epidemiology of bladder cancer. A second look. *Cancer* 1977; **40**: 1246–68.

60 Schwartz GG, Flamant R, Lellouch J, Denoix PF. Results of a French survey in the role of tobacco, particularly inhalation, in different cancer sites. *J Natl Cancer Inst* 1961; **26**: 1085–108.

61 Morrison H, Buring JE, Verhoek WG *et al.* An international study of smoking and bladder cancer. *J Urol* 1984; **131**: 650–4.

62 Vineis P, Estève J, Terracini B. Bladder cancer and smoking in males: Types of cigarettes, age at start, effect of stopping and interaction with occupation. *Int J Cancer* 1984; **34**: 165–70.

63 Schwartz GG, Denoix PF, Anguera G. Cancer sites associated with tobacco and alcohol in humans. *Fr Bull Cancer* 1957; **44**: 336–61.

64 Dunham LJ, Rabson AS, Stewart HL, Frank AS, Young JL. Rates, interview, and pathology study of cancer of the urinary bladder in New Orleans, Louisiana, *J Natl Cancer Inst* 1968; **41**: 683–709.

65 Cartwright RA, Adib R, Appleyard I *et al.* Cigarette smoking and bladder cancer: An epidemiological inquiry in West Yorkshire. *J Epidemiol Commun Health* 1983; **37**: 256–63.

66 Habuchi T, Takahashi R, Yamada H *et al.* Influence of cigarette smoking and schistosomiasis on *p53* gene mutation in urological cancer. *Cancer Res* 1993; **53**: 3795–9.

67 Zhang ZF, Sarkis AS, Cordon Cardo C *et al.* Tobacco smoking, occupation, and p53 nuclear overexpression in early stage bladder cancer. *Cancer Epidemiol Biomarkers Prev* 1994; **3**(1): 19–24.

68 Uchida T, Wada C, Ishida H *et al.* p53 mutations and prognosis in bladder tumors. *J Urol* 1995; **153**(4): 1097–104.

69 Tyrrell AB, MacAirt JG, McCaughey WTE. Occupational and non-occupational factors associated with vesical neoplasms in Ireland. *J Irish Med Assoc* 1971; **64**: 213–17.

70 McLaughlin JK, Blot WJ, Mandel JS *et al.* Etiology of cancer of the renal pelvis. *J Natl Cancer Inst* 1983; **71**: 287–91.

71 Vineis P, Simonato L. Proportion of lung and bladder cancers in males resulting from occupation: a systematic approach. *Arch Environ Health* 1991; **46**: 6–15.

72 Sorahan T, Lancashire RJ, Sole G. Urothelial cancer and cigarette smoking: findings from a regional case-controlled study. *Br J Urol* 1994; **74**(6): 753–6.

73 Anton Culver H, Lee Feldstein A, Taylor TH. The association of bladder cancer risk with ethnicity, gender and smoking. *Ann Epidemiol* 1993; **3**(4): 429–33.

74 Hartge P, Silverman DT, Schairer C, Hoover RN. Smoking and bladder cancer risk in blacks and whites in the United States. *Cancer Causes Control* 1993; **4**(4): 391–4.

75 Salminen E, Pukkala E, Teppo L. Bladder cancer and the risk of smoking-related cancers during follow-up. *J Urol* 1994; **152**: 1420–3.

76 Begg CB, Zhang ZF, Sun M, Herr HW, Schantz SP. Methodology for evaluating the incidence of second primary cancers with application to smoking-related cancers from the Surveillance, Epidemiology, and End Results (SEER) program. *Am J Epidemiol* 1995; **142**(6): 653–65.

77 Hirayama T. Diet and cancer. *Nutr Cancer* 1979; **1**: 67–81.

78 Jensen OM. *Cancer morbidity and Causes of Death Among Danish Brewery Workers,* Lyon: International Agency for Research on Cancer 1980.

79 Pell S, D'Alonzo CA. A five-year mortality study of alcoholics. *J Occup Med* 1973; **15**: 120–5.

80 Robinette CD, Hrubec Z, Fraumeni JF Jr. Chronic alcoholism and subsequent mortality in World War II veterans. *Am J Epidemiol* 1979; **109**: 687–700.

81 Williams RR, Horm JW. Association of cancer sites with tobacco and alcohol consumption and socioeconomic status of patients: interview study from the Third National Cancer Survey. *J Natl Cancer Inst* 1977; **58**: 525–47.

82 Mommsen S, Aagaard J, Sell A. An epidemiological case-control study of bladder cancer in males from a predominantly rural district. *Eur J Cancer Clin Oncol* 1982; **18**: 1205–10.

83 Thomas DB, Uhl CN, Hartge P. Bladder cancer and alcoholic beverage consumption. *Am J Epidemiol* 1983; **118**: 720–7.

84 Brownson RC, Chang JC, Davis JR. Occupation, smoking, and alcohol in the epidemiology of bladder cancer. *Am J Publ Health* 1987; **77**: 1298–1300.

85 Harris RE, Chen Backlund JY, Wynder EL. Cancer of the urinary bladder in blacks and whites. A case-control study. *Cancer* 1990; **66**(12): 2673–80.

86 Claude J, Kunze E, Frentzel-Beyme R *et al.* Life-style and occupational risk factors in cancer of the lower urinary tract. *Am J Epidemiol* 1986; **124**: 578–89.

87 Akdas A, Kirkali Z, Bilir N. Epidemiological case-control study on the etiology of bladder cancer in Turkey. *Eur Urol* 1990; **17**(1): 23–6.

88 IARC (International Agency for Research on Cancer) Alcohol drinking. *Monogr Eval Carcinog Risk Hum* **44**, Lyon: IARC, 1988.

89 Longnecker MP. Alcohol consumption and risk of cancer in humans: an overview. *Alcohol* 1995; **12**: 87–96.

90 Nomura A, Heilbrun LK, Stemmermann GN. Prospective study of coffee consumption and the risk of cancer. *J Natl Cancer Inst* 1986; **76**: 587–90.

91 LeGrady D, Dyer AR, Shekell RB, Stamler J, Liu K, Paul O, Lepper M, MacMillan Shryock A. Coffee consumption and mortality in the Chicago Western Electric Company study. *Am J Epidemiol* 1987; **126**: 803–12.

92 IARC (International Agency for Research on Cancer) Coffee, tea, mate, methylxanthines (caffeine, theophylline, theobromine) and methylglyoxal. *Monogr Eval Carcinog Risk Hum* 1991; **51**, Lyon: IARC

93 Viscoli CM, Lachs MS, Horwitz RI. Bladder cancer and coffee drinking: a summary of case-control research. *Lancet* 1983; **341**(8858): 1432–7.

94 Moran EM. Epidemiological factors of cancer in California. *J Environ Pathol Toxicol Oncol* 1992; **11**: 303–7.

95 D'Avanzo B, La Vecchia C, Franceschi S *et al.* Coffee consumption and bladder cancer risk. *Eur J Cancer* 1992; **28**: 1480–4.

96 Vena JE, Freudenheim J, Graham S *et al.* Coffee, cigarette smoking, and bladder cancer in western New York. *Ann Epidemiol* 1993; **3**: 586–91.

97 Etherton GM, Kochar MS. Coffee: facts and controversies. *Arch Fam Med* 1993; **2**: 317–22.

98 IARC (International Agency for Research on Cancer). Overall evaluations of carcinogenicity: an updating of IARC Monographs volumes 1 to 42. *Monogr Eval Carcinog Risks Hum (Suppl)* 1987; **7**: 1–440.

99 Cohen SM, Johansson SL. Epidemiology and etiology of bladder cancer. *Urol Clin North Am* 1992; **19**: 421–8.

100 Shirai T. Etiology of bladder cancer. *Semin Urol* 1993; **11**: 113–26.

101 Brooks DR, Geller AC, Chang J, Miller DR. Occupation, smoking, and the risk of high-grade invasive bladder cancer in Missouri. *Am J Ind Med* 1992; **21**: 699–713.

102 La Vecchia C, Negri E, D'Avanzo B, Franceschi S. Occupation and the risk of bladder cancer. *Int J Epidemiol* 1990; **19**: 264–8.

103 Silverman DT, Levin LI, Hoover RN. Occupational risks of bladder cancer among white women in the United States. *Am J Epidemiol* 1990; **132**: 453–61.

104 Dolin PJ, Cook Mozaffari P. Occupation and bladder cancer: a death-certificate study. *Br J Cancer* 1992; **66**: 568–78.

105 Zheng W, McLaughlin JK, Gao YT *et al.* Bladder cancer and occupation in Shanghai, 1980–1984. *Am J Ind Med* 1992; **21**: 877–85.

106 Badawi AF, Mostafa MH, Probert A, O'Connor PJ. Role of schistosomiasis in human bladder cancer: evidence of association, aetiological factors, and basic mechanisms of carcinogenesis. *Eur J Cancer Prev* 1995; **4**: 45–59.

107 Rosin MP, Saad el Din Zaki S, Ward AJ, Anwar WA. Involvement of inflammatory reactions and elevated cell proliferation in the development of bladder cancer in schistosomiasis patients. *Mutat Res* 1994; **305**: 283–92.

108 El Bolkainy MN, Mokhtar NM, Ghoneim MA, Hussein MH. The impact of schistosomiasis on the pathology of bladder carcinoma. *Cancer* 1981; **48**(12): 2643–8.

109 Cannon J, Linke CA, Cos LR. Cyclophosphamide-associated carcinoma of urothelium: modalities for prevention. *Urology* 1991; **38**(5): 413–16.

110 Sigal SH, Tomaszewski JE, Brooks JJ, Wein A, LiVolsi VA. Carcinosarcoma of bladder following long-term cyclophosphamide therapy. *Arch Pathol Lab Med* 1991; **115**: 1049–51.

111 Pathak AB, Advani SH, Gopal R, Nadkarni KS, Saikia TK. Urinary bladder cancer following cyclophosphamide therapy for Hodgkin's disease. *Leuk Lymphoma* 1992; **8**(6): 503–4.

112 Ellis M, Lishner M. Second malignancies following treatment in non-Hodgkin's lymphoma. *Leuk Lymphoma* 1993; **9**(4–5): 337–42.

113 Boffetta P, Kaldor JM. Secondary malignancies following cancer chemotherapy. *Acta Oncol* 1994; **33**: 591–8.

114 Kaldor JM, Day NE, Kittlemann B *et al.* Bladder tumours following chemotherapy and radiotherapy for ovarian cancer: a case-control study. *Int J Cancer* 1995; **63**: 1–6.

115 Radis CD, Kahl LE, Baker GL *et al.* Effects of cyclophosphamide on the development of malignancy and on long-term survival of patients with rheumatoid arthritis. A 20-year follow-up study. *Arthritis Rheum* 1995; **38**: 1120–7.

116 Travis LB, Curtis RE, Glimelius B *et al.* Bladder and kidney cancer following cyclophosphamide therapy for non-Hodgkin's lymphoma. *J Natl Cancer Inst* 1995; **87**: 524–30.

117 McCredie M, Coates MS, Ford JM *et al.* Geographical distribution of cancers of the kidney and urinary tract and analgesic nephropathy in Australia and New Zealand. *Aust N Z J Med* 1990; **20**: 684–8, 694.

118 McCredie M, Stewart JH, Ford JM, MacLellan RA. Phenacetin-containing analgesics and cancer of the bladder or renal pelvis in women. *Br J Urol* 1983; **55**: 220–4.

119 McCredie M, Stewart JH, Ford JM. Analgesics and tobacco as risk factors for cancer of the ureter and renal pelvis. *J Urol* 1983; **130**: 28–30.

120 Moller-Jensen O, Knudsen JP, Sørensen BL, Clemmesen J. Artificial sweeteners and absence of bladder risk in Copenhagen. *Int J Cancer* 1983; **32**: 577–82.

121 Elcock M, Morgan RW. Update on artificial sweeteners and bladder cancer. *Regul Toxicol Pharmacol* 1993; **17**(1): 35–43.

122 Steinmetz KA, Potter JD. Vegetables, fruit, and cancer. I. Epidemiology. *Cancer Causes Control* 1991; **2**(5): 325–57.

123 Shibata A, Paganini-Hill A, Ross RK, Henderson BE. Intake of vegetables, fruits, beta-carotene, vitamin C and vitamin supplements and cancer incidence among the elderly: a prospective study. *Br J Cancer* 1992; **66**(4): 673–9.

124 Parkin DM, Muir CS, Whelan S *et al. Cancer Incidence in Five Continents*, Vol VI (IARC Scientific Publication No. 120). Lyon: International Agency for Research on Cancer, 1992.

125 Muir CS, Waterhouse JAH, Mack T, Powell J, Whelan S (eds) *Cancer Incidence in Five Continents*, Vol V (IARC Scientific Publication No. 88). Lyon: International Agency for Research on Cancer, 1987.

CHAPTER 2

Bladder cancer as a molecular disease

G. Dalbagni and W.R. Fair

Introduction

Over 50,000 new cases of bladder cancer are diagnosed every year in the US and are responsible for more than 10,000 deaths annually [1]. Seventy percent of bladder tumours are superficial at initial presentation, i.e. confined to the mucosa or submucosa (Ta, T1, Tis). Approximately 50–70% of these tumours will recur with 10–30% showing grade and stage progression [2]. Identifying those patients whose tumours will progress is obviously critical in selecting appropriate therapy and reducing mortality. Thirty percent of bladder-tumour patients present initially with muscle-invasive and or metastatic disease. Of these, 50% will ultimately succumb to metastatic disease despite aggressive local therapy [3]. The optimal management of human bladder cancer requires early detection of the tumour and an accurate assessment of its biological potential.

Despite the recent advances in diagnostic modalities, we still lack the ability to predict the behaviour of bladder tumours. Recent efforts to investigate the role of tumour-suppressor genes in bladder-tumour progression have led to the identification of tumour markers that may potentially complement existing modalities and improve our diagnosis, assessment and management of bladder cancer.

Genetic alterations follow a sequence of events leading to cancer progression. Certain genotypes correlate with clinicopathological parameters of poor clinical outcome such as stage, grade, vascular invasion and nodal status. These genetic alterations result in activation of oncogenes or inactivation of tumour-suppressor genes.

A normal regulatory gene that is stimulatory or results in cell proliferation when activated is called a proto-oncogene and is a normal component of the cell (Fig. 2.1). When this gene is altered, it is called an oncogene and results in uncontrolled cell proliferation. The second category of genes are inhibitory genes which result in cell inhibition. These are called tumour-suppressor genes and if altered result in uncontrolled cell proliferation (Fig. 2.2).

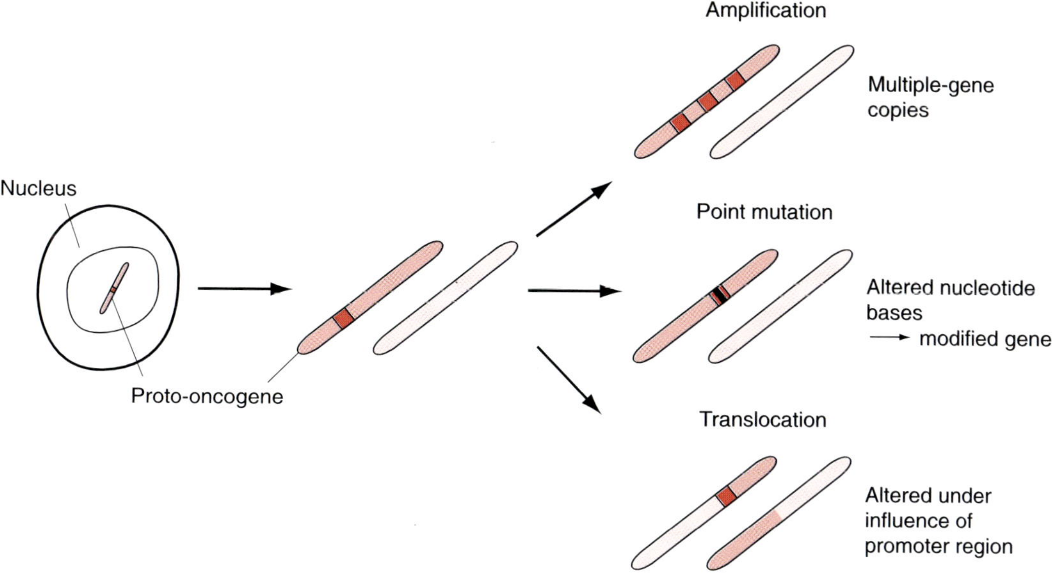

Figure 2.1. Oncogene activation.

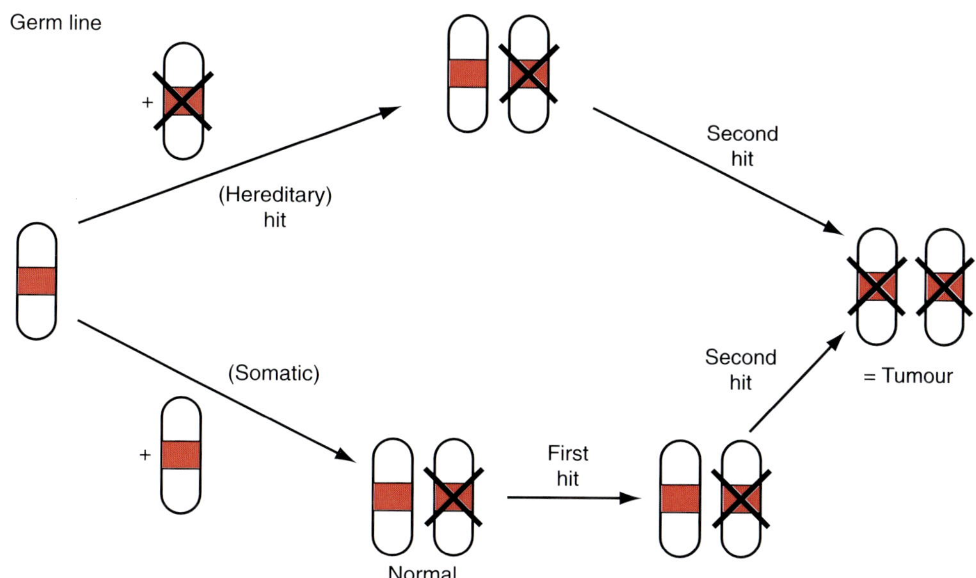

Figure 2.2. Tumour-suppressor gene.

Genetic alterations in bladder cancer

We adopted the following strategy to detect genetic alterations in bladder tumours. Primary-bladder tumours obtained from radical cystectomy specimens or from endoscopic resection were obtained. Polymorphic probes located on nine different chromosomal arms were used to detect loss of heterozygocity (LOH). Densitometry using an Ultrascan XL laser densitometer was performed. The ratio of alleles in tumour and normal samples was determined. The non-deleted allele in the tumour was used to normalize the densitometric tracing. LOH was defined as a greater than 40% decrease in signal intensity of an allele [4].

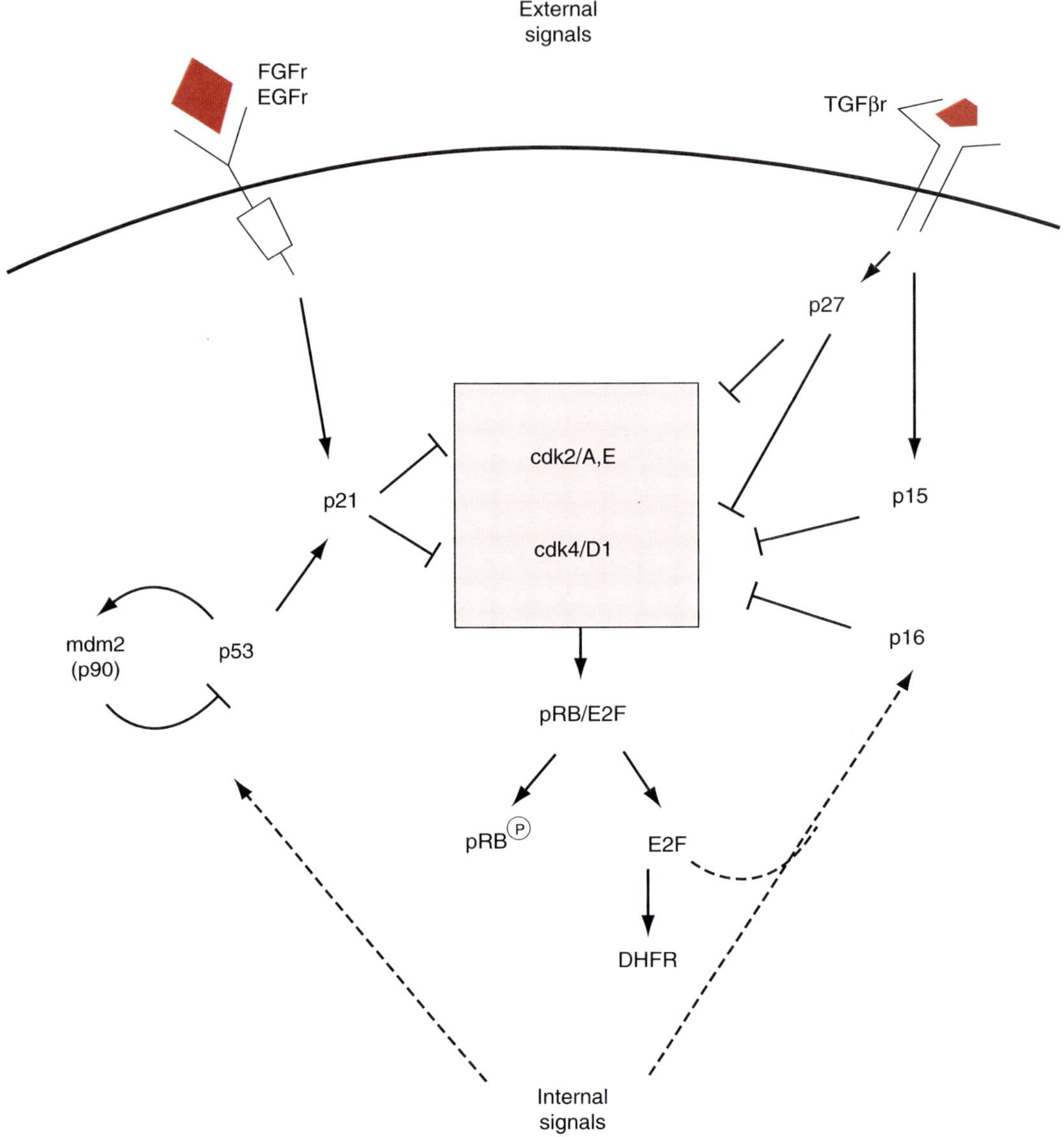

Figure 2.3. Cell cycle regulation. Cordon-Cardo C. Mutations of cell cycle regulators. Biological and clinical implications for human neoplasia. Am J Path 147: 545–60, 1995. Reproduced with permission.

Allelic deletion of *3p* was not present in any of the informative superficial papillary lesions, while 18 of 33 invasive tumours had such an alteration. The difference was statistically significant.

Allelic deletions were identified in 11 out of 40 informative cases. The data indicate that *5q* deletions do occur in bladder cancer and suggest that a tumour-suppressor gene located on chromosome 5 might be involved in the transition from papillary superficial Ta to locally invasive transitional cell carcinoma (TCC). The *adenomatous polyposis coli* (APC) gene might be such a gene. Mutations of the APC were also found to be mutated in the bladder carcinoma cell line SV-HUC.

All the deletions were detected in the muscle-invasive tumours, suggesting the participation of *6q* LOH in bladder-cancer progression.

Loss of heterozygocity of *9q* was detected in 60% of the informative cases (22/37). All Ta tumours and 9 out of 10 T1 showed *9q* alterations. However, only 43% of (10 out of 23) muscle invasive tumours had *9q* deletions. There was a statistically significant difference when comparing *9q* LOH between T1 vs T2–4 (*p* = 0.021). This finding suggests that two different pathways exist in the transition from superficial non-invasive and early invasive-bladder tumours to muscle-invasive lesions. One may postulate that muscle-invasive tumours showing *9q* alterations develop from Ta/T1 lesions. Alternatively, T2+ tumours without such abnormality may develop from a different early lesion, most likely cis.

Allelic deletion of *13q* was detected in 6 out of 24 informative cases. This corroborates previously reported data in which alteration of the *Rb* gene was detected in a small percentage of cases. Discrepancies between genetic studies and altered pattern of *Rb* expression might be due to transcriptional or translational modifications.

Allelic deletion of *17p* has been detected in 21 out of 47 informative cases with a statistically significant difference when comparing different stages. Deletions were not identified among Ta while 21 out of 38 invasive tumours exhibited *17p* LOH (Table 2.1).

Only *3p* correlated with vascular invasion. No association was found between allelic deletion and the nodal status. This is surprising in view of the fact that on *17q* lies the *nm23* gene which is involved in metastasis of breast cancer and melanoma. This lack of association between *nm23* deletion and nodal status may be due to a defect at the post-transcription or post-translational level, or might be due to the heterogeneity of the tumour in which the metastatic clonal population did have an *nm23* deletion which could not be detected by our technique.

Table 2.1 Association between allelic deletion and stage.

	3p	*5q*	*6q*	*9q*	*11p*	*13q*	*17p*	*17q*	*18q*
Stage*									
Cis	0/0	0/1	0/0	0/1	0/0	0/0	0/1	0/1	0/0
Ta/Pa	0/8	0/3	0/1	3/3	1/4	1/3	0/8	1/8	0/5
T1/P1	3/8	3/10	0/5	9/10	3/8	1/5	3/7	3/7	0/5
T2+/P2+	15/25	8/26	6/19	10/23	7/18	4/16	18/31	6/37	6/20
Total	18/41	11/40	6/25	22/37	11/30	6/24	21/47	10/53	6/30

*Expressed as number of deletions/number of informative cases.

p53 mutations and bladder cancer

The *p53* gene has been mapped to *17p13.1.* and encodes a 53 Kd nucleoprotein which appears to be involved in cell-cycle regulation and act as a check point arresting cells in G1. DNA damage resulting from exposure to a mutagenic agent for example, leads to an increase of the level of *p53* which will result in cell-cycle arrest and allows the DNA damage to be repaired. *p53* might also induce apoptosis or programmed cell death [5,6]. Mutations in the *p53* gene will result in the inactivation of its encoded product and lead to cell proliferation in the presence of DNA damage with the subsequent accumulation of genetic alterations.

Genetic alterations of the *p53* gene, such as intragenic mutations, homozygous deletions, and structural rearrangements, are frequent events in bladder cancer [5,6]. Sidranski *et al.* [7] identified genetic alterations of the *p53* gene in 11 of 18 invasive-bladder carcinomas. Furthermore, by using the polymerase chain reaction (PCR), mutations were detected in the urine samples of three patients. Fujimoto *et al.* [8] investigated structural alterations of the *p53* gene using single-strand conformation polymorphism (SSCP) in 25 bladder tumours. This technique is based on the fact that the presence of mutations will result in a change in the conformation of the DNA molecule and thus will migrate at a different rate in a polyacrylamide gel. They found mutations in 6 of 12 invasive carcinomas, but in only 1 of 13 superficial bladder tumours. Moreover, mutations were not identified in any of the 10 grade-1 and -2 lesions, while 8 of 15 grade-3 bladder carcinomas were found to have intragenic mutations.

We have defined chromosome 17 alterations in human bladder tumours and correlated p53 nuclear overexpression with *17p* deletions [9]. In this study, we made the assumption that nuclear overexpression as detected by immunohistochemistry reflects the presence of mutations in the majority of cases. This assumption was based on the fact that the presence of a mutation confers upon the gene-product a half-life 4–20 times longer than the wild-type p53 [10]. This increased half-life is partially due to conformational changes of the molecule [10]. Thus an increase in the steady-state level of the mutated protein leads to a positive nuclear staining by IHC, whereas the short half-life of the wild-type product precludes its detection using this technique. We studied 60 bladder tumours with a panel of mouse monoclonal antibodies (PAb1801, PAb240 and PAb1620) to the mutant and the wild-type p53 proteins using immunohistochemistry (Table 2.2). p53 nuclear overexpression correlated with grade (p = 0.027), stage (p = 0.008), vascular invasion (p = 0.021) and the presence of nodal metastases (p = 0.007). Nuclear overexpression of p53 was seen in superficial as well as in invasive tumours, whereas loss of heterozygocity was seen only in invasive tumours.

We also examined the hypothesis that p53 nuclear overexpression reflects the presence of mutations. We evaluated the sensitivity and specificity of immuno-histochemistry in detecting mutations, when compared to SSCP and sequencing [11]. Forty-two patients with bladder tumours in whom paired normal and tumour tissues were available were used for this study. Nuclear immunoreactivities were observed in 26 of 42 bladder tumours that were analysed. Abnormal shifts in mobility were noted in 14 of the 42 cases in distinct exons, with one tumour revealing three mutations. There was a strong association between p53 nuclear overexpression and detection of *p53* mutations by SSCP and sequencing (p < 0.001). By using receiver-operating curve statistical analysis, the accuracy of detecting *p53* mutations by IHC was estimated to be 90.3%. It was concluded that IHC is a highly sensitive and specific method that could be used in a clinical setting to detect mutations in the *p53* gene.

Data from the previously discussed studies pointed to the importance of *17p* abnormalities and the implication of the *p53* gene in bladder cancer. The aim of the next series of analyses was to investigate the possibility that altered patterns of *p53* expression correlated with tumour progression in patients with bladder cancer.

A cohort of patients with early invasive disease (T1), were studied retrospectively. Forty-three bladder tumours were evaluated by immunohistochemistry, using the mouse monoclonal antibody PAb1801 on deparaffinized tissue sections. The data were then correlated with clinicopathological variables, including grade, vascular invasion, the presence of associated carcinoma *in situ*, age and sex. The median follow-up for these patients was 119 months. None of the normal urothelial cells and stromal cells showed p53 nuclear overexpression. However, patients with T1 bladder tumours could be stratified into two groups. Eighteen patients (42%) had undetectable or less than 20% tumour cells with positive nuclear staining (Group A), while the remaining 25 patients (58%) had more than 20% tumour cells with nuclear immunoreactivity (Group B). Patients in Group B had a significantly shorter progression-free interval ($p < 0.001$). Disease-progression rates were 20.5% per year for Group B and 2.5% for Group A [12].

The prevalence and clinical relevance of *p53* nuclear overexpression were investigated in 54 patients with Ta bladder carcinomas, who did not receive any prior adjuvant therapy [13]. The median follow-up was 110 months. The same threshold for the scoring of IHC was used as in the previous study. The patients were stratified into Group A (< 20% positive tumour cells), and Group B (> 20% positive tumour cells). Tumour progression was observed in 5 of 42 patients in Group A, while 7 of 12 patients of Group B progressed ($p = 0.002$). Nuclear overexpression of p53 was the only independent variable associated with death due to bladder cancer in this cohort ($p = 0.004$).

Analysis of p53 nuclear overexpression in 33 patients with carcinoma *in situ* revealed a similar trend. These patients did not receive any adjuvant therapy. The median follow-up for this cohort of patients was 124 months, and 16 patients developed disease progression during that period. The association of the p53 phenotype and tumour progression was evaluated by multivariate analysis. Disease progression occurred in 3 of 18 patients with p53-negative phenotype (<20% cells positive), while 13 of 15 p53-positive patients (>20% cells positive) progressed. Moreover, death specifically due to bladder cancer was associated with altered patterns of *p53* expression [14].

A similar study examined the role of p53 as a prognostic marker in muscle-invasive tumours. Ninety bladder tumours from 111 patients treated with neo-adjuvant MVAC were evaluated. The median follow-up was 5.8 years. Patients with p53 overexpression had a significantly higher proportion of cancer deaths. The long-term survival in the p53 overexpressors was 7 of 17 (41%) vs 20 of 26 (77%) in the non-expressors [15].

Lipponen [16] independently reported a similar analysis in 212 unselected patients with bladder tumours, using immunohistochemistry and 20% positive nuclear staining as the cut-off value. However, the primary antibody was a purified rabbit polyserum (NCL-CM1-1:150 dilution). The mean follow-up time was greater than 10 years. The tumours were staged as follows: Ta ($n = 39$), T1 ($n = 57$), T2 ($n = 65$), T3 ($n = 34$) and T4 ($n = 17$). The grades were assigned as follows: 78 tumours were grade 1, 91 grade 2 and 43 grade 3. A positive p53 phenotype was detected in 62 tumours, 38 of those displaying over 20% tumour-cell staining. Nuclear overexpression of p53 was associated with tumour grade ($p = 0.014$). Progression was significantly related to *p53* nuclear overexpression. However, in a multivariate analysis, overexpression of p53 had no independent prognostic value over clinical stage and mitotic index.

Based on the data from these studies, *p53* nuclear overexpression, as detected by the monoclonal antibody PAb1801, seems to predict tumour behaviour. It may be useful for the selection of therapy in patients with superficial as well as invasive tumours.

During proliferation, the cell progresses through the cell cycle, which is under the control of different protein complexes. These protein complexes are composed of cyclins and cyclin-dependent kinases (CDK). The CDK-inhibitory molecules are a new family of proteins that exert their function through the inactivation of the catalytic operative units (Fig. 2.3).

The wild-type *p53* inhibits cell proliferation by interfering with the CDK2-cyclin complex through the induction of *p21*, a CDK-inhibitory molecule.

Conceptually, any mechanism that results in the deregulation of the cell cycle might result in tumorigenesis or tumour progression. Detailed analysis of the alterations in the cell cycle in bladder cancer are the current focus of laboratory investigation.

References

1   Silverberg E, Boring CC, Squires TS. Cancer statistics 1990. *CA* 1990; **40**: 1.

2   Catalona WJ, Dresner SM, Haaff EO *et al.* Management of superficial bladder cancer. In: Skinner DG, Lieskofsky G (eds) *Diagnosis and management of genitourinary cancer*. Philadelphia: WB Saunders, 1988; 281–94.

3   Whitmore WF Jr. Toward the rational management of bladder cancer. An overview. *Urology* 1988; **31**: 5–11.

4   Dalbagni G, Presti J, Reuter V, Fair WR, Cordon-Cardo C. Genetic alterations in bladder cancer. *Lancet* 1993; **342**: 469–71.

5   Levine AJ, Momand J, Finlay CA. The *p53* tumour suppressor gene. *Nature* 1991; **351**: 453–6.

6   Vogelstein B, Kinzler K. p53 function and dysfunction. *Cell* 1992; **70**: 523–6.

7   Sidransky D, von Eschenbach A, Tsai YC *et al.* Identification of the *p53* gene mutations in bladder cancers and urine samples. *Science* 1991; **252**: 706–9.

8   Fujimoto K, Yamada Y, Okajima E *et al.* Frequent association of *p53* gene mutation in invasive bladder cancer. *Cancer Res* 1992; **52**: 1393–8.

9   Dalbagni G, Presti JC Jr, Reuter VE *et al.* Molecular genetic alterations of chromosome 17 and p53 nuclear overexpression in human bladder cancer. *Diagnos Mol Pathol* 1993; **2**: 4–13.

10 Rivas CI, Wisniewski D, Strife A *et al.* Constitutive expression of p53 protein in enriched normal human marrow blast cell populations. *Blood* 1992; **79**: 1982–6.

11 Cordon-Cardo C, Dalbagni G, Saez GT *et al.* *p53* mutations in human bladder cancer: genotypic versus phenotypic patterns. *Int J Cancer* 1994; **56**: 347–53.

12 Sarkis AS, Dalbagni G, Cordon-Cardo C *et al.* Nuclear overexpression of p53 protein in transitional cell bladder carcinoma: a marker for disease progression. *J Nat Cancer Inst* 1993; **85**: 53–9.

13 Sarkis AS, Zhang Z-F, Cordon-Cardo C *et al.* p53 nuclear overexpression and disease progression in Ta bladder carcinoma. *Int J Oncol* 1993; **3**: 355–60.

14 Sarkis AS, Dalbagni G, Cordon-Cardo C *et al.* Association of p53 nuclear overexpression and tumor progression in carcinoma *in situ* of the bladder. *J Urol* 1994; **152**: 388–92.

15 Sarkis AS, Bajorin D, Reuter *et al.* The prognostic value of p53 nuclear overexpression in patients with invasive bladder cancer treated with neoadjuvant MVAC. *J Clin Oncol* 1995; **13**: 1384–90.

16 Lipponen PK. Overexpression of p53 nuclear oncoprotein in transitional cell bladder cancer and its prognostic value. *Int J Cancer* 1993; **53**: 365–70.

CHAPTER 3

Current issues in pathology of superficial bladder cancer

W.M. Murphy

Introduction

The term 'superficial bladder cancer' defines a group of neoplasms with widely varying pathological features and capacities for aggressive behaviour. Neoplasms in this category include low-grade transitional-cell tumours, intermediate- and high-grade non-invasive and superficially-invasive transitional-cell carcinomas, flat, non-invasive carcinoma *in situ* and even invasive, nodular transitional-cell carcinomas that have not yet invaded the detrusor muscle. Some lesions are benign, some are cytologically malignant but biologically non-aggressive, and some are both malignant and aggressive. The inclusion of an array of disparate neoplasms in a single category creates the need to subcategorize in order to optimize the approach to patient management. This discussion deals with the following issues.

- classification based on cellular features and patient outcomes;
- detection and monitoring;
- prognostic factors.

Classification

Neoplasms comprising 'superficial bladder cancer' can be divided into lesions of low- and high-aggressive potential based upon their cytological features as well as empirical observations of patient outcome (Table 3.1). The lowest grade, papillary transitional-cell tumours are so biologically innocuous that they should be considered benign and labelled transitional-cell papilloma.

Transitional-cell papilloma

Transitional-cell papilloma is an exophytic tumour that may comprise as much as 25% of all transitional-cell neoplasms [1]. These tumours have been classified as grade 1 transitional-cell carcinoma; grade-A transitional-cell carcinoma; and grade-1a transitional-cell carcinoma in other schemes [2,3]. These tumours most often occur at the bladder base and nearly 70% are single lesions [4]. Histologically, four to several layers of transitional cells are arranged on a delicate fibrovascular stalk. Rarely, these

Table 3.1 Histological classification of bladder tumours.

Low aggressive potential
   Transitional-cell papilloma
   Primary CIS
   Low-grade TCC with gland-like lumina
   Verrucous carcinoma
   Villous tumour
High aggressive potential
   High-grade TCC — with or without invasion
   CIS associated with high-grade TCC
   TCC, nested type
   TCC, sarcomatoid type
   TCC, micropapillary type
   TCC, with mixed or heterologous components
   Non-transitional-cell carcinomas — all types

TCC, transitional-cell carcinoma
CIS, carcinoma *in situ.*

cells may be completely normal in their phenotype but more commonly they are slightly atypical (Fig. 3.1). DNA synthesis, as evaluated by multiple parameters including assessment of nucleolar organizer regions and *Ki67*, has not varied significantly from normal in the cells of transitional-cell papillomas [5,6]. Neither do

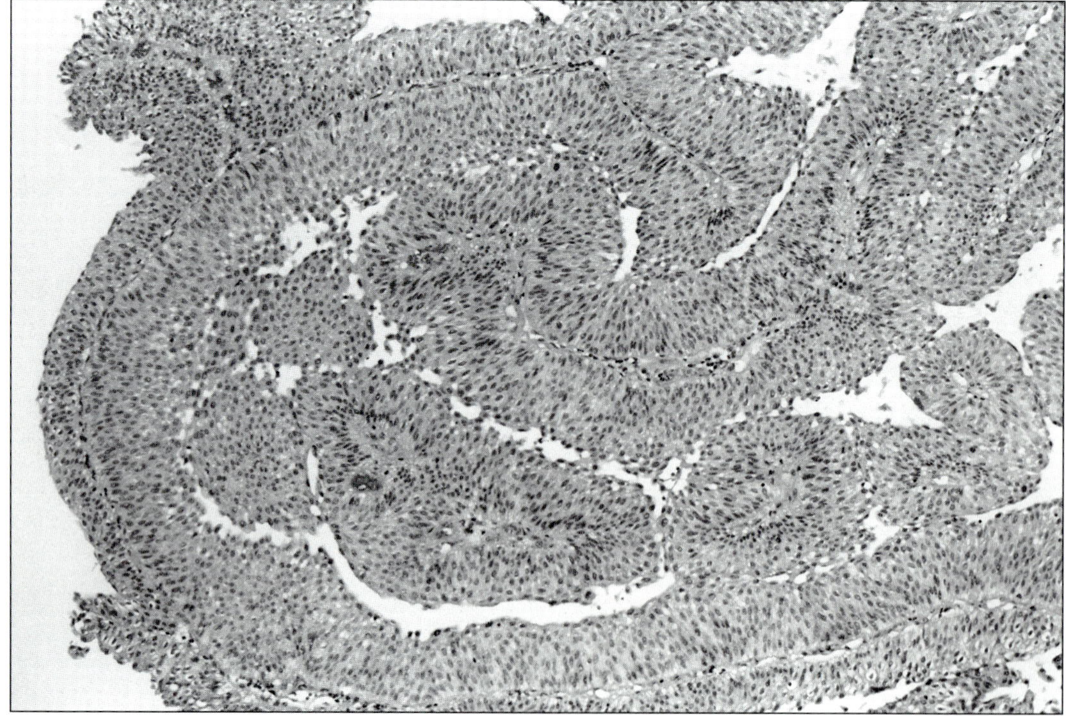

Figure 3.1. Transitional cell papilloma.

the cells of these lesions harbour significant genetic abnormalities [7]. DNA diploidy has been documented in almost 95% of cases examined [8,9,10]. In fact, the cells of transitional-cell papillomas are closely akin to normal in nearly every respect. In cytological samples of urine or bladder washings, disaggregated cells from transitional-cell papillomas can be recognized as significantly abnormal in only 30–60% of cases, again reflecting their benign cellular phenotype [10,11].

The natural course of patients with transitional-cell papillomas has been incompletely documented. Tumours most likely grow slowly and sporadically and, if untreated, at least some lesions can achieve large size and become the source of significant bleeding and infection. The frequency with which this occurs is unknown since approximately 50% of patients have no recurrences after primary resection and many individuals are undoubtedly lost to follow-up. Neither invasion into the muscular wall nor metastases have been well documented for transitional-cell papillomas [12]. The 10-year actuarial survival in one series was 98% and all deaths from bladder cancer occurred 9–15 years after patients presented with a transitional-cell papilloma [1]. It should be emphasized that the prognosis for patients presenting with a transitional-cell papilloma is very good. A more aggressive carcinoma has developed in less than 10% of cases in most series. In contrast to previous thinking, there seems to be no direct relationship between the number and frequency of recurrences and the likelihood of developing a more aggressive tumour. Nonetheless, patients with transitional-cell papillomas are at increased risk, compared to the general population, for the development of an aggressive transitional-cell carcinoma and a small percentage of these individuals have died of bladder cancer.

Transitional-cell carcinomas of intermediate and high grade have the capacity to invade and metastasize and should be considered true carcinomas [1,13]. The histological and cytological distinction between intermediate- and high-grade

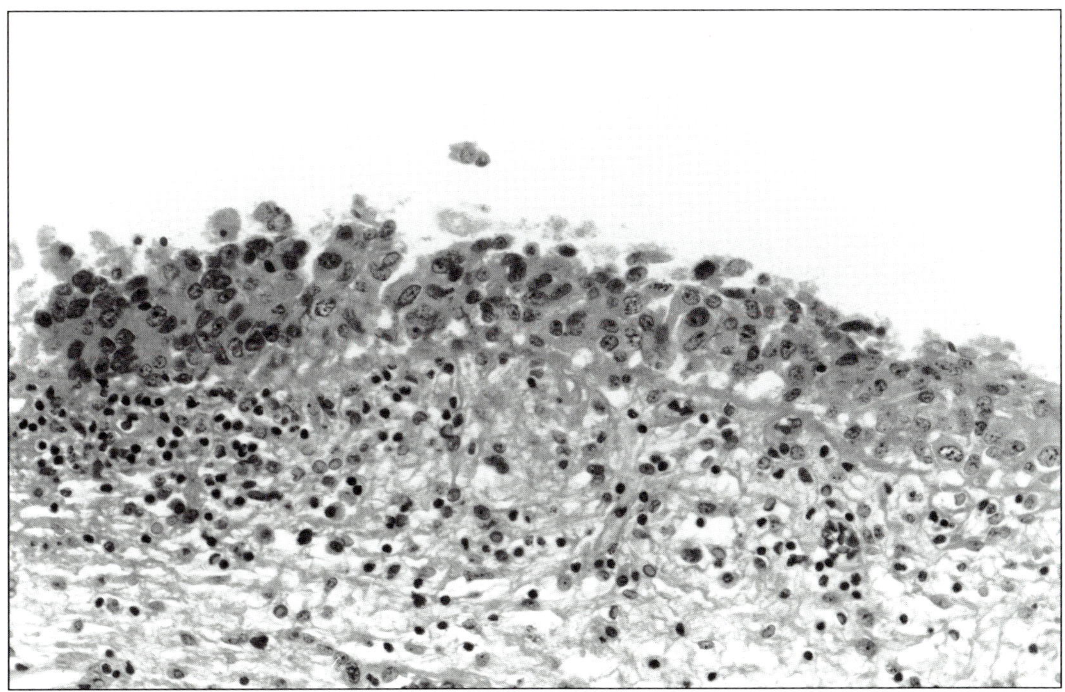

Figure 3.2. Urothelial carcinoma in situ.

transitional-cell carcinomas is vague and poorly reproducible among pathologists. As a practical matter, the majority of transitional-cell carcinomas are of high cytological grade and almost all cancer-related deaths occur among patients who present with high-grade transitional-cell carcinoma [1,13,14]. These lesions can invade the lamina propria as well as the detrusor muscle while still maintaining a papillary component. The notion that almost all invasive tumours arise as nodular lesions is often stated but poorly documented.

At least two issues regarding sub-staging of superficial bladder cancers, on the basis of lamina proprial invasion have been raised: (1) involvement of thin-walled blood vessels beneath the epithelium, and (2) transgression of the 'muscularis mucosae'. While vascular invasion into vessels in the lamina propria can certainly occur, a cautious approach to interpretation is advised. Many of the spaces immediately beneath the bladder epithelium are fixation artifacts rather than true vessels [15]. The possibility of sub-staging T1 lesions on the basis of transgression of the muscularis mucosae is intriguing but probably not practical. Most importantly, the muscularis mucosae (if defined as an anatomical barrier composed of smooth muscle cells like that of the colon) does not exist in the human urinary bladder. Instead, a loosely arranged, non-planar aggregation of thick-walled blood vessels and wispy smooth muscle fibres is present. The muscle fibres may be well developed in 6–20% of cases, but almost never form a continuous layer [16,17]. Accurate assessment is often impossible in bladder biopsies and transurethral resections. Very superficial invasion can be distinguished from invasion to the detrusor but assessment of the area between these points is very likely to be irreproducible among pathologists, since the anatomical structures themselves are quite variable.

Urothelial carcinoma in situ

Urothelial carcinoma *in situ* is a controversial subject upon which no general agreement exists (Fig. 3.2). Many authors believe that the lesion is itself aggressive and that patients with carcinoma *in situ* (CIS) are at the threshold of having an invasive carcinoma. Observations from several other groups indicate that CIS is an indolent lesion lacking the ability to invade [18,19,20]. The problem is compounded by the fact that nearly all carcinomas *in situ* arise in patients who already have high-grade transitional-cell carcinomas, whether these high grade TCCS have been previously resected or are occurring concomitantly. In such cases, the prognosis probably relates more to the invasive neoplasm than to the *in situ* component. Patients presenting with CIS as their initial lesion (primary CIS) have a very low observed death rate from bladder cancer and a much lower rate of progression than those having CIS in association with invasive transitional-cell carcinoma (secondary CIS). Further, both the antigenic composition and chromosomal abnormalities of CIS differ from those of invasive carcinoma [21,22]. Expression of the suppressor gene *p53* is more variable in CIS than one would expect [23]. The cells of CIS apparently prefer to live in an intraepithelial environment, not invading even when their basement membranes are ruptured mechanically by biopsy forceps. Despite a low potential for aggressive behaviour, patients with CIS have a serious disease that requires constant monitoring, even when the CIS is not associated with a previous or coincident invasive carcinoma.

Detection and monitoring

Clinical and laboratory tests for the detection and monitoring of bladder cancer have been developed to determine the presence of neoplasia, localize the process and gauge its extent, and evaluate its biological potential. No single method can adequately fulfil all of these requirements and new techniques are constantly being investigated. Methods for detection and monitoring can be considered in three basic categories: (1) established tests with an extensive data base grounded in years of empirical observation and comparative studies; (2) promising techniques with limited data bases of empirical observation lacking long-term monitoring; (3) methods whose practical value is curtailed by limited clinical applications, inconsistent results, lack of specificity, or an insufficient database. This discussion will deal with only items (1) and (2).

Established methods for detection and monitoring include bi-manual palpation, cystoscopy with or without biopsy, random or selected-site biopsies, and urinary cytology. Each is an important factor and these methods should be considered complementary rather than mutually exclusive. Of course, histological examination is the gold standard, since bladder cancer is defined in histological terms. Urinary cytology as a diagnostic procedure actually antedates histology and has recently been widely accepted as a monitoring tool [11,24,25]. Bladder washings, especially when multiple specimens are taken, are associated with the highest diagnostic yield, but random voided urines are also useful [26]. Many pathologists find urinary cytology particularly difficult and may tend to undercall the lesions. Therefore, a pathological diagnosis of 'suspicious' should be given more attention than it otherwise might when this term is used to describe a urinary specimen. The urinary cytological method is capable of detecting well over 90% of all true bladder carcinomas, given adequate samples and in competent hands. Urinary cytology is not particularly diagnostic for non-malignant lesions, such as transitional-cell papillomas (grade-1 carcinoma in other systems). Urinary cytology is especially helpful for monitoring patients having received topical therapy, since the epithelial changes occurring after topical therapy can confound cystoscopic evaluation. The most frequently employed topical agent, bacillus Calmette–Guérin (BCG), causes no urothelial changes that would confound the pathological interpretation of carcinoma [25]. Topical alkylating agents such as Mitomycin C can cause bizarre nuclear changes but these are essentially confined to superficial cells and should not cause significant confusion among pathologists aware of the effects of topical alkylating agents. A positive urinary cytology in association with a negative cystoscopy should lead the urologist to examine the prostatic ducts, ureters and urethra for residual neoplasm.

The total amount of DNA in urothelial cells can be assessed using either flow or image cytometry. Results are usually expressed as 'DNA ploidy' although that terminology actually indicates the number of chromosomes in a nucleus. The clinical value of cytometry for DNA ploidy is inversely proportional to the proficiency of pathologists with urinary cytology [27,28,29]. In general, cells with hyperchromatic, pleomorphic nuclei are DNA aneuploid. Pathologists using classification schemes such as the World Health Organization (WHO), where over 50% of lesions are grouped into an intermediate category, benefit from subcategorization using cytometry. Those lacking proficiency in urinary cytology also benefit. Cytometry for DNA ploidy has been useful in certain practice situations but is not generally recommended for routine monitoring [30].

Quantitative nuclear morphometry has been extensively studied in a limited number of institutions [31,32]. A vast array of means, coefficients, and indices can be calculated after measuring only a few actual parameters, such as nuclear perimeter and nuclear diameters in various planes. Despite its potential virtues, especially in diagnostic precision, quantitative morphometry has not achieved widespread clinical acceptance.

The infrastructure and genetic composition of bladder neoplasms has been assessed using antibodies to a variety of cellular constituents [21,33,34,35,36]. (Table 3.2) Antibodies can be separated into four types based upon the antigens to which they react: blood group antigens, cytokeratins, nuclear-matrix proteins, and glycoproteins. They have been used in four basic ways:

- to identify early changes of neoplasia in urothelium;
- to distinguish epithelial cells from stromal elements, often in the lamina propria of small bladder biopsies with recurrent transitional-cell carcinoma;
- to differentiate metastatic transitional-cell carcinomas from other tumours;
- to identify malignant transitional cells in urinary specimens.

In clinical settings, direct application of antibodies to cells in urinary or tissue specimens can be efficacious in certain situations, e.g. increasing the level of certainty when evaluating tissues for invasive carcinoma, detection of low- and high-grade neoplastic cells in urinary specimens, and detection of the presence of a transitional-cell carcinoma in urinary specimens that lack recognizable tumour cells. Use of these

Table 3.2 Antibodies (AB) and transitional-cell neoplasia.

Antibody	Sensitivity
Blood group ABH	Normal TC
Blood group T, LeX	TCC, high grade
CEA	Reactive TC, TCC
486P 3/12	TCC, all grades
M344	TCC, low grade > high grade
19A211	TCC, low grade > high grade
BL2-10DI	TCC, low grade > high grade
BLCA-8	TCC
DD23	TCC
CK 7, 8, 13, 18. 19	Normal, TCC
CK 20	TCC
GPs-Om5	Normal, TCC
—T138	TCC, high grade > low grade
—T43	TCC
—MO145	Normal, TCC low grade
—G4	Normal, TCC
—others	Mostly TCC high grade
NMPs	Nuclear matrix proteins from neoplasms and regenerating epithelium

TCC, transitional-cell carcinoma.

antibodies for detection and monitoring has been successful in only a very few hands; they are not in widespread use.

Genes and gene products can be assessed by a variety of techniques, including light microscopy after appropriate immunohistochemical reactions. This is a very rapidly changing field and the clinical significance of any particular finding cannot be assured. Even the conceptual underpinning for identification of genes, i.e. that changes in single genes can cause single diseases, is undergoing modification among cancer biologists [37]. For transitional-cell carcinomas, the most important genetic abnormalities apparently occur in suppressor genes rather than proliferation genes. Abnormal expression of the *p53* gene, for example, has been associated with the presence of high-grade transitional-cell carcinoma and may be valuable in certain situations, where the malignancy of the cells in tissue or urinary specimens is in doubt. The value of *p53* in superficial bladder cancer is controversial [38,39]. It is important to recall that a significant percentage of patients with high-grade transitional-cell carcinomas suffer progressive disease in the absence of demonstrable abnormalities in the *p53* gene.

Chromosomal abnormalities are manifested either by abnormal numbers or abnormal structural changes [40]. The most important chromosomes in bladder cancer seem to be 5, 9, 11, and 17 although a high frequency of abnormalities in chromosomes 1, 3, 7, and y has also been documented. With the exception of chromosome 9, these abnormalities almost all occur among high-grade tumours and the possibility of an epiphenomenon is strong. Interestingly, chromosome 9 is the site of the blood group antigens as well as of a relatively recently described suppressor gene called *p16* (MTS) [41,42].

Cell kinetics, like genetic constitution, is a rapidly evolving area. Determinations of cell turnover are rarely important to detection and monitoring of bladder neoplasms and the subject is included here primarily for completeness. The rate of DNA synthesis can be assessed in many different ways [5,6]. Few studies of programmed cell death (apoptosis) have been applied to transitional-cell neoplasms, but the scant information available seems to indicate no clinical value [43,44].

Prognostic factors

A vast array of pathological features has been considered important in predicting the outcome of patients with bladder neoplasms (Table 3.3). Most have failed to stand the test of time, very likely because human cancer is an incredibly complex phenomenon whose mechanisms vary among individuals. Modern technology allows us to search the genome for key events but there may be no common genetic pathways for bladder neoplasms. Those who would study prognostic factors should be aware of the following mitigating phenomena:

- prognostic factors, i.e. features of disease that predict its outcome, are often confused with biological markers, i.e. features of neoplasms that allow their detection or describe their metabolic functions;
- when addressing prognostic factors, results are often reported in the literature using known outcomes for comparison when the actual outcome will not have been known at the time the putative prognostic factor was measured;

Table 3.3 Prognostic factors in bladder cancer.

Established value
  Tumour type
  Grade (TCC) only)
  Stage —
      Detrusor-muscle depth
      Vessels
      Prostate gland/seminal vesicles
      Urethra, ureters
      Specimen margins (cystectomy)
      Metastases
  Positive cytology
Possible value
  Associated CIS
  Genes (*p53*, *p16*)
  Proliferation/synthesis (MIB1, PCNA)
  Receptors (adhesion molecules)
  Morphometry
  Cytometry (DNA ploidy)
  Muscularis mucosae
  Angiogenesis
Unproven value
  CEA
  Blood group antigens (? except Lewis X)
  Surface morphology (SEM)
  Apoptosis

- most adverse prognostic factors are determined from tumours that have already progressed and these features cannot be distinguished from epiphenomena, i.e. non-causative features arising simultaneously or subsequently to the factors responsible for the progression;
- the constant pressure to deliver data tends to favour reports with short follow-ups, justified with statistical methods that require little actual outcome information, so that a great deal of assumption is built into the statistical conclusions;
- even studies reporting results in terms of multivariate analyses have examined only a small number of the many factors touted to have prognostic value;
- the prognostic value of any particular test can be inflated if the observers are not proficient with older methods used for comparison or if the classification scheme includes a broad range of dissimilar lesions within a single grade or type;
- many reports measure outcome only in terms of patient status at last contact and do not also include interval changes during follow-up;
- all prognostic factors are determined for populations of patients and may not be applicable to any particular individual;
- regardless of the number of prognostic factors reported, patients with bladder neoplasms can follow only a limited number of courses — they can be alive with

no evidence of disease throughout their course; alive with disease but unaffected by it; alive with disease and limited by it; dead from other causes with or without disease; or dead from disease.

It has become customary to separate prognostic factors into three categories: (1) features of known value accepted by tradition, consensus, or controlled trials — these factors should be included in every appropriate pathology report; (2) features of possible value that lack an appropriate database or general agreement among experts — these factors may be evaluated and reported depending upon the resources of the individual group practice; (3) features of unproven value either because of the paucity of data or because of lack of consensus after extensive study. Some of the tests used to detect and monitor superficial bladder cancers have also been considered to have prognostic value. A positive cytology after topical chemotherapy, for example, tends to identify patients who will eventually have an adverse outcome when compared to patients with similar tumours treated in a similar way but having negative cytology [45,46]. Factors detected by newer modalities of testing, such as abnormalities in the *p53* gene or its products, may have prognostic value but results have been conflicting [22,29].

In summary, current issues in the pathology of superficial bladder cancer have centered upon classification, detection and monitoring, and prognostic factors. Most studies tend to advocate the value of one system or factor over all others but it is very likely that the secret to superficial bladder neoplasia is multifactorial. Each test only examines a part of the problem and one needs to create a paradigm to incorporate the results of multiple tests into a scheme for improving patient management. The pathologist is often central to this process and should be considered a medical consultant with special expertise in the interpretation of technical findings as well as the biology of bladder neoplasia. An important issue that is rarely assessed is the measurement of benefits to any particular individual from any particular treatment regimen. In an age of dwindling medical resources, it can no longer be assumed that any treatment is better than none. Nor can it be assumed that patients will benefit when treated upon principles that might apply to groups rather than to individuals. Our challenge for the future is to design a paradigm that will be flexible enough to incorporate variations in testing for individual patients, in order to determine treatment regimens that will benefit the patient receiving the therapy, rather than a hypothetical group of individuals that might be treated in a similar fashion.

References

1   Jordan AM, Weingarten J, Murphy WM. Transitional cell neoplasms of the urinary bladder: can biologic potential be predicted from histologic grading? *Cancer* 1987; **60**: 2766–74.

2   Mostofi FK, Sorbin LH, Torloni H. Histological typing of urinary bladder tumours. *International Classification of Tumours* 19. Geneva: WHO 1973.

3   Malmström P-U, Busch C, Norlén BJ. Recurrence, progression and survival in bladder cancer: A retrospective analysis of 232 patients with ≥5-year follow-up. *Scand J Urol Nephrol* 1987; **21**: 185–95.

4   Prout GR Jr, Barton BA, Griffin PP *et al.* Treated history of noninvasive grade 1 transitional cell carcinoma. *J Urol* 1992; **148**: 1413–19.

5   Cairns P, Suarez V, Newman J, Croker J. Nucleolar organizer regions in transitional cell tumors of the bladder. *Arch of Path Lab Med* 1989; **113**: 1250–2.

6   Okamura K, Miyake K, Koshikawa T, Asai J. Growth fractions of transitional cell carcinoma of the bladder defined by the monoclonal antibody Ki-67. *J Urol* 1990; **144**: 875–8.

7   Miyamoto H, Shuin T, Ikeda I *et al.* Loss of heterozygosity at the p53, RB, DCC and APC tumor suppressor gene loci in human bladder cancer. *J Urol* 1996; **155**: 1444–7.

8   Tribukait B. Flow cytometry in assessing the clinical aggressiveness of genito-urinary neoplasms. *World J Urol* 1987; **5**: 108–22.

9   Murphy WM, Chandler RW, Trafford RM. Flow cytometry of deparaffinized nuclei compared to histological grade for the pathological evaluation of transitional cell carcinomas. *J Urol* 1986; **135**: 694–7.

10 Rife CC, Farrow GM, Utz DC. Urine cytology of transitional cell neoplasms. *Urol Clin N Am* 1979; **6**: 599–612.

11 Murphy WM, Soloway MS, Jukkola AF *et al.* Urinary cytology and bladder cancer — the cellular features of transitional cell neoplasms. *Cancer* 1984; **53**: 1555–65.

12 Melamed MR. Papillary tumors of the bladder. *J Cell Biochem* 1992; **161**(Suppl.): S44–70.

13 Kaubisch S, Lum BL, Reese J *et al.* Stage T1 bladder cancer: grade is the primary determinant for risk of muscle invasion. *J Urol* 1991; **146**: 28–31.

14 Kaye KW, Lange PH. Mode of presentation of invasive bladder cancer: Reassessment of the problem. *J Urol* 1982; **128**: 31–3.

15 Larsen MP, Steinberg GD, Brendler CB, Epstein JI. Use of *Ulex europaeus* agglutinin I (UEA1) to distinguish vascular and "pseudovascular" invasion in transitional cell carcinoma of bladder with lamina propria invasion. *Mod Pathol* 1990; **3**: 83–8.

16 Keep JC, Piehl M, Miller A, Oyasu R. Invasive carcinoma of the urinary bladder: evaluation of tunica muscularis mucosae involvement. *Am J Clin Pathol* 1989; **91**: 575–9.

17 Ro JY, Ayala AG, El-Naggar A. Muscularis mucosa of urinary bladder: importance for staging and treatment. *Am J Surgical Pathol* 1987; **11**: 668–73.

18 Farrow GM, Utz DC, Rife CC, Greene LF. Clinical observations on 69 cases of *in situ* carcinoma of the urinary bladder. *Cancer Res* 1977; **37**: 2794–8.

19 Orozco RE, Martin AA, Murphy WM. Carcinoma *in situ* of the urinary bladder: clues to host involvement in human carcinogenesis. *Cancer* 1994; **74**: 115–22.

20 Frazier HA, Robertson JE, Dodge RK, Paulson DF. The value of pathologic factors in predicting cancer-specific survival among patients treated with radical cystectomy for transitional cell carcinoma of the bladder and prostate. *Cancer* 1993; **71**: 3993–4001.

21 Bander NH. Monoclonal antibodies in urologic oncology. *Cancer* 1987; **60**: 658–67.

22 Spruck CH III, Ohneseit PF, Gonzalez–Zulueta M *et al.* Two molecular pathways to transitional cell carcinoma of the bladder. *Cancer Res* 1994; **54**: 784–8.

23 Hudson MA, Herr HW. Carcinoma *in situ* of the bladder. *J Urol* 1995; **153**: 564–72.

24 Raab SS, Slagel DD, Jensen CS *et al.* Transitional cell carcinoma: cytologic criteria to improve diagnostic accuracy. *Mod Pathol* 1996; **9**: 225–32.

25 Murphy WM, Beckwith JB, Farrow GM. Tumors of the kidneys, bladder and related urinary structures. In: Rosai J (ed) *Atlas of Tumor Pathology* (3rd series Fascicle). Washington DC: Armed Forces Institute of Pathology, 1994; 193–248.

26 Morrison DA, Murphy WM, Ford KS, Soloway MS. Surveillance of stage O, grade I bladder cancer by cytology alone — is it acceptable? *J Urol* 1984; **132**: 672–4.

27 Amberson JB, Laino JP. Image cytometric deoxyribonucleic acid analysis of urine specimens as an adjunct to visual cytology in the detection of urothelial cell carcinoma. *J Urol* 1993; **149**: 42–50.

28 Badalament RA, O'Toole RV, Keyhani-Rofagha S *et al.* Flow cytometric analysis of primary and metastatic bladder cancer. *J Urol* 1990; **143**: 912–6.

29 Murphy WM, Emerson LD, Chandler RW *et al.* Flow cytometry vs. urinary cytology in the evaluation of patients with bladder cancer. *J Urol* 1986; **136**: 815–19.

30 Wheeless LL, Badalament RA, deVere White RW, *et al.* Consensus review of the clinical utility of DNA cytometry in bladder cancer. *Cytometry* 1993; **14**: 478–81.

31 Blomjous CE, Vos W, Schipper NW *et al.* The prognostic significance of selective nuclear morphometry in urinary bladder carcinoma. *Hum Pathol* 1990; **21**: 409–13.

32 van der Poel HG, Schaafsma HE, Vooijs GP *et al.* Quantitative light microscopy in urological oncology. *J Urol* 1992; **148**: 1–13.

33 Sheinfeld J, Reuter VE, Melamed MR *et al.* Enhanced bladder cancer detection with the Lewis X antigen as a marker for neoplastic transformation. *J Urol* 1990; **143**: 285–8.

34 Heinzer H, Huland E, Mönk M, Huland H. Distribution of 486P 3/12 antigens, ABO(H) blood group antigen and T antigen in cystectomy specimens from patients with stage T2 transitional cell carcinoma of the bladder. *J Urol* 1992; **148**: 802–5.

35 Miettinen M. Keratin 20: Immunohistochemical marker for gastrointestinal, urothelial, and Merkel cell carcinomas. *Mod Pathol* 1995; **8**: 384–8.

36 Sarosdy MF, deVere White RW, Soloway MS *et al.* Results of a multicenter trial using the BTA test to monitor for and diagnose recurrent bladder cancer. *J Urol* 1995; **154**: 379–84.

37 Farber E, Rubin H. Cellular adaptation in the origin and development of cancer. *Cancer Res* 1991; **51**: 2751–61.

38 Sidransky D, Von Eschenbach A, Tsai YC *et al.* Identification of *p63* gene mutations in bladder cancers and urine samples. *Science* 1991; **252**: 706–9.

39 Têtu B, Fradet Y, Allard P, *et al.* Prevalence and clinical significance of HER-2/neu, p63, and Rb expression in primary superficial bladder cancer. *J Urol* 1996; **155**: 1784–8.

40 Sandberg AA. Chromosome changes in early bladder neoplasms. *J Cell Biochem* 1992; **161**(Suppl.): S76–90.

41 Yeager T, Stadler W, Belair C *et al.* Increased p16 levels correlate with pRb alterations in human urothelial cells. *Cancer Res* 1995; **55**: 493–7.

42 Poddighe PJ, Ramaekers FCS, Smeets AW *et al.* Structural chromosome 1 aberrations in transitional cell carcinoma of the bladder: interphase cytogenetics combining a centromeric, telomeric, and library DNA probe. *Cancer Res* 1992; **52**: 4929–34.

43 King ED, Matteson J, Jacobs SC, Kyprianou N. Incidence of apoptosis, cell proliferation and bcl-2 expression in transitional cell carcinoma of the bladder: association with tumor progression. *J Urol* 1996; **155**: 316–20.

44 Lipponen PK, Aaltomaa S. Apoptosis in bladder cancer as related to standard prognostic factors and prognosis. *J Pathol* 1994; **173**: 333–9.

45 Cant JD, Murphy WM, Soloway MS. Prognostic significance of urine cytology on initial follow-up after intravesical Mitomycin C for superficial bladder cancer. *Cancer* 1986; **57**: 2119–22.

46 Herr HW, Badalament RA, Amato DA *et al.* Superficial bladder cancer treated with bacillus Calmette–Guérin: A multivariate analysis of factors affecting tumor progression. *J Urol* 1989; **141**: 22–9.

CHAPTER 4

Natural history and prognosis of 'untreated' and 'treated' superficial bladder cancer

K. Kurth

Introduction

The term 'superficial bladder carcinoma' describes a type of transitional-cell carcinoma of the bladder with such common characteristics as: (1) limitation of the growth to the epithelial layer (Tis, Ta) or to the lamina propria (T1), (2) treatment mainly by the transurethral route and (3) a smaller risk of dying from this type of bladder tumour than from muscle-invasive tumours. Biologically the three types of superficial bladder tumours differ remarkably; on the one hand the lesions (TaG1, G2) show, during the course of the disease, neither morphologically nor in their behaviour, the sequelae of a truly malignant tumour. On the other hand the lesion which has already broke through the basal membrane shows its invasive property (T1). Cytologically the flat tumour (Tis) and the superficial grade-3 tumour show anaplastic abnormalities within the bladder epithelium (such as increased cellularity, nuclear crowding, disturbances of cellular polarity, polymorphism, irregularity in size and shape of cells, variation in chromatin pattern of nuclei, displaced or abnormal mitotic figures and giant cells) [1]. Wolf *et al.* [2] proposed not to apply the term carcinoma to Ta grade-1 and grade-2 tumours, because of the lack of evidence that this lesion has the biological relevance of a 'true' bladder carcinoma. The National Bladder Cancer Collaborative Group (US) (NBCCG) found little data to support the use of the term papilloma to describe even stage Ta, grade-1 tumours without reservation [3]. Whereas stage and grade-progression rates are low for Ta grade 1 and 2, these are only being reported for patients whose tumours have been treated. No evidence is available to indicate that if tumours were left alone they would not eventually undergo stage progression. With this in mind, considering the 50–90% recurrence rate (single v multiple tumours) at 5 years, it is wise to classify stage Ta grade-1 papillary tumours as transitional-cell carcinomas, rather than benign lesions, until more refined markers of prognosis and classification are available [4].

Regardless of treatment there is a 10–30% difference in survival between patients presenting with tumours of the Ta category compared to those with T1 tumours [5,6].

Carcinoma *in situ* is the most harmful type of superficial bladder carcinoma, it is considered to be the precursor of invasive cancer and may coexist with non-invasive papillary cancer.

Surveillance after transurethral resection (TUR) of superficial bladder carcinoma

The predilection for superficial transitional-cell carcinoma of the bladder (STCCB) to be recurrent, multiple and to progress to $\geq$ T2 in a low percentage (overall $\approx$ 15%) is well known [7]. The frequency of recurrences based on retrospective studies is variable and depends on the characteristics of the population included (Table 4.1).

The National Bladder Cancer Collaborative Group A (NBCCGA) organized a prospective study in 1972 (protocol 1) to answer among others the following questions: (1) what treatment modalities are generally used for patients with STCCB?, (2) what is the rate of recurrence and progression in this group? and (3) are stage, size or number of tumours predictors of recurrence [8,9]? To accomplish these goals all bladder-cancer patients were entered into a surveillance protocol. Data from this protocol have provided a unique opportunity to review the history of patients presenting with bladder cancer for the first time and to study the recurrence and progression patterns in the absence of interventions other than TUR and fulguration techniques [9]. Resected tissue specimens were reviewed in one institution and

Table 4.1 Recurrence in patients with primary Ta/T1 bladder tumours treated by resection and fulguration only.

Study	Stage/grade		Patients (N)	Recurrence (%)	Follow-up
Fitzpatrick et al. [11]	Ta	G1+2	414	46	mean 59 months
			(188)	(54)	$\geq$ 5 yrs
			(59)	(55)	$\geq$ 10 yrs
	Multiple		65	69	
	$\geq$ 10 Gm		81	80	
Prout et al. [3] (NBCCG)	Ta	G1	178	61	median 58 months
Cutler et al. [10] (NBCCG)	Ta	G1–3	118	54	$\geq$ 36 months
	T1	G1–3	70	56	
Lutzeyer et al. [16]	Ta	G1–2	194	52	$\geq$ 36 months
	T1	G1–3	80	69	
	Ta	G1	144	42	
	Ta	G2	41	55	
	Solitary Ta	G1	-	29	
	Solitary Ta	G2	-	50	
	Multiple Ta	G1	-	94	
	Multiple Ta	G2	-	3/3	
Gilbert et al. [17]	Ta	G3	23	44	$\geq$ 5 yrs
	T1	G3	25	44	
Holmäng et al. [22]	Ta/T1		176	80	$\leq$ 20 yrs

therefore provided a consistency of histopathological diagnosis not available in most studies. Of 1071 patients registered 249 presented initially with tumours confined to the bladder mucosa or lamina propria and were treated by TUR and fulguration only before the first new occurrence of the tumour. Since 42 patients received intravesical chemotherapy after the first new occurrence and before progression was demonstrated 207/249 patients were eligible for tumour progression analysis after TUR only. In the analysis reported in 1983 duration of interval free of disease was significantly less for patients with grade-3 tumours than for grade-1 or 2-disease ($p < 0.01$), T1 tumours recurred faster than Ta ($p < 0.01$), multiple tumours (≥ 4) faster than single tumours ($p < 0.01$) and the tumour-free interval for patients with tumours ≥ 5 cm was significantly less than for patients with tumours < 5 cm [9].

Median time to first recurrence was 31 months compared to 13 months from successful treatment of the first recurrence to diagnosis of the second recurrence. The corresponding figure from second to third recurrence was 12 months [10].

The tendency for progression significantly increased when tumour invaded the lamina propria (Ta vs T1 $p < 0.001$, Table 4.2), time to invasion was longer for patients with grade 1 compared to grade 2 ($p < 0.05$) and for grade 2 compared to grade 3 ($p < 0.001$) [30].

A striking observation in patients with Ta grade 1 was reported by Prout *et al.* [3]. Whereas patients with a single TaG1 tumour started after 'TUR only' with a recurrence

Table 4.2 Progression to $\geq$ T2 in patients with primary Ta/T1 bladder tumours treated by resection and fulguration only.

Study	Stage/grade		Patients (N)	Progression (%)	Follow-up
Heney *et al.* [9]		0	5	0	median
(NBCCG)	Ta	1	85	2	39 months
		2	50	6	
		3	4	25	
	T1	1	7	0	
		2	29	21	
		3	27	48	
Fitzpatrick [11]	Ta	1 + 2	414	4.6	$\geq$ 10 yrs 59 pts
					$\geq$ 5 yrs 188 pts
					< 5 yrs 226 pts
Prout *et al.* [3]	Ta	1	178	1.6	median 58 months
(NBCCG)					
Gilbert *et al.* [17]	Ta	3	23	30	$\geq$ 5 yrs
	T1	3	25	16	
Kaubisch *et al.* [30]	T1		51	27	median 78 months
		1*		0	
		2*		22	
	3* + 4*			50	

*grading following Broders [31]

per month of 0.032 in year 1 of follow-up, this recurrence-rate decreased steadily through the years of follow-up to a low of 0.018 recurrences per month in year 5. Multiple tumour patients maintained a fairly constant rate of recurrences, starting with a rate of 0.060 recurrences per month in year 1 of follow-up and ending with the same rate in year 5. Transurethral resection or fulguration after biopsy was used as initial therapy in all 178 patients. Intravesical chemotherapy was never given to 123 patients (69%) and out of 55 patients (31%) 14 patients (8%) received intravesical chemotherapy initially and 41 patients (22%) at some time distant from the initial evaluation (Table 4.1). Although not analysed further in this report, one can assume that mainly multiple tumours were adjuvantly treated, thus the decrease in the recurrence-rate of single tumours can not be explained by adjuvant measures. Clinical information and pathological specimens in this study were collected from all patients with primary bladder cancer, according to the stipulations of the aforementioned NBCCG protocol 1 [8].

Fitzpatrick *et al.* [11] reported on 414 patients with primary Ta grade-1 and -2 tumours. Initially, partipating patients were only treated by TUR of the bladder tumour [11]. At a mean of 5.5 years after the initial diagnosis 35 patients (8.4%) were treated with intravesical epodyl. Follow-up was for 5 or more years in 188 patients and for less than 5 years in 226 patients. After the initial resection 220 of 414 patients (53.1%) had no further recurrence. Considering the length of follow-up no further recurrences developed in 86 (45.7%) of the 188 patients followed-up for 5 or more years and 26 (44%) of the 59 patients followed-up for 12 or more years. The findings at the first control cystoscopy 3 months after 'complete' resection of all tumours were identified as an important prognostic factor. Patients free of tumour at 3 months had an 80% chance of having no further recurrence, whereas in patients with a recurrence at 3 months only 10 percent had no further recurrences thereafter. Whether a 'true' recurrence (or an incomplete initial resection and residual disease?) at the same site was seen or whether it was a new occurrence at a different site (overlooked during initial resection?) was not differentiated by the authors. Several authors confirmed the prediction value of the first check cystoscopy 3 months after TUR [6,12,13]. Reading *et al.* [13] analysed all newly diagnosed cases of superficial bladder cancer presenting to a single urology department and combining the two prognostic factors, which according to Parmar *et al.* [12] are of greatest predictive value; these are: (1) the number of tumours at diagnosis (single or more than one), and (2) whether there was tumour recurrence or not at the first-check cystoscopy 3 months later. Combining these two factors three distinct groups of patients were identified: Group 1 (good risk): patients who had a solitary tumour at diagnosis and no recurrence at first-check cystoscopy. Group 2 (medium risk): patients either with a solitary tumour at the time of diagnosis and recurrence at their first check or, alternatively, multiple tumours at diagnosis but no recurrence at 3 months. Group 3 (poor risk): patients with multiple tumours at diagnosis and recurrent tumour at the first-check cystoscopy. A retrospective study was undertaken of 232 consecutive patients with newly diagnosed Ta/T1 bladder cancer treated by TUR of the visible tumour at diagnosis. Intravesical chemotherapy was not given at the time of diagnosis, but used for those patients with multiple recurrences [13]. Mean or median follow-up is not reported by the authors, but after one year 75, 50 and 20% are free of recurrence in group 1, 2 and 3, respectively. Thus the reproducibility and clinical relevance of the prognostic factors tested was convincingly demonstrated.

That multiple tumours and large tumours at presentation are poor prognostic factors is confirmed by many authors (Table 4.1).

Before intravesical chemo- or immunotherapy became popular several authors reported large series of patients treated only by either the transurethral route or occasionally by open surgery. Because of different shortcomings they cannot, or can only partly, be included in this review of natural disease of STCCB; tumour category Ta and T1 were pooled [14,15], the type of progression (progression to T1 or $\geq$ T2) was not described [16], and frequency of recurrences and progression were only related to grade and not to stage [17].

Barnes *et al.* [14] reported on 114 patients who had TUR for cure of bladder tumours and in whom one or more recurrences were observed [14]. In this retrospective study stage 0 (Ta) and stage A (T1) were both designated stage A. The authors stated 'it is difficult, if not impossible, to differentiate 0 from A', however, such a statement should not be true for today's pathologists as long as they receive properly resected and handled tissue samples [18]. Admittedly authors applying the Tumour Node Metastasis (TNM) system, until the third edition in 1978 did not differentiate between Ta and T1 tumours, they were all listed as T1 [15,19]. Frequency of tumour progression cannot be listed when progression from Ta to T1 and to $\geq$ T2 is not differentiated [16]. Gilbert *et al.* [17] reported on 365 patients treated by conservative operative techniques, TUR and fulguration being the most common. Except for grade-3 tumours depth of tumour growth was not mentioned, the natural history of papillary transitional-cell carcinoma of the bladder (including muscle invasive lesions) was discovered solely on the basis of grading of the transurethrally resected fragments. Although it may be true that — as stated by the author —'the results of treatment often are compared on the basis of clinical or pathological staging, each of these methods is subject to considerable error', one cannot expect with certainty that grading by pathologists is always conducted in a more reliable way. Both the European Organization for Research and Treatment of Cancer-Genitourinary Group (EORTC-GU) and the MRC (Medical Research Council) Genito-Urinary Group reported on remarkable differences in staging and grading when local and central pathology were compared [12,20,21].

That translation of old findings into the actually used definitions for stage and grade of superficial transitional-cell carcinoma is possible was demonstrated by a Swedish group [22]. A retrospective analysis was conducted on 176 patients, with primary stage Ta- and T1-bladder cancer, treated between 1963 and 1972. All patients except one were followed-up until death or for at least 20 years. The histological material was reviewed by one pathologist in 1977 and in 1993. Autopsy was carried out in 82 (50.3%) of 163 cases in which the patients died; more than 80% of the patients died in hospitals or extended-care facilities. The majority of patients had undergone cystoscopy within 1 year of death. All but one patient underwent endoscopy every year, or every other year, even when the recurrence among them was diagnosed in 1973. Thus progression to $\geq$ T2, death due to bladder cancer or death due to any concurrent disease were not assumed but were based on complete follow-up with endoscopic examination. Important findings were: (1) 22% of patients died of bladder cancer, if followed for a sufficient interval (Table 4.3); (2) the larger the number and volume of the recurrent tumour, the shorter the survival; (3) all patients with four or more primary tumours either underwent cystectomy or died with or of bladder cancer; and (4) patients with recurrences more than 4 years after the

Table 4.3 Death due to bladder cancer in patients with primary superficial transitional-cell carcinoma Ta/T1 treated by resection and fulguration#.

Study	Stage/grade	Patients (*N*)	DCB (%)	Death (%)	Follow-up
Holmäng *et al.* [22]	Ta G1–3*	77	9 (11)		≥ 20 yrs
				124/176 (70)	
	T1 G2–G4*	99	30 (30)		

DBC = death due to bladder cancer; Death = death due to intercurrent disease.
*grading following Bergkvist *et al.* [32].
#13/176 with multiple tumours at every cystoscopy and one with recurrent Tis were treated with thiotepa. All went on with further recurrences and 10 died of bladder cancer.

primary operation continued to have recurrent tumours until death unless cystectomy was performed. Two additional observations are of interest. Only three upper-tract cancers were found among 176 patients followed from the primary operation until death or for at least 20 years. Whereas routine follow-up intravenous pyelograms (IVPs) were performed at various intervals for all patients the upper-tract tumour was detected by this method in only one patient. Thus the authors stated routine IVPs are neither cost-effective nor necessary in this group (Ta/T1) of patients.

Summarizing the discovered natural disease in patients with superficial transitional-cell carcinoma of the bladder category Ta and T1 one can conclude that: (1) the highest occurrence of recurrences is observed in patients with multiple and large tumour volume. When the treatment of the primary is complete and the first-check cystoscopy shows neither a true recurrence nor a new occurrence the risk for new occurrences decreases; recurrent tumours are more often located at the site of the bladder dome than primary (supporting the hypothesis of tumour implantation) [23]; (2) progression to ≥ T2 is more often observed in patients with increasing numbers of positive cystoscopies, in grade-3 tumours and in tumours of category T1; and (3) with increasing duration of follow-up more patients will eventually die due to bladder carcinoma (11% with tumours staged Ta, 30% staged T1, globally 22%), including TaG1–2 tumours. The risk of dying increases with larger number and volume of the recurrent tumour.

There is evidence that the majority of tumours becoming muscle invasive display this invasiveness at first diagnosis [24].

This review will not deal with CIS, but it is obvious that papillary Ta/T1 tumours associated with CIS or severe dysplasia will do worse [25]. Advances in the field of molecular genetics have suggested that mutations in specific loci resulting in the loss of tumour suppressor genes (*Rb*-gene, *p53*) are associated with tumour recurrence and progression [26]. Genetic alteration of *3p*, *11p*, *17p* and *18q* are rare events in low-grade, superficial tumours, whereas they are common in high-grade and invasive-bladder cancer. In superficial bladder tumours loss of heterozygocity on chromosome *17p* or *p53* gene mutation seems to be rare (20% and 23%) compared to muscle-invasive tumours [27,28]. With further evidence of the predictive value of molecular markers by studies applying molecular genetic methods, these methods may enter common clinical usage and allow to identify better those patients who will most likely progress and die due to a lesion which started superficially [29].

Natural disease of adjuvantly treated transitional-cell carcinoma of the bladder, stage Ta/T1

Numerous randomized studies have demonstrated the advantage of adjuvant intravesical treatment after TUR to decrease the recurrence rate of superficial bladder cancer compared with TUR alone [20,33,34,35,36] (Table 4.4). However, in some controlled studies only a marginal benefit, or no advantage at all, was demonstrated [15]. Factors that may explain a different outcome are [37,38,39]: (1) the time lapse between tumour resection and initiation of intravesical chemotherapy (early instillation after 24 hours or less is better than delayed instillation) [40]; (2) small

Table 4.4 Recurrence observed in randomized, controlled studies after adjuvant treatment of TaT1 bladder cancer or after resection alone.

Study	Drug	Stage/grade	Control (%)	TUR + drug (%)	Follow-up	p value
Kurth *et al.* [7]	Ethoglucid 1.13 g weekly for 4 wks + monthly for 11 months.	Ta/T1 G1–3	47/72 (65)	74/170 (44)	median 3.4 yrs	<0.001
	Doxorubicin 50 mg weekly for 4 wks + monthly for 11 months.	Ta/T1 G1–3	47/72 (65)	86/184 (49)	median 3.4 yrs	< 0.001
	(Ta: Doxo vs Etho vs Control p = 0.05 T1: Doxo vs Etho vs Control p < 0.001)					
Rübben *et al.* [37]	Doxorubicin 50 mg 1. Twice weekly for 6 wks	Ta/T1 G1–3	32/82 (39)	36/79 (45)	≥ 3 yrs	> 0.1
	2. Twice weekly for 6 wks, Twice monthly for 4.5 months, then monthly for a total of 1 year	Ta/T1 G1–3	32/82 (39)	25/59 (43)	≥ 3 yrs	> 0.1
Oosterlinck *et al.* [20]	Epirubicin 80 mg single instillation	single Ta/T1 G1–3	72/205 (38)	55/194 (29)	mean 24 months	0.02
Pagano *et al.* [55]	BCG-Pasteur 75 mg weekly for 6 wks (22 had second course)	Ta/T1 multiple tumours	52/63 (83)	18/70 (26)	mean 21 months	< 0.001
Rübben *et al.* [51]	BCG-Connaught 120 mg weekly for 6 wks, then monthly for 4 months	Ta/T1 G1–3	17/40 (42)	13/37 (35)	median 18.3 months	n.s.

sample size of a trial without the discriminating power to detect small differences in a group of patients with low- or intermediate-risk for recurrence [37]; (3) an inappropriate treatment schedule (single instillation or one instillation at resection followed by four instillations together with cystoscopic examination at 3-month intervals in patients who also had multiple, $\geq$ 5 cm and T1 tumours) [38]; or (4) an ineffective drug at the dose or schedule used [15,39].

Recently a combined analysis of EORTC and MRC randomized clinical trials for the prophylactic treatment of Ta/T1 bladder cancer was performed. The purpose of this study was to compare immediate vs no (or delayed after off study) adjuvant prophylactic treatment after TUR with respect to a patient's disease-free interval, time to progression to $\geq$ T2, duration of survival and progression-free survival [41]. A total of 2535 patients met the inclusion criteria. Meta-analysis techniques were used, e.g. a formal statistical methodology to combine the results of separate, but similar studies in a quantitative manner. All trials were randomized, Phase III studies assessing the adjuvant prophylactic treatment of primary or recurrent, transitional cell, TaT1 bladder cancer. This includes studies with cytotoxic drugs given intravesically or oral agents. Because neither the European Organization for Research and Treatment of Cancer (EORTC) nor the MRC conducted any trials in which TUR alone was compared to TUR plus bacillus Calmette–Guérin (BCG) trials with BCG were not included. Updated follow-up information on the endpoints mentioned above was collected by the EORTC. After a median duration of follow-up for the disease-free interval of 4.6 years (range 3 months to 13 years) the difference in favour of adjuvant treatment was statistically significant ($p < 0.01$). As in this analysis treatment results were only compared within a given trial and the results then combined across all trials, the statistical heterogeneity of results across trials is assessed and at no time are patients in different trials being compared. The use of proper meta-analysis techniques allows for assessment of trials which vary according to the mode of administration, dose, duration of instillations, interval between instillations, duration of treatment and the prognosis of the patient being included. This method is preferable to a simple summing-up of treatment results disregarding all variations [42]. Trials in which cytostatics were compared in their ability to reduce the recurrence rate have failed to demonstrate the definitive superiority of one agent over another [40,43,44]. Some authors [45,46,47,48] would consider intravesical BCG and not chemotherapy to be the first-line treatment of choice in the adjuvant treatment of TaT1 bladder cancer, especially in high-risk patients (two recurrences or more per year, multifocal T1, CIS). Most randomized Phase III trials, including predominantly high-risk patients, indicate the superiority of BCG over chemotherapeutic agents with respect to the recurrence rate [45,47,49].

In two larger trials, including relatively few patients with high-risk tumour no significant difference for the disease-free interval was seen in the comparison of BCG and Mitomycin C [50,51,52]. In controlled studies comparing TUR alone with TUR followed by BCG, adjuvant immunotherapy in all trials except one [51] was significantly effective in preventing recurrence [53,54,55] (Table 4.4). These studies with the exception of the trial reported by Pagano *et al.* [55] were of small sample size.

However, for high-risk patients BCG is regarded as the most effective intravesical agent for prevention of recurrence. Some authors suggest that BCG prevents tumour death from bladder cancer [45,46,49]. Because only 10–15% of all TaT1 bladder cancer can be expected to progress, individual trials have only a very low power to detect differences with respect to muscle invasion. In the aforementioned combined analysis of EORTC and MRC trials [41] for time to progression (> T1), no statistically significant difference was observed comparing adjuvant treatment, not including BCG, with TUR alone. In a randomized controlled study comparing long-term intravesical instillation of Mitomycin C, 40 mg, and BCG (Pasteur strain), the latter was superior regarding recurrence prophylaxis, since patients given BCG had fewer recurrences and a significantly longer time to treatment failure compared to those treated with Mitomycin C. No statistically significant difference was observed regarding progression. Tumour progressed to > T1 in 15/125 patients in the BCG and 15/125 in the Mitomycin C group (13.2%) after a median follow-up of 39 months [56]. Long-term treatment was chosen in this study (both drugs weekly for 6 weeks, then monthly for up to 1 year and every 3 months during year 2). In a Dutch study reported by Vegt *et al.* [57], progression to > T1 was observed in 8 (6%) of the Mitomycin C group, 7 (5%) of the group treated with BCG-Tice and 8 (6%) treated with the RIVM-BCG. Treatment duration for BCG was weekly for 6 consecutive weeks and for Mitomycin C (30 mg) once a week for 4 weeks and thereafter once a month for a total of 6 months. In this study (later updated by Witjes *et al.* [50]) at no time was a statistically significant difference found for any of the endpoints tested except for Mitomycin C, which was more effective than Tice BCG therapy ($p = 0.01$) in preventing new recurrences.

In the controlled, randomized study [58] reporting equal frequency of muscle-invasive and/or metastatic disease, both were significantly delayed by BCG treatment compared to resection alone (p = 0.012). Cystectomies were required in 18/43 (42%) control and 11/43 (26%) BCG-treated patients. Median time to cystectomy was 8 months for control and 24 months for BCG-treated patients. Based on initial treatment (19 patients of the control group [44%] had crossover to BCG after local failure), survival was improved by BCG therapy ($p = 0.03$) (median follow-up 6 years). Only high-risk patients were treated in this study, but after a long-term follow-up the results suggested that intravesical BCG can delay disease progression, prolong the period of bladder preservation, and increase overall survival [58].

Long-term follow-up was more easily achieved in this unicentre study than may be the case for larger multicentre studies. Long-term follow-up studies for trials comparing BCG with different cystostatics are urgently needed to confirm not only the superiority of BCG over cytostatics, as reported by several authors, but more importantly to confirm prevention, or at least the delay to muscle-invasive disease, of superficial TaT1 transitional-cell carcinoma of the bladder. The EORTC and MRC demonstrated that long-term follow-up was possible for patients recruited in their trial [41], however, considering the mobile society in the US it may be more difficult for large co-operative study groups, such as the SWOG which conducted several important BCG trials, to follow-up patients long enough for observation of possible differences in the endpoints of: (1) time to progression to > T1, or (2) death due to bladder carcinoma. Another important question that needs to be answered is what is the treated natural history of patients with superficial bladder tumours, stage TaT1, managed with BCG and who failed BCG? Klein *et al.* [59] examined this issue in a small group of patients. They reviewed the management and survival of 41 patients who failed BCG within the bladder or prostatic urethra and who subsequently were treated with a variety of secondary therapies. Of the 41 patients 6 (15%) died. A multivariate statistical model revealed that patients with early prostatic urethral involvement and the presence of stage T1 tumour at diagnosis had the highest risk of death from bladder cancer. The reason for change in therapy at failure of BCG had no impact on survival. Not all patients recurring after BCG were destined to precede to muscle invasion or metastases, some patients may be managed safely by repeated endoscopic resection and intravesical therapy with cystectomy delayed until objective progression is evident.

Summarizing, the adjuvantly treated natural history of patients with superficial bladder tumours stage TaT1, the following conclusions can be drawn: (1) intravesical chemotherapy with widely used drugs (Mitomycin C, doxorubicin, epirubicin, Epodyl and thiotepa) is superior to TUR alone. This effect is still demonstrable after long-term follow-up [7,41]; (2) no benefit in progression-free survival by intravesical chemotherapy compared to TUR alone/or delayed intravesical therapy could be observed [41]; (3) BCG is superior to intravesical chemotherapy in preventing new recurrences in patients at high risk [45,49,56], such superiority was not observed in trials including only few patients at high risk [52,57,60]; (4) the superiority of BCG over intravesical chemotherapy, in prevention of muscle-invasive disease, is not yet convincingly demonstrated [56,57]; and (5) the natural history of BCG-failed treatment of superficial TaT1 bladder carcinoma is not yet sufficiently investigated.

Recently Kurth *et al.* [6] reported on factors affecting recurrence and progression in superficial bladder tumours. Data from two trials (excluding control arm) were pooled to facilitate analysis of prognostic factors. The results from 576 patients, all of whom were receiving intravesical chemotherapy, were analysed. No association was found between the adjuvant group assigned and either recurrence, invasion or survival. Thus, the drugs selected were equally effective [43,61]. Patients characteristics, percentage of patients with recurrence, invasion, death due to any cause or death due to malignant disease are shown in Table 4.5. The relative importance of factors contributing to recurrence, invasion and survival were investigated by performing a multivariate analysis. Based on the most important prognostic factors and their association with invasion and death, an index was computed reflecting the risk of both invasion and death due to malignant disease, respectively. The index was used to assign patients to one of three prognostic groups (Table 4.6).

Three main factors determined a patient's prognosis: tumour size, G-grade and prior recurrence rate per year. Risk groups were suggested based on the computed index (Table 4.6). In this prognostic model only 36/576 stage-TaT1 patients (6.2%) belonged to the high-risk group (progression to > T1 in 41.6% and death by cancer 36.1%), 281/576 patients (48.7%) were estimated low risk (progression to > T1 7.1%, death by cancer 4.3%) or intermediate risk (progression to > T1 17.4%, death by cancer 12.8%). Any additional treatment to favourably influence the natural history in patients with superficial transitional-cell carcinoma of the bladder may be decided depending on the risk group to which the patient belongs.

Table 4.5 Patient characteristics.

Coding	Patients		% of patients			
	Number	%	Recurrence	Invasion	Death	MD
Overall	576	100	54	13	22	10
Age						
(1) ≤ 60	154	27	57	9	8	5
(2) 61–79	379	66	52	15	26	12
(3) ≥ 80	43	7	53	9	44	19
Sex						
Female	97	17	52	9	15	4
Male	479	83	54	14	24	11
Size of largest tumour (cm)						
(1) < 1.5	347	61	53	9	18	7
(2) 1.5–3	133	23	55	19	29	15
(3) ≥ 3	94	16	55	22	29	14
Number of tumours						
(1) ≤ 6	474	82	50	12	21	9
(2) ≥ 7	102	18	69	18	29	17
T category						
(1) Ta	310	54	54	9	21	9
(2) T1	266	46	53	18	24	11
G category						
(1) G1	236	44	47	6	16	4
(2) G2	247	46	59	17	26	14
(3) G3	56	10	61	30	25	16
Time from diagnosis (yrs)						
(1) primary	219	38	43	14	25	8
(2) 1 or less	99	17	61	12	22	14
(3) 2 or 3	109	19	64	16	25	16
(4) > 3	147	25	56	11	18	7
Prior recurrence rate/year						
(1) primary	219	38	43	14	24	8
(2) < 1	128	22	51	9	16	6
(3) 1–3	183	32	63	13	20	11
(4) > 3	44	8	73	23	41	27
Trigone involvement						
(1) No	492	85	52	11	21	9
(2) Yes	84	15	65	24	30	18
Right or left ureteral orifice						
(1) No	422	73	56	13	23	11
(2) Yes	154	27	47	14	21	7
Right or left wall						
(1) No	235	41	46	10	20	8
(2) Yes	341	59	59	15	24	12
Anterior wall						
(1) No	504	87	53	13	21	10
(2) Yes	72	13	56	15	31	15
Posterior wall						
(1) No	353	61	48	14	20	9
(2) Yes	223	39	62	12	26	13
Dome						
(1) No	415	72	47	12	21	9
(2) Yes	161	28	70	15	25	14
Neck						
(1) No	124	78	51	9	20	8
(2) Yes	452	22	65	21	33	18
First cystoscopy after entry						
(1) Negative	480	83	44	10	21	8
(2) Positive	96	17	100	27	30	21
% positive cystoscopies after entry						
(1) 30 or less	435	76	—	6	18	6
(2) > 30	141	24	—	37	37	25

MD = death due to malignant disease.
Reprinted from European Journal of Cancer, 1995 pp. 1840–1846, with kind permission from Elsevier Science Ltd, The Boulevard, Langford Lane, Kidlington, OX5 1GB, UK.

Table 4.6 Risk index for patients in various subgroups.

Tumour size	Primary, RR < 1			1–3			> 3		
(G-grade)	< 1.5	1.5–3	> 3	< 1.5	1.5–3	> 3	< 1.5	1.5–3	>3
G1	**1**	**1**	**1**	**1**	**2**	**2**	**2**	**2**	**3**
	0	0.48	0.97	0.51	1.0	1.5	1.0	1.5	2.0
	0	0.44	0.87	0.89	1.3	1.8	1.8	2.2	2.7
	77	36	26	71	6	4	12	2	0
G2	**1**	**2**	**2**	**2**	**2**	**3**	**3**	**3**	**3**
	0.84	1.3	1.8	1.4	1.8	2.3	1.9	2.4	2.8
	0.73	1.2	1.6	1.6	2.1	2.5	2.5	3.0	3.4
	71	38	38	53	19	3	13	9	1
G3	**2**	**2**	**2**	**2**	**3**	**3**	**3**	**3**	**3**
	1.7	2.2	2.7	2.2	2.7	3.2	2.7	3.2	3.7
	1.5	1.9	2.3	2.4	2.8	3.3	3.3	3.7	4.1
	12	10	15	9	4	2	2	2	0

Each cell gives the risk group, the risk index pertaining to invasion and death from malignant disease as well as the number of patients.

RR, recurrence rate per year.

Risk index, odds ratio estimated from the Cox model including only three factors: Tumour size (TS), G-grade (G) and RR.

The estimated Cox models are: for invasion: 0.51 RR + 0.84 G + 0.48 TS; for death: 0.89 RR + 0.73 G + 0.44 TS. The bold numbers in the table refer to the risk group: (1) 254 patients; (2) 218 patients; (3) 36 patients.

Reprinted from European Journal of Cancer, 1995 pp. 1840–1846, with kind permission from Elsevier Science Ltd, The Boulevard, Langford Lane, Kidlington, OX5 1GB, UK.

References

1   Kurth KH, Schellhammer PF, Okajima E *et al.* Current methods of assessing and treating carcinoma *in situ* of the bladder with or without involvement of the prostatic urethra. *Int J Urol* 1995; **2**(2): 8–22.

2   Wolf H, Kakizoe T, Smith P *et al.* Bladder tumors. Treated natural history. In: Niijima T, Aso Y, Koontz W, Prout G, Denis L (eds) *Consensus Development In Clinical Bladder Cancer Research.* Jersey, Channel Islands; Scientific Communication International (S.C.I.), 1993; 219–53.

3   Prout GR Jr, Barton BA, Griffin PP, Friedell GH for the National Bladder Cancer Collaborative Group. Treated history of noninvasive grade 1 transitional cell carcinoma. *J Urol* 1992; **148**: 1413–19.

4   Messing EM. Editorial Comment on [3] Prout GR Jr, Barton BA, Griffin PP, Friedell GH for the national bladder cancer group. Treated history of non-invasive grade 1 transitional cell carcinoma. *J Urol* 1992; **148**: 1413–19.

5   Anderström C, Johansson S, Nilsson S. The significance of lamina propria invasion on the prognosis of patients with bladder tumors. *J Urol* 1980; **124**: 23–5.

6   Kurth KH, Denis L, Bouffioux Ch *et al.* Factors affecting recurrence and progression in superficial bladder tumours. *Eur J Cancer* 1995; **31A**(11): 1840–6.

7   Kurth KH, Tunn U, Ay R *et al.* Adjuvant chemotherapy of superficial transitional cell bladder carcinoma: long term results of an European Organization for Research and Treatment of Cancer randomized trial comparing doxorubicin, ethoglucid and transurethral resection alone. Accepted *J Urol* 1996.

8   National Bladder Cancer Collaborative Group A. Surveillance, initial assessment, and subsequent progress of patients with superficial bladder cancer in a prospective longitudinal study. *Cancer Res* 1977; 37: 2907–10.

9   Heney NM, Ahmed S, Flanagan MJ *et al.* Superficial bladder cancer: progression and recurrence. *J Urol* 1983; **130**: 1083–6.

10 Cutler SJ, Heney NM, Friedell GH. Longitudinal study of patients with bladder cancer: factors associated with disease recurrence and progression. In: Bonney WW, Prout GR Jr (eds) *Bladder Cancer.* AUA Monographes. Baltimore: The Williams & Wilkins Co, 1982; vol 1, chap 4, p. 35.

11 Fitzpatrick JM, West AB, Butler MR, Lane V, O'Flynn JD. Special bladder tumors (stage pTa, grades 1 and 2): the importance of recurrence pattern following initial resection. *J Urol* 1986; **135**: 920–2.

12 Parmar MKB, Freedman LS, Hargreave TB, Tolley DA. Prognostic factors for recurrence and follow-up policies in the treatment of superficial bladder cancer: report from the British Medical Research Council Subgroup on superficial bladder cancer (Urological Cancer Working Party). *J Urol* 1989; **142**: 284–8.

13 Reading J, Hall RR, Parmar MKB. The application of a prognostic factor analysis for TaT1 bladder cancer in routine urological practice. *Br J Urol* 1995; **75**: 604–7.

14 Barnes R, Hadley H, Dick A, Johnston O, Dexter J. Changes in grade and stage of recurrent bladder tumors. *J Urol* 1977; **118**: 177–8.

15 Schulman CC, Robinson M, Denis L *et al.* Prophylactic chemotherapy of superficial transitional cell bladder carcinoma: an EORTC randomized trial comparing thiotepa, and epipodophyllotoxin (VM26) and TUR alone. *Eur Urol* 1982; **8**: 207–12.

16 Lutzeyer W, Rübben H, Dahm H. Prognostic parameters in superficial bladder cancer: an analysis of 315 cases. *J Urol* 1982; **127**: 250–2.

17 Gilbert HA, Logan JL, Kagan AR *et al.* The natural history of papillary transitional cell carcinoma of the bladder and its treatment in an unselected population on the basis of histologic grading. *J Urol* 1978; **119**: 488–92.

18 Kurth KH, Soloway MS, Herr H *et al.* Surgical techniques in the management of patients with superficial bladder cancer. In: Niijima T, Aso Y, Koontz W, Prout G, Denis L (eds) *Consensus Development In Clinical Bladder Cancer Research.* Jersey, Channel Islands: Scientific Communication International (S.C.I.), 1993; 116–23.

19 UICC. TNM classification of malignant tumors (International Union Against Cancer, Geneva 1978) 3rd edn., 113–17.

20 Oosterlinck W, Kurth KH, Schröder F *et al.* A prospective European Organization for Research and Treatment of Cancer Genitourinary Group randomized trial comparing transurethral resection followed by a single intravesical instillation of epirubicin or water in single stage Ta, T1 papillary carcinoma of the bladder. *J Urol* 1993; **149**: 749–52.

21 Kurth KH, Schröder FH, Debruyne F *et al.* Long-term follow-up in superficial transitional cell carcinoma of the bladder: prognostic factors for time to first recurrence, recurrence rate, and survival. Final results of a randomized trial comparing doxorubicin hydrochloride, ethoglucid and transurethral resection alone. *Prog Clin Biol Res* 1989; **303**: 481–90.

22 Holmäng S, Hedelin H, Anderström C, Johansson SL. The relationship among multiple recurrences, progression and prognosis of patients with stages Ta and T1 transitional cell cancer of the bladder followed for at least 20 years. *J Urol* 1995; **153**: 1823–7.

23 Heney NM, Nocks BN, Daly JJ *et al*. Ta and T1 bladder cancer: location, recurrence and progression. *Br J Urol* 1982; **54**(2): 152–7.

24 Kaye KW, Lange PH. Mode of presentation of invasive bladder cancer. Reassessment of the problem. *J Urol* 1982; **128**: 31–3.

25 Althausen AF, Prout GR Jr, Daly JJ. Non-invasive papillary carcinoma *in situ*. *J Urol* 1976; **116**: 575–80.

26 Presti JC Jr, Reuter VE, Galan T, Fair WR, Cordon-Cardo C. Molecular genetic alterations in superficial and locally advanced human bladder cancer. *Cancer Res* 1991; **51**(19): 5405–9.

27 Uchida T, Wada C, Ishida H *et al*. p53 mutations and prognosis in bladder tumors. *J Urol* 1995; **153**: 1097–104.

28 Nakopoulou L, Constantinides C, Papandropoulos J *et al*. Evaluation of overexpression of p53 tumor suppressor protein in superficial and invasive transitional cell bladder cancer: comparison with DNA ploidy. *Urology* 1995; **46**(3): 334–40.

29 Tanka HJ, Florijn RJ, Vrolijk J, Raap AK. Molecular cytogenetics: unraveling of the genetic composition of individual cells by fluorescence *in situ* hybridization and digital imaging microscopy. *World J Urol* 1995; **13**(3): 138–42.

30 Kaubisch S, Lum BL, Reese J, Freiha F, Torti FM. Stage T1 bladder cancer: grade is the primary determinant for risk of muscle invasion. *J Urol* 1991; **146**: 28–31.

31 Broders AC. Epithelioma of the genito-urinary organs. *Ann Surg* 1922; **75**: 574.

32 Bergkvist A, Ljungqvist A, Moberger G. Classification of bladder tumours based on the cellular pattern. Preliminary report of a clinical–pathologic study of 300 cases with a minimum follow-up of eight years. *Acta Chirurgica Scand* 1965; **130**: 371–78.

33 Kurth KH, Schröder FH, Tunn U *et al*. Adjuvant chemotherapy of superficial transitional cell bladder carcinoma: preliminary results of a European Organization for Research on Treatment of Cancer randomized trial comparing doxorubicin hydrochloride, ethoglucid and transurethral resection alone. *J Urol* 1984; **132**: 258–62.

34 Koontz WW, Prout GR Jr, Smith W, Frable W, Minnis JE. The use of intravesical thiotepa in the management of non-invasive carcinoma of the bladder. *J Urol* 1981; **125**: 307–12.

35 Byar D, Blackard C, the Veterans Administration Cooperative Urological Research Group. Comparisons of placebo, pyridoxine, and topical thiotepa in preventing recurrence of stage 1 bladder cancer. *Urology* 1977; **10**(6): 556–61.

36 Tolley DA, Hargreave TB, Smith PH *et al*. Effect of intravesical Mitomycin C on recurrence of newly diagnosed superficial bladder cancer: interim report from the Medical Research Council Subgroup on Superficial Bladder Cancer (Urological Cancer Working Party). *Br Med J* 1988; **296**: 1759–61.

37 Rübben H, Lutzeyer W, Fischer N *et al*. Natural history and treatment of low and high risk superficial bladder tumors. *J Urol* 1988; **139**: 283–5.

38 MRC Working Party on Urological Cancer, London. The effect of intravesical thiotepa on the recurrence rate of newly diagnosed superficial bladder cancer. An MRC study. *Br J Urol* 1985; **57**: 680–5.

39 Flamm J, Donner G, Oberleitner S, Hausmann R, Havelec L. Adjuvant intravesical mitoxantrone after transurethral resection of primary superficial transitional cell carcinoma of the bladder. A prospective randomised study. *Eur J Cancer* 1995; **31A**(2): 143–6.

40 Bouffioux Ch, Kurth KH, Bono A *et al*. Intravesical adjuvant chemotherapy for superficial transitional cell bladder carcinoma: results of 2 European Organization for Research and Treatment of Cancer randomized trials with Mitomycin C and doxorubicin comparing early versus delayed instillations and short-term versus long-term treatment. *J Urol* 1995; **153**: 934–41.

41 Pawinski A, Sylvester R, Kurth KH *et al*. A combined analysis of EORTC and MRC randomized clinical trials for the prophylactic treatment of TaT1 bladder cancer. *J Urol* 1996; **156**: 1934–41.

42 Lamm DL, v.d. Meijden APM, Akaza H *et al*. Intravesical chemotherapy and immunotherapy: how do we assess their effectiveness and what are their limitations and uses? *Int J Urol* 1995; **2**(2): 23–35.

43 Bouffioux Ch, Denis L, Oosterlinck W *et al*. Adjuvant chemotherapy of recurrent superficial transitional cell carcinoma: results of a European Organization for Research on Treatment of Cancer randomized trial comparing intravesical instillation of thiotepa, doxorubicin and cisplatin. *J Urol* 1992; **148**: 297–301.

44 Huland H, Klöppel G, Feddersen I *et al*. Comparison of different schedules of cytostatic intravesical instillations in patients with superficial bladder carcinoma: final evaluation of a prospective multicenter study with 419 patients. *J Urol* 1990; **144**: 68–72.

45 Lamm DL, Blumenstein BA, Crawford ED *et al*. A randomized trial of intravesical doxorubicin and immunotherapy with baccille Calmette–Guérin for transitional-cell carcinoma of the bladder. *N Engl J Med* 1991; **325**: 1205–9.

46. Herr HW, Schwalb DM, Zhang ZF *et al*. Intravesical bacillus Calmette–Guérin therapy prevents tumor progression and death from superficial bladder cancer; ten-year follow-up of a prospective randomized trial. *J Clin Oncol* 1995; **13**(6): 1404–8.

47 Martinez-Pineiro JA, Jimenez Léon J, Martinez-Pineiro L Jr *et al*. Bacillus Calmette–Guérin versus doxorubicin versus thiotepa: a randomized prospective study in 202 patients with superficial bladder cancer. *J Urol* 1990; **143**: 502–6.

48 Rintala E, Jauhiainen K, Alfthan O *et al*. Intravesical chemotherapy (Mitomycin C) versus immunotherapy (bacillus Calmette-Guérin) in superficial bladder cancer. *Eur Urol* 1991; **20**: 19.

49 Lamm DL, Blumenstein BA, Crawford ED *et al*. Randomized intergroup comparison of bacillus Calmette–Guérin immunotherapy and Mitomycin C chemotherapy prophylaxis in superficial transitional cell carcinoma of the bladder. *Urological Oncol* 1995; **1**: 119–26.

50 Witjes WPJ, Witjes JA, Oosterhof GON, Debruyne FMJ on behalf of the Dutch South East Cooperative Urological Group. Update on the Dutch Cooperative trial: mitomycin versus bacillus Calmette–Guérin-Tice versus bacillus Calmette-Guérin RIVM in the treatment of patients with pTa-pT1 papillary carcinoma and carcinoma *in situ* of the urinary bladder. *Sem Urologic Oncol* 1996; **14**(1): 10–16.

51 Rübben H, Graf-Dobberstein C, Ostwald R *et al*. Prospective randomized study of adjuvant therapy after complete resection of superficial bladder cancer; Mitomycin C vs BCG Connaught vs TUR alone. In: DeKernion JB (ed) *Immunotherapy for Urological Tumours*: Churchill-Livingstone, 1990; 27–36.

52 Debruyne FMJ, v.d. Meijden APM, Witjes JA *et al*. Bacillus Calmette-Guérin versus Mitomycin C intravesical therapy in superficial bladder cancer. Results of randomized trial after 21 months of follow-up. Urology (Suppl.) 1992; 40: S11–15.

53 Lamm DL. Bacillus Calmette–Guérin in immunotherapy for bladder cancer. *J Urol* 1985; **134**: 40–47.

54 Herr HW, Pinsky CM, Whitmore WF Jr *et al*. Experience with intravesical bacillus Calmette–Guérin therapy of superficial bladder tumors. *Urology* 1985; **25**: 119–23.

55 Pagano F, Bassi P, Milani C *et al*. A low dose bacillus Calmette–Guérin regimen in superficial bladder cancer therapy: is it effective? *J Urol* 1991; **146**: 32–5.

56 Lundholm C, Norlén BJ, Ekman P *et al*. A randomized prospective study comparing long-term intravesical instillations of Mitomycin C and bacillus Calmette–Guérin in patients with superficial-bladder carcinoma. *J Urol* 1996; **156**: 372–6.

57 Vegt PDJ, Witjes JA, Witjes WPJ *et al*. A randomized study of intravesical mitomycin C, bacillus Calmette–Guérin Tice and bacillus Calmette–Guérin RIVM treatment in pTa–pT1 papillary carcinoma and carcinoma *in situ* of the bladder. *J Urol* 1995; **153**: 929–33.

58 Herr HW, Laudone VP, Badalament RA *et al*. Bacillus Calmette–Guérin therapy alters the progression of superficial bladder cancer. *J Clin Oncol* 1988; **6**(9): 1450–5.

59 Klein EA, Rogatko A, Herr HW. Management of local bacillus Calmette–Guérin failures in superficial bladder cancer. *J Urol* 1992; **147**: 601–5.

60 Krege S, Giani G, Meyer R, Otto T, Rübben H, and participating clinics. A randomized multicenter trial of adjuvant therapy in superficial bladder cancer: transurethral resection only versus transurethral section plus Mitomycin C versus transurethral resection plus bacillus Calmette–Guérin. *J Urol* 1996; **156**: 962–6.

61 Kurth KH, Schröder FH, Debruyne FMJ. Long-term follow-up in superficial transitional cell carcinoma of the bladder: prognostic factors for time to first recurrence, recurrence rate, and survival. In: Murphy GP, Khoury S (eds) Therapeutic progress in urological cancers. *Prog Clin Biol Res* 1989; **303**: 481–90.

CHAPTER 5

Prognostic factors: back to the future

Y. Fradet

Introduction

The management of superficial bladder cancer is a constant challenge due to a heterogeneous natural history and to various therapeutic options. Papillary superficial (Ta, T1) tumours, representing 75% of primary cases, will recur 60% of times within 18 months of first resection. Since pathological information cannot accurately predict recurrence, check cystoscopies are performed at 3-month intervals in all patients, resulting in cost and morbidity. Clearly, the availability of sensitive and specific diagnostic and prognostic tests would significantly improve the management of the disease. It is also not possible to identify which patient will respond favourably to intravesical immuno- or chemotherapy, or to megadose vitamins. Moreover, progression from superficial to muscle-infiltrating cancer occurs in approximately 10% of patients and the accurate identification of high-risk tumours would justify a more aggressive treatment.

Modern cancer-patient care requires improvement in cancer control, but decrease in morbidity and costs have also become essential components of the equation. As with business and military activities, medicine is being revolutionized by technology and knowledge. The quantum leap forward of Toffler's third wave, based on information and technology, was overwhelming in the decisive military demonstration of the 'Desert Storm' operation. By analogy, third-wave medicine will allow specialized and more effective interventions on specific targets. Tumour markers, which have mostly been viewed as laboratory tools for academic medicine, will be central to knowledge-based management of bladder cancer. They will help better define the target and monitor the intervention resulting in improved therapy. One only has to consider the effect prostate specific antigen (PSA) has had on the management of prostate cancer to appreciate the extent of potential for change in bladder-cancer management. The following discussion will review the most promising tumour biomarkers currently under study, their contribution to the understanding of molecular pathways of bladder carcinogenesis and their emerging role in managed care for the year 2000.

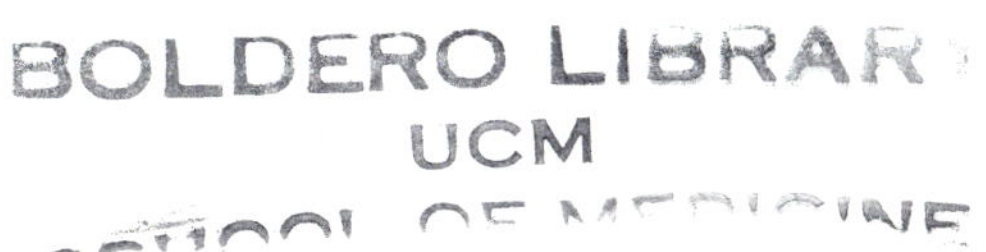

Conventional markers

Pathology and cytology

The management of superficial bladder cancer is currently dependent on diagnostic and prognostic tests that are totally dependent on visual subjective interpretation; the cystoscopic assessment by the urologist on one hand, and the histological and cytological interpretation of resected material or shed exfoliated cells in urine or bladder irrigation by the pathologist. Certainly, the most important indicator of unfavourable prognosis is the stage and grade of the tumour. Although histological criteria have been carefully defined [1,2], several studies have shown a low reproducibility between different observers and even with the same observers at different times [3–6]. Thus, in multicentre studies, central-pathology review has become an absolute requirement for standardization process [7]. Furthermore, pathological criteria continue to evolve, as for example, with new subclassification of T1 disease, based on depth of invasion in relation to the muscularis mucosae, a criteria that had limited clinical testing up to now. Urinary cytology, the only widely used non-invasive diagnostic test for bladder cancer, is also very subjective despite established morphological criteria. This test has never been subjected to large clinical studies as is required for new diagnostic tests. In a recently conducted double blind study in 861 patients, including 190 bladder-tumour patients and a variety of controls, cytology was found to have a specificity of 99% but a low sensitivity of 34% [8], consistent with results also recently reported from trials in North America and in Europe [9,10]. The implications of this finding is that cytology is useful when positive, particularly in patients with no visible tumour to suspect carcinoma *in situ* (CIS), but has little value in the diagnosis and monitoring of the most common papillary superficial tumours.

DNA analysis

Flow cytometry, and more recently image-analysis systems, have been introduced to measure tumour-cell DNA content in an attempt to develop a more quantitative pathology test. Both techniques are based on the quantification of specific dyes incorporated into DNA. Tumours are defined as diploid (normal DNA content) or aneuploid when compared with normal control lymphocytes. As assessed in a recent consensus conference, tumour-DNA cytometry provides prognostic information on the risk of progression in patients with superficial (Ta, T1, Tis) bladder cancer [11] but not in those with muscle-invasive cancers (T2–T4). Moreover, aneuploidy was not predictive of a higher recurrence rate in a recent study of 350 newly diagnosed Ta, T1 tumours [12]. On the other hand, in bladder-irrigation specimens, the presence of a clear non-tetraploid aneuploid DNA population is diagnostic of recurrent tumour or CIS. However, the sensitivity of DNA analysis of exfoliated cells to detect bladder tumours has been at best comparable and more often lower than urinary cytology. In a recent study of over 1500 specimens obtained at different times from 237 patients followed for bladder tumours. DNA-flow cytometry on bladder-wash specimens was less sensitive than urinary cytology to detect and even predict tumour recurrence [13]. A less invasive DNA analysis on voided urine samples has not been extensively studied, but recent results would suggest that it has no additional value over urinary cytology alone [8]. More recent information using image-analysis systems suggests that nuclear features referred to as karyometric analysis may have increased sensitivity in predicting recurrences in patients treated for Ta, T1 tumours [14].

Tumour markers and molecular pathways of carcinogenesis

Tumour biology has evolved very rapidly in recent years resulting in the identification of numerous genes and gene-products potentially involved in bladder carcinogenesis [15]. These discoveries have been driven mostly by technological advances in immunology, molecular biology and genetics which have made it possible to develop tests using a minimal amount of clinical material such as tumour biopsies or voided urine samples. Immunoassays, the polymerase chain reaction (PCR) and other sophisticated molecular-biology techniques have had a tremendous impact on the development of tests that can be used in routine clinical practice. A definite role for tumour markers is emerging and it is thus important to understand the nature of the markers, the feasibility of their clinical testing, the clinical problems they may help to resolve, the extent of their clinical validation and the steps required before their introduction into clinical practice.

Genetic markers

Chromosomal anomalies are a hallmark of cancer cells which can be grossly assessed by measuring total-DNA content. However, further insights may be gained by using the technique of fluorescent *in situ* hybridization (FISH). Probes to DNA sequences specific for each chromosome are hybridized to tumour nuclei obtained directly from tumour biopsies or bladder irrigations. By counting fluorescent spots, one can estimate numerical changes in given chromosomes or even in specific chromosomal arms [16,17]. The loss of specific chromosome segments have also been studied by a molecular biology technique referred to as restriction fragment-length polymorphism (RFLP) which exploits the difference in specific genes of the length of alleles from both parents. The power of this approach has been increased tremendously by studying microsatellite DNA using PCR techniques that essentially allow cytogenetics study of a few cells cut from a tumour or a small biopsy specimen. Using these two techniques, several chromosomal anomalies have been consistently observed at high frequency in bladder cancer specimens [18–20]. Several studies have shown that deletions of chromosome *9q* (long arm) are more common in Ta bladder tumours while *9p* short-arm deletions may be more frequent in T1 cancers. Deletions on *17p* chromosome where the suppressor gene *p53* is located are observed in 50–60% of CIS.

Loss of chromosomal material in association with tumour phenotype has allowed us to identify tumour-suppressor genes. These genes encode an interactive network of molecules co-ordinating the cell cycle and the cell-repair pathways. The most extensively studied tumour-suppressor genes are the *p53* and the retinoblastoma gene (*Rb*) [21,22]. Both gene products can be detected using antibodies; the anomalous expression of *Rb* will result in loss of nuclear staining, while *p53* will result in positive-nuclear staining both occurring with increasing frequency in invasive cancers. As shown in Fig. 5.1, *Rb* is influenced by complex protein interactions involving cyclin-dependent kinases (CDK) which once activated, will phosphorylate the *Rb* protein resulting in the release of the transcriptor factor E2F which activates cell

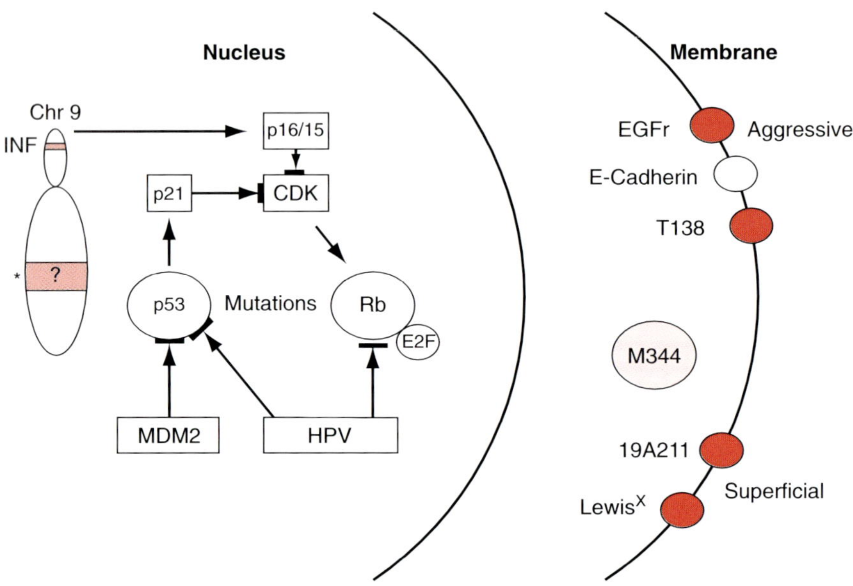

Figure 5.1. Schematic representation of nuclear and membrane tumour markers suspected to be of clinical relevance in bladder cancer management. The Rb protein plays a central role in controlling cell growth at the transition from G1 to S phase. Rb phosphorylation, which releases the transcription factor E2F, is induced by cyclin-dependent kinases (CDK) which are in turn negatively regulated by a family of proteins (p21, p16, p15). p53 is a suppressor protein induced by DNA-damage to stop cell division in order to allow cell repair or induce cell death. p53 exerts its inhibition on Rb via the p21-CDK pathway. The MDM2 oncogene can inactivate p53 and both p53 and Rb can be inactivated by gene mutations or by viral oncoproteins of the human papillomavirus (HPV). Two bladder cancer suppressor genes are suspected on chromosome 9: 9p21 appears to code for p16 inhibitory protein and the 9q gene remains unidentified. Interferon (IFN) genes are also located on the frequently deleted 9p region. Also represented on the right are phenotypic changes in membrane and cytoplasmic proteins that have been associated with distinct biological behaviour of bladder cancer (aggressive and superficial).

division. The *p16* and *p15* are products of suppressor-genes found on chromosome *9p* and inhibit the activation of CDK complexes while *p53* inhibition of *Rb* is exerted through the p21 protein. *P53* also induces cell death by apoptosis in response to DNA damage, a suspected important mechanism for the action of chemotherapeutic agents. The action of *p53* and *Rb* may be inhibited by viral proteins produced by human papilloma viruses (HPV) type-16. Several studies have reported detection of HPV DNA by molecular techniques in approximately one-third of bladder cancers [23,24]. The prognostic significance of this finding remains unknown. A newly described proto-oncogene, the *MDM2*, has also been shown to bind to *p53* and inactivate its physiological role. The *MDM2*-gene product was detected in 32% of bladder cancers, mostly Ta,T1 tumours [25]. The gene responsible for the production of the interferon is located on chromosome *9p* in the region frequently deleted in superficial bladder tumours. This observation may be particularly relevant to bladder cancer which is known to respond to therapy based on immunological-response modifiers, such as BCG, interferon and bropirimine.

Phenotypic markers

For many years, loss of ABH blood-group antigen expression was the only tumour marker in bladder cancer [26]. Monoclonal antibodies have provided better reagents allowing immunopathology studies on formalin-fixed material. The National Cancer Institute (NCI) Bladder Tumour Marker Network studied 131 patients with primary Ta,T1 tumours and long follow-up [27]. Loss of expression of ABH was observed in 40% of cases, irrespective of the recurrence or progressor status of the patients, thus suggesting no benefit from the study of these antigens. Lewis[X] antigen on the other hand was expressed in over 90% of the tumours. This may result in increased detection of tumour cells and exfoliated cells of the urine [28]. However, Lewis[X] is also expressed on polymorphonuclear cells as well as normal umbrella cells thus limiting its clinical utility.

Cell cycle control mechanisms are also under the influence of external cell stimulation through receptors such as the receptor for epidermal growth factor (EGFR). Studies have suggested that increased expression of EGFR on superficial bladder tumours is a good predictor of progression to muscle-invasive cancers [29]. Other factors such as angiogenic factors and autocrine motility factors are also known to be produced in higher stage bladder cancer, but their exact prognostic significance remains unknown. Recent studies have shown that loss of normal membrane E-cadherin expression (a molecule involved in cell adhesion) correlates with increasing grade and stage of tumour as well as with shortened patient survivals [30].

Several bladder-cancer markers were defined by monoclonal antibodies, and few were found to react with the Lewis[X] blood-group antigen. Three other antigens identified by our group have been shown to have both prognostic and diagnostic potential in several clinical studies. The antigen defined by monoclonal antibody T138 is a membrane molecule expressed in 15% of superficial tumours and 60% of invasive cancers [31,32]. Several studies have shown that expression of T138 antigen is associated with poor clinical outcome in patients with bladder cancer [33]. The two other antigens defined by monoclonal antibodies M344 and 19A211 are mostly expressed in superficial papillary-bladder tumours. The M344 reacts with a high molecular weight cytoplasmic mucin expressed in 70% of Ta,T1 tumours, 25% of T and 15% of muscle-invasive cancers [34,35]. No normal tissue, including urothelium, was found to express M344. The antigen recognized by 19A211 is expressed on a bladder cancer carcinoembryonic antigen (CEA) molecule and another low molecular weight molecule of unknown specificity [36–38]. It is expressed on a majority of superficial tumours and approximately 50% of invasive cancers. Both antigens are also expressed in normal-appearing urothelium adjacent or at distant site from bladder tumours [39]. Thus, M344 and 19A211 appear to be promising biomarkers for detection and monitoring of superficial bladder tumours, but also as early indicators of a premalignant state [40].

Molecular pathways

Molecular patterns are beginning to emerge that may provide fingerprints of tumours with two distinct biological potentials and originating from two carcinogenic pathways, as clinically suspected [41,42]. Genetic susceptibility, in addition to the influence of specific carcinogens, may lead to papillary tumours that are most frequently diploid, or to CIS — mostly aneuploid and likely to evolve towards muscle-invasive cancer. *9q* deletion is a common feature of papillary tumours, which also frequently express MDM2, M344 and 19A211 antigens. These tumours are genetically more stable and thus likely to be diagnosed at a superficial stage. The other patterns is associated with high-grade CIS which has frequent *p53* mutations and genetic instability resulting in numerous anomalies. These tumours are likely to cumulate alterations such as loss of *Rb* expression, expression of T138 and/or lack E-cadherin expression. Because of their genetic instability, these cancers are mostly diagnosed at an advanced stage and are more likely to metastasize. A superficial bladder-tumour phenotype may thus provide indications on its molecular origin and on its potential for rapid or slow cancer progression.

Clinical utility of tumour biomarkers

When assessing the utility of tumour markers in clinical management, several points must be considered. First, the test must be feasible on all tumour samples or biological samples, such as voided urine or blood test, to avoid selection bias that may hamper interpretation of results. Second, rigorous clinical studies must be performed to determine the independent value of markers above known clinical parameters. The vast majority of published series on tumour markers have been done on selected small populations and show some correlation with grade and stage. These studies should be considered as Phase I or II by analogy with phases of clinical trials. Promising tumour markers must undergo well-designed Phase III studies to determine the independent value of any of these tests above existing clinical parameters using multivariate analysis. It is also important to determine which level of confidence would be required for the clinician to modify its treatment plan. For example, what probability of cancer progression in what length of time would trigger recommending a radical cystectomy in a patient with superficial bladder cancer — 50%, 60% or more? The following section outlines, according to clinical utilities, the main tumour biomarkers under current investigation for superficial tumours as well as those perceived as possible in the near future (summarized in Table 5.1).

Prognosis of recurrence

Several epidemiological studies have shown that the number and size of the tumours, as well as tumour stage and grade, were the most important clinical predictors of recurrence. One limitation of the more recent studies is the difficulty in truly assessing the natural history of resected bladder tumours without the influence of intravesical therapy, which is frequently used. A recent study performed in the Province of Quebec in 382 newly diagnosed Ta, T1 primary tumours confirmed results of other studies showing that the number of tumours and their size, and the tumour stage and grade were the most important adverse tumour characteristics (ATCs) to predict recurrence [43]. Based on these ATCs, a management algorithm was developed as illustrated in Fig. 5.2 to allow a more objective basis for clinical decision [44]. It is noteworthy, that less than 1% of these patients received any form of intravesical therapy between their initial transurethral resection (TUR) and the first tumour recurrence thus providing a good assessment of the natural evolution. Approximately 20% of patients have no ATC: the 1-year risk of recurrence is 21% and no patient

Table 5.1 Biomarkers of clinical utility in managing superficial bladder tumours.

Prognosis of recurrence	
Tests on tumours	M344, T138, p53
Tests on exfoliated cells	Quanticyte
	M344, 19A211, Lewis^X
Tests on shed urinary proteins	NMP22
Prognosis of progression to T2$^+$	
Tests on tumours	p53, T138, E-cadherin
	Ploidy
Diagnostic tests	
Immunocytology	M344, 19A211, Lewis^X
Shed urinary markers	BTA, FDP, FGF
Predictors of tumour response	Interferon genes
	BCG resistance genes
	Ki-67
	Drug resistance markers

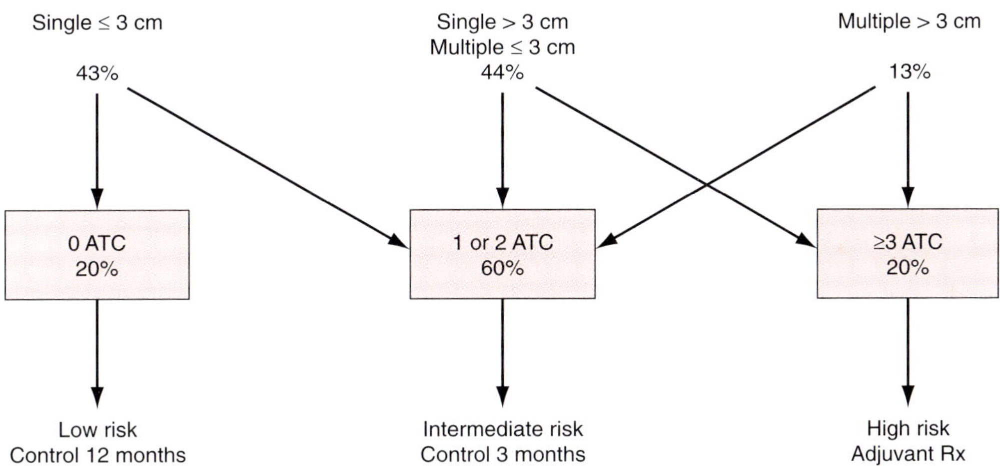

Figure 5.2 Management algorithm for patients with primary Ta, T1 bladder tumours based on pathological characteristics. The four adverse tumour characteristics (ATC) are number, size, grade 2 or 3, stage T1.

progressed after 3 years. The intermediate-risk category comprises 60% of patients that have 36% 1-year risk of recurrence and 1% progression. Finally, 20% of patients are in the high-risk category with a 66% 1-year recurrence risk and a 9% risk of progression over 3 years. While low-risk patients could be followed yearly, intermediate-risk patients require close monitoring and high-risk patients need aggressive adjuvant intravesical treatment at first diagnosis.

The clinical utility of any new marker to predict tumour recurrence must thus take into account the contribution of proper pathological assessment. In this Quebec study, the tumour markers T138, M344 and *p53* were found to provide additional independent predictive value above and beyond that provided by the ATC. Expression of T138 was associated with a significantly increased risk ratio (RR 1.6 ± 0.3) for earlier recurrence, while expression of M344 was associated with an increased tumour rate (RR 1.67 ± 0.3). These two parameters were found to be independent predictors in multivariate analysis. Patients with *p53* positive tumours also recurred more rapidly [45]. An important observation was that *p53* and T138 were usually not coexpressed, suggesting independent prognostic value. Cumulative-risk indices combining significant clinical and tumour biomarker parameters will better define indications for follow-up schedules and intravesical therapy. A first-check cystoscopy at 3 months will nevertheless remain standard to monitor completeness of resection and lack of early recurrence.

After tumours have been resected, the risk of recurrence is mostly dependent on the field changes that will lead to new tumour formation. Monitoring of field changes at this time may be provided by analysis of exfoliated cells obtained by bladder irrigation at the time of cystoscopy. The Nijmegen group has shown increased precision in predicting recurrence using the karyometric analysis (Quanticyte) [14]. Studies are also in progress to determine the value of M344 and 19A211 tests on irrigations and voided urine samples in a multi-institution study of the Bladder-Marker Network. Preliminary data suggests that patients with no tumour seen, but with positive tumour marker test, have approximately 75% risk of tumour recurrence within 6 months compared to less than 20% in those patients with negative markers [40]. Consistent with this observation, mapping studies of the bladder have shown the frequent occurrence of M344 positive cells in histologically normal bladder mucosa of patients with bladder tumours [39]. Results of a very limited trial also suggest that the NMP22 test, which measures shed nuclear-matrix proteins in the urine, may be helpful in predicting patient recurrence after TUR. However, the true utility of such a test cannot be determined until properly designed studies have shown its additional value above that provided by the adverse tumour characteristics described above.

Prognosis of progression

Four markers have been associated with increased risk of cancer progression in superficial bladder cancer: EGFR [29], T138 [33,46], E-cadherin [30] and *p53* [47,48]. All these markers were studied in a select group of patients. The presence of *p53* mutations as measured by immunostaining with pAb1801 showed a marked increase in risk of progression in a study of 43 T1 tumours, 54 Ta tumours and 33 patients with CIS of the bladder. Similarly, in a subgroup of 45 patients with T1 cancer probability of progression was 62% for patients with p53-positive tumours compared to 7% in *p53*-negative tumours. In at least three different studies, expression of T138 in bladder cancer was associated with high metastatic potential. In the first study of 68 patients, cancer death was observed in 35% of patients with diploid, T138-positive tumours compared to 0% for diploid, T138-negative and 60% for aneuploid T138 positive [33]. In addition, four of five patients with T138-positive Ta,T1 tumours later progressed to invasive and metastatic cancer. In a more recent study of 55 bladder cancers, comparing T138 and EGFR, only tumour stage (p = 0.0001) and T138 (p = 0.006) had an independent prognostic value in multivariate analysis [46]. Preliminary results show no correlation between T138 and E-cadherin with *p53* anomalies, suggesting that these three markers may be complementary (unpublished data).

Diagnosis and monitoring

Urinary cytology is reasonably sensitive to detect high-stage cancers, but has a low 10–30% sensitivity for the most common low-stage tumours. Thus, cystoscopy remains the main diagnostic tool for the investigation of symptomatic patients and for the follow-up of tumour patients. The first likely improvement in non-invasive diagnosis will consist in immunocytological tests. Studies using anti-Lewis[X] antibodies have shown improved sensitivity over cytology alone [28], but careful interpretation is required since Lewis[X] antigen is also expressed on normal umbrella cells and inflammatory cells. In a prospective study of 250 bladder irrigations, M344 and 19A211 antibodies were positive in 95% of Ta,T1 tumours with positive urinary cytology, but also 80% of cytology negative ones [40]. The antibody test was also predicting recurrence in patients with no tumour seen at control cystoscopy. Both antigens are well preserved on exfoliated cells of urine. Immunocytology with M344 and 19A211, using a suboptimal immunoperoxidase technique, was performed in a double-blind study of 861 patients including 190 bladder tumour patients. The combination of these two antibodies resulted in an increased sensitivity from 34% with cytology alone to 72% with cytology and the two antibodies [8]. Results of a study by immunofluorescence on urine cells with M344 antibody alone showed up to 85% sensitivity and 95% specificity for tumour detection [49]. There is thus good hope that optimized testing, with these combinations of antibodies using fluorescence techniques, will bring the sensitivity of tumour detection to a level that would allow the clinician to safely use these techniques to monitor non-invasively patients followed for bladder tumours.

Other tumour markers shed as soluble antigens in urine have also been studied. The BTA developed by 'BARD Diagnostics' and recently approved by the Food and Drug Administration (FDA), is measuring basement-membrane antigens using latex agglutination assay. The results of studies have shown a sensitivity comparable to cytology, although some cytology positive specimens were negative with bladder tumour antigen (BTA) and vice versa. Overall, sensitivity for detecting superficial bladder tumours remains well below 50% when combining BTA and cytology [9]. The Auratek, which measures fibrinogen degradation products (FDP) in the urine has been reported to have a higher sensitivity, reaching close to 70% in a recent American Urological Association (AUA) report [10]. Other potential shed-tumour markers are the acid-FGF (fibroblastic growth factor) and basic-FGF which have both been studied in very limited clinical populations [50]. More recently, microsatellite DNA markers were used to detect loss of heterozygocity and genomic instability in cells shed in urine compared to cells obtained from a blood sample from the same patient [51]. These results, in a very limited population of 20 tumour patients and five controls, were highly publicized and suggested that 95% sensitivity of tumour detection could be reached. Although promising, several technical issues must be resolved and, more importantly, properly designed clinical trials must be performed before consideration can be given to the routine use of such an approach in clinical practice. Nevertheless, it is clear from this discussion that several potential tests are emerging and that in the very near future diagnosis and monitoring of bladder cancer using non-invasive tests is likely to become a reality.

Predicting response to intravesical therapy

Bladder-tumour patients at high risk of recurrence can be effectively treated by intravesical immunotherapy with bacille Calmette-Guérin (BCG) or by intravesical chemotherapy with agents such as Mitomycin C or Adriamycin. However, not all patients respond to either one of these therapies and a proper identification of those likely to respond or not would save costs and morbidity in addition to optimizing therapy with the most appropriate agent. Several drug-resistance mechanisms have been identified that could provide markers to predict response or monitor induction of resistance to chemotherapy. It is also possible that tumours with the highest proliferative rate are more sensitive to the effect of chemotherapeutic agents. The use of markers such as Ki-67 to measure proliferation rate of tumour cells may be useful in this regard. The response to intravesical instillation of BCG is variable and not predictable from one patient to the other. The recent discovery of genes responsible for the natural resistance to BCG and other intracellular parasites may provide a means to better identify patients unlikely to respond to this therapy [52]. Similarly, the finding of frequent deletions of the short arm of chromosome 9 in bladder tumours may also be associated with changes in the interferon genes which may be associated with different sensitivity to intravesical intron A and oral bropirimine therapy. Clearly, there is a need and a potential for tumour markers in guiding intravesical therapy, but we are looking in to the future as no study with any of these markers has yet been reported with the exception of studies on multidrug resistance gene (MDR).

Bioeconomy of bladder cancer management

Improving the management of bladder cancer must meet three objectives: (1) improving cancer control, (2) decreasing morbidity, and (3) decreasing costs of the various interventions (Fig. 5.3). The improved knowledge gained by use of tumour markers and tests developed from them will be a key element in this process. Improved cancer control will result from the prevention of tumour recurrence, and the identification of high-risk superficial tumours better treated by early radical surgery. Effective screening may become possible with more sensitive and specific diagnostic tests, an approach that could substantially reduce the incidence of invasive bladder cancer as suggested by home screening studies using Haemastix [53]. Decreased morbidity is likely to result at first from a decrease in the need for check cystoscopies with the appropriate use of clinical and tumour-marker parameters, as well as more sensitive non-invasive diagnostic tests to allow safe monitoring of bladder-tumour patients. Similarly, targeting intravesical therapy to those patients most likely to recur and to respond to a given form of treatment will minimize side-effects.

Preliminary studies in a cohort of workers exposed to carcinogens have shown that the M344 test may be very sensitive to detect early cancer [54]. Such a test could identify a premalignant state and help monitor preventive interventions which would be the ultimate in avoiding morbidity. The economic realities have brought managed care and global costs into the practice of medicine. While new tests will increase costs, their down-stream effect on diagnostic interventions and treatments may result in significant dollar savings. By helping targeting therapy to those patients most likely to respond, tumour-marker tests will improve the cost-effectiveness of these therapies while decreasing the overall costs.

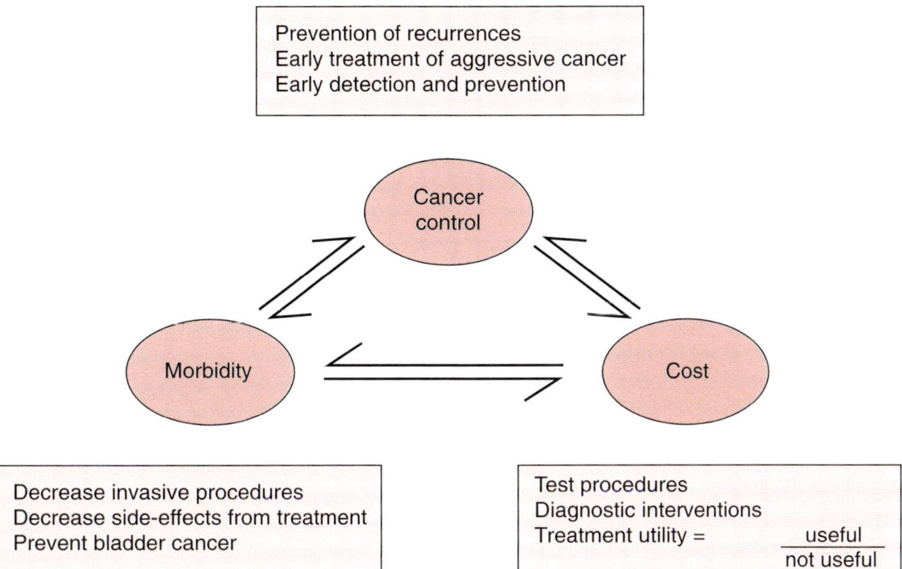

Figure 5.3 Bio-economy model of bladder cancer management representing the three main endpoints to measure improvements: cancer control, patient morbidity and cost.

There is, however, a long road ahead after the initial report of striking results with the use of any biomarkers and the implementation of such tests in routine clinical practice. The clinician anxious to use these tests must realize how many variables may greatly affect the precision of the tests and thus the significance of the results. In that regard, *p53* is perhaps one of the most dangerous markers at this time since some surgeons may be tempted to treat patients with superficial tumours aggressively based on the *p53* phenotype of the tumour. The results of a *p53* assay will be dependent on the type of antibody used for the assay, the conditions under which the tissue biopsy has been handled and fixed, and also the sample preparation using microwave and other antigen-retrieval techniques, not even mentioning the possible variability from the reading of the slides. Cumulating these variables may lead to completely opposite results on the same clinical samples. Such meticulous considerations are part of the culture of clinical biochemistry laboratories, but to a lesser extent of pathology laboratories which practise classically a more subjective science. In that regard, specialized reference laboratories offering services nationwide may provide an intermediate step to offer earlier some of these new tests in a well-controlled environment before optimized reagents and standard-operating procedures are developed and approved by regulatory agencies. Such agencies like the FDA are taking on a more active role in ensuring the quality of the tests and their proper use in the management of cancer patients in order to produce more good than harm.

Possible therapeutic applications

The urinary bladder lends itself to easy access for intravesical therapy. As such, it provides a unique opportunity to test the tumoricidal effect of new treatments in a more or less isolated environment. Targeting EGFR with EGF (epidermal growth factor) coupled with TP40 toxin was shown to be effective in treating CIS of the bladder [55]. Studies have also shown that monoclonal antibodies can be used to target radioactive agents in bladder tumours by intravesical instillation [56]. Some antigens may have more appropriate characteristics than others for successful targeting of cytotoxic agents in bladder cancer [57,58].

Other possible therapies currently under investigation are based on gene transfer. The objective is to reintroduce in to cancer cells and premalignant cells normal genes such as *p53* or *Rb* using viral vectors or liposomes. Another approach that may be of value in the future is the development of vaccines [59]. Bladder cancer is one of the most sensitive cancers to non-specific immunotherapy. The identification of tumour-associated antigens, specific for malignant and premalignant lesions of the bladder, may provide a basis for the construction of vaccines using a variety of available viral vectors [60].

Conclusion

Rapid progress has been made in recent years in identifying molecular pathways of bladder carcinogenesis. A constellation of new markers have been studied and some are clearly showing promise as prognostic or diagnostic tests. Appropriately designed Phase III studies should provide the information required to base treatment decisions on tumour-marker tests. Moreover, the new molecules identified, coupled with the power of biotechnology, may lead to a new generation of therapeutic products. Knowledge-based management of bladder cancer will be part of the 'new civilization' that will emerge at the turn of this century.

References

1   Hermanek P, Sobin LH. TNM Classification of Malignant Tumors. International Union Against Cancer, 4th edn. Heidelberg: Springer-Verlag, 1987.

2   Koss LG. Tumors of the urinary bladder. In: Hartmann WH, Sobin LH (eds) *Atlas of Tumor Pathology*, 2nd edn. Fascicle 11. Washington DC: Armed Forces Institute of Pathology, 1975.

3   Ooms ECM, Anderson WAD, Alons CL *et al.* Analysis of the performance of pathologists in the grading of bladder tumors. *Hum Pathol* 1983; **14**: 140–3.

4   Eble JN, Young RH. Benign and low grade papillary lesions of the urinary bladder: a review of the papilloma–papillary carcinoma controversy, and a report of five typical papillomas. *Semin Diagn Pathol* 1989; **6**: 351–71.

5   Abel PB, Henderson D, Bennett MK *et al.* Differing interpretations by pathologists of the pT category and grade of transitional cell cancer of the bladder. *Br J Urol* 1988; **62**: 339–42.

6   Lynch CF, Platz CE, Jones MP *et al.* Cancer registry problems in classifying invasive bladder cancer. *J Nat Cancer Inst* 1991; **83**: 429–33.

7   Witjes JA, Kiemeney LALM, Schaafsma HE, Zandberg A, Debruyne FMJ. The influence of review pathology on study outcome of a randomised multicentre superficial bladder cancer trial. *Br J Urol* 1994; **73**: 172–6.

8   Fradet Y, Veltri RW, Simard P *et al.* Improved detection of bladder cancer by immunocytology with monoclonal antibodies M344 and 19A211. *Can J Urol* 1996; **3**: A40.

9   Sarosdy MF, deVere White RW, Soloway MS *et al.* Results of a multicenter trial using the BTA test to monitor for and diaganose recurrent bladder cancer. *J Urol* 1995; **154**: 379–84.

10 Schmetter BS, Habichi K, De Jager R *et al.* AURATEK FDP: a multicenter trial evaluation of a novel diagnostic method for bladder cancer. *Proc Am Urol Assoc* 1995; **153**: 457A (Abst. 915).

11 Wheeless LL, Badalament RA, White RWD, Fradet Y, Tribukait B. Consensus review of the clinical utility of DNA cytometry in bladder cancer. *Cytometry* 1993; **14**: 478–81.

12 Têtu B, Allard P, Fradet Y, Roberge N, Bernard P. Prognostic significance of nuclear DNA content and S phase fraction by flow cytometry in primary superficial bladder cancer. *Human Pathol* 1996; **27**: 922–6.

13 Grégoire M, Fradet Y, Bois R *et al.* Diagnostic accuracy of urinary cytology and DNA flow cytometry and cytology on bladder washings during follow-up for bladder tumors. *J Urol* 1997 (in press).

14 van der Poel HG, Oosterhof GON, Debruyne FMJ, Schalken JA. Image analysis in superficial transitional cell carcinoma of the bladder. *Semin Urol* 1993; **11**: 164–70.

15 Fradet Y, Cordon-Cardo C. Tumor markers in the management of bladder cancer. In: Raghavan D, Scher HL, Leibel SA, Langer PH (eds) *Principles and Practice of Genitourinary Oncology.* Philadelphia: J.B. Lippincott Company 1996: 231–8.

16 Hopman AH, Moesker O, Smeets AW *et al.* Numerical chromosome 1, 7, 9, and 11 aberrations in bladder cancer detected by *in situ* hybridization. *Cancer Res* 1991; **51**: 644–51.

17 Waldman FM, Carroll PR, Kerschmann R *et al.* Centromeric copy number of chromosome 7 is strongly correlated with tumor grade and labeling index in human bladder cancer. *Cancer Res* 1991; **51**: 3807–13.

18 Miyao N, Tsai YC, Lerner SP *et al.* Role of chromosome 9 in human bladder cancer. *Cancer Res* 1993; **53**: 4066–70.

19 Cairns P, Tokino K, Eby Y, Sidransky D. Homozygous deletions of 9P21 in primary human bladder tumors detected by comparative multiplex polymerase chain reaction. *Cancer Res* 1994; **54**: 1422–4.

20 Orlow I, Lianes P, Lacombe L *et al.* Chromosome 9 allelic losses and microsatellite alterations in human bladder tumors. *Cancer Res* 1994; **54**: 2848–51.

21 Levine AJ, Momand J, Finlay CA. The *p53* tumour suppressor gene. *Nature* 1991; **351**: 453–6.

22 Cordon-Cardo C, Dalbagni G, Richon VM. Significance of the retinoblastoma gene in human cancer. *Princ Pract Oncol* 1992; **6**: number 9.

23 LaRue H, Simoneau M, Fradet Y. Human papillomavirus in transitional cell carcinoma of the urinary bladder. *Clin Cancer Res* 1995; **1**: 435–40.

24 Furihata M, Inoue K, Ohtsuki Y *et al.* High-risk human papillomavirus infections and overexpression of p53 protein as prognostic indicators in transitional cell carcinoma of the urinary bladder. *Cancer Res* 1993; **53**: 4823–7.

25 Lianes P, Orlow I, Zhang ZF *et al.* Altered patterns of MDM2 and TP53 expression in human bladder cancer. *J Nat Cancer Inst* 1994; **86**: 1325–30.

26 Sheinfeld J, Reuter VE, Fair WR, Cordon-Cardo C. Expression of blood group antigens in bladder cancer: current concepts. *Semin Surg Oncol* 1992; **8**: 308–15.

27 Sarkis AS, Charytonowicz E, Cordon-Cardo C *et al.* Blood group antigen expression in bladder tumors. An immunohistochemical study of low-grade bladder lesions. *J Exp Clin Cancer Res* 1994; **13**: 139–44.

28 Sheinfeld J, Reuter VE, Melamed MR *et al.* Enhanced bladder cancer detection with the Lewis X antigen as a marker of neoplastic transformation. *J Urol* 1990; **143**: 285–8.

29 Neal DE, Sharples I, Smith K *et al.* The epidermal growth factor receptor and the prognosis of bladder cancer. *Cancer* 1990; **65**: 1619–25.

30 Bringuier PP, Umbas R, Schaafsma HE *et al.* Decreased E-cadherin immunoreactivity correlates with poor survival in patients with bladder tumors. *Cancer Res* 1993; **53**: 3241–5.

31 Fradet Y, Cordon-Cardo C, Thomson T *et al.* Cell surface antigens of human bladder cancer defined by mouse monoclonal antibodies. *Proc Nat Acad Sci* 1984; **81**: 224–8.

32 Fradet Y, Cordon-Cardo C, Whitmore WF Jr., Melamed MR, Old LJ. Cell surface antigens of human bladder tumors: definition of tumor subsets by monoclonal antibodies and correlation with growth characteristics. *Cancer Res* 1986; **46**: 5183–8.

33 Fradet Y, Tardif M, Bourget L, Robert J and the Laval University Urology Group. Clinical cancer progression in urinary bladder tumors evaluated by multiparameter flow cytometry with monoclonal antibodies. Laval University Urology Group. *Cancer Res* 1990; **50**: 432–7.

34 Fradet Y, Islam N, Boucher L *et al.* Polymorphic expression of a human superficial bladder tumor antigen defined by mouse monoclonal antibodies. *Proc Nat Acad Sci* 1987; **84**: 7227–31.

35 Bergeron A, Champetier S, LaRue, H, Fradet Y. MAUB, a new mucin antigen associated with bladder cancer. *J Biol Chem* 1996; **271**: 6933–41.

36 Fradet Y, LaRue H, Parent-Vaugeois C *et al.* Monoclonal antibody against a tumor-associated sialoglycoprotein of superficial papillary bladder tumors and cervical condylomas. *Int J Cancer* 1990; **46**: 990–7.

37 Cordon-Cardo C, Wartinger DD, Melamed MR, Fair W, Fradet Y. Immunopathologic analysis of human urinary bladder cancer. Characterization of two new antigens associated with low-grade superficial bladder tumors. *Am J Pathol* 1992; **140**: 375–85.

38 Bergeron A, LaRue H, Fradet Y. Identification of a bladder tumor-associated glycoform of the carcinoembryonic antigen by monoclonal antibody 19A211. *Cancer Res* 1996; **56**: 908–15.

39 Rao JY, Hemstreet GP, Hurst RE *et al.* Alterations in phenotypic biochemical markers in bladder epithelium during tumorigenesis. *Proc Nat Acad Sci* 1993; **90**: 8287–91.

40 Fradet Y, Lafleur L, LaRue H. Strategies of chemoprevention based on antigenic and molecular markers of early and premalignant lesions of the bladder. *J Cellular Biochem* 1992; **161**: 85–92.

41 Fradet Y, Cordon-Cardo C. Critical appraisal of tumor markers in bladder cancer. *Sem Urol* 1993; **11**: 145–53.

42 Spruck CH, Ohneseit PF, Gonzalez Zulueta M *et al.* Two molecular pathways to transitional cell carcinoma of the bladder. *Cancer Res* 1994; **54**: 784–8.

43 Allard P, Fradet Y, Têtu B, Bernard P. Tumor-associated antigens as prognostic factors for recurrence in 382 patients with primary transitional cell carcinoma of the bladder. *Clin Cancer Res* 1995; **1**: 1195–202.

44 Allard P, Fradet Y, Bernard P, Têtu B. An algorithm to determine the prognosis of patients with primary superficial Ta and T1 bladder cancer. *Can J Urol* 1996; **3**: A40. Abst. 31.

45 Têtu B, Fradet Y, Allard P *et al.* Prevalence and clinical significance of HER-2/neu, P53 and Rb expression in primary superficial bladder cancer. *J Urol* 1996; **155**: 1784–8.

46 Ravery V, Colombel M, Popov Z *et al.* Prognostic value of epidermal growth factor-receptor, T138 and T43 expression in bladder cancer. *Br J Cancer* 1995; **71**: 196–200.

47 Sarkis AS, Dalbagni G, Cordon-Cardo C *et al.* Nuclear overexpression of p53 protein in transitional cell bladder carcinoma: a marker for disease progression. *J Nat Cancer Inst* 1993; **85**: 53–9.

48 Esrig D, Elmajian D, Groshen S *et al.* Accumulation of nuclear p53 and tumor progression in bladder cancer. *N Engl J Med* 1994; **331**: 1259–64.

49 Bonner RB, Hemstreet GP, Fradet Y *et al.* Bladder cancer risk assessment with quantitative fluorescence image analysis of tumor markers in exfoliated bladder cells. *Cancer* 1993; **72**: 2461–8.

50 Chopin DK, Caruelle JP, Colombel M *et al.* Increased immunodetection of acidic fibroblast growth factor in bladder cancer, detectable in urine. *J Urol* 1993; **150**: 1126–30.

51 Mao L, Schoenberg MP, Scicchitano M *et al.* Molecular detection of primary bladder cancer by microsatellite analysis. *Science* 1996; **271**: 659–62.

52 Cellier M, Govoni G, Vidal S *et al.* Human natural resistance-associated macrophage protein: cDNA cloning, chromosomal mapping, genomic organization, and tissue-specific expression. *J Exp Med* 1994; **180**: 1741–52.

53 Messing EM, Young TB, Hunt VB *et al.* Comparison of bladder cancer outcome in men undergoing hematuria home screening versus those with standard clinical presentations. *Urology.* 1995; **45**: 387–97.

54 Bi WF, Rao JY, Hemstreet GP, Fang *et al.* Field molecular epidemiology: feasibility of monitoring for the malignant bladder cell phenotype in a benzidine-exposed occupational cohort. *J Occup Med* 1993; **35**: 20–7.

55 Goldberg MR, Heimbrook DC, Russo P *et al.* Phase I clinical study of the recombinant oncotoxin TP40 in superficial bladder cancer. *Clin Cancer Res* 1995; **1**: 57–61.

56 Bamias A, Bowles MJ, Krausz T, Williams G, Epenetos AA. Intravesical administration of indium-111-labelled HMFG2 monoclonal antibody in superficial bladder carcinomas. *Int J Cancer* 1993; **54**: 899–903.

57 de Harven E, Fradet Y, Connelly JG *et al.* Antibody drug carrier for immunotherapy of superficial bladder cancer — ultrastructural studies. *Cancer Res* 1992; **52**: 3131–7.

58 Battelli MG, Polito L, Bolognesi A *et al.* Toxicity of ribosome-inactivating proteins-containing immunotoxins to a human bladder carcinoma cell line. *Int J Cancer* 1996; **65**: 485–90.

59 Boon T, Coulie P, Marchand M *et al.* Genes coding for tumor rejection antigens: perspectives for specific immunotherapy. In: DeVita VT, Hellman S, Rosenberg SA (eds) *Important Advances in Oncology*. Philadelphia: J.B. Lippincott Company, 1994; 53–69.

60 Saad F, Bergeron A, LaRue H, Lafleur L, Fradet Y. Biochemical characteristics and immunotherapeutic potential of a human epithelial mucin of superficial transitional cell bladder carcinoma. *J Urol* 1992; **147**: 371A.

CHAPTER 6

Towards a better knowledge of bladder cancer

W.R. Fair

The excellent papers thus far point out the major factors involved in the epidemiology, natural history, and prognosis of superficial bladder cancer. Although much was reviewed, the concept of bladder neoplasia set forth by Dr Murphy deserves reiteration (Table 6.1).

The most important concept is that the behaviour of these tumours is generally determined before their clinical detection [1]. While clinicians recognize that recurrence is a much more common phenomenon in patients with superficial bladder tumours than progression, and that the number of recurrences does not increase the likelihood of progression, the concept that the behaviour of tumours is determined by the molecular biology of the lesion, and is set before the lesion is detected, is one that is foreign to most clinicians. However, it is mandatory that this concept be understood before a rational clinical approach can be evolved.

The excellent discussion of the molecular biology of bladder cancer by Dr Guido Dalbagni underscores the rapid events that have recently occurred in our understanding of the aetiology and biology of superficial bladder cancer, especially the relationship among proto-oncogenes, oncogenes and suppressor genes. This research elucidates the delicate balance that exists among factors favouring tumour development and progression, and those factors inhibiting the formation of new tumours or the progression of already established tumours (Fig. 6.1). Oncogenes, when stimulated, work to decrease regulation of cell growth, decrease cell differentiation and decrease cell adhesion. Inhibition of suppressor genes will act to increase angiogenesis, increase invasiveness and increase the propensity for metastases.

Table 6.1 Concepts of bladder neoplasia.

Behaviour set before detection
Clinical lesions are late events in tumour growth
Progression and grade is unusual
Recurrence does not equal progression

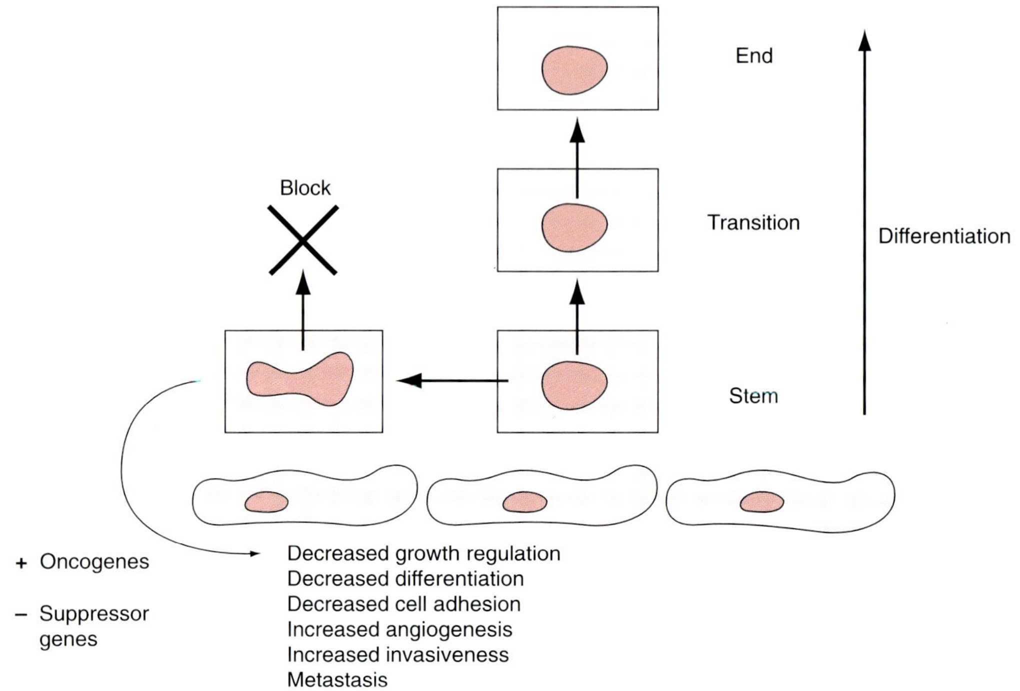

Figure 6.1. The opposing actions of oncogenes and suppressor genes.

Dr Karl Heinz Kurth presents an excellent review of the natural history and prognosis of untreated and treated superficial bladder cancer, and again, underscores the observation that recurrence of superficial disease — especially Ta disease — does not necessarily indicate future progression, and the primary goal of treatment should be to inhibit progression rather than recurrence of superficial tumours, most of which present no risk to the life of the patient. In contrast, the T1 tumour, especially when occurring after resection and intravesical therapy, is occasioned by a rate of progression, defined as the development of muscle-invading disease or distant-metastatic disease, in the order of 9–25% [2,3,4]. There appears to be general agreement that transurethral resection (TUR) alone, while providing excellent local control, does not prevent the development of new tumours, and intravesical therapy combined with TUR offers the greatest hope in altering the natural history of these lesions.

Dr Yves Fradet has reviewed the prognostic factors associated with recurrence and progression. This topic, along with the discussion on molecular biology of bladder cancer referenced above, underscored the promise of molecular biology providing us with an increasing knowledge of molecular events leading up to the development and progression of superficial bladder cancers, as well as potential strategies for prevention or treatment. Although progress has been substantial, at present the *results* of molecular biology remain primarily a *promise* for the clinician, as the development of effective clinical strategies may lag a decade or more behind laboratory observations. In this regard, we should consider the elegant studies on the carcinogenesis of colon carcinoma by Vogelstein and Kinzler [5] and associates. Although much has been learned about the biology of colon cancer, an effective strategy based on inhibition of oncogenes due to stimulation of suppressor genes remains to be evolved. As illustrated in Fig. 6.2, similar progress has been made in

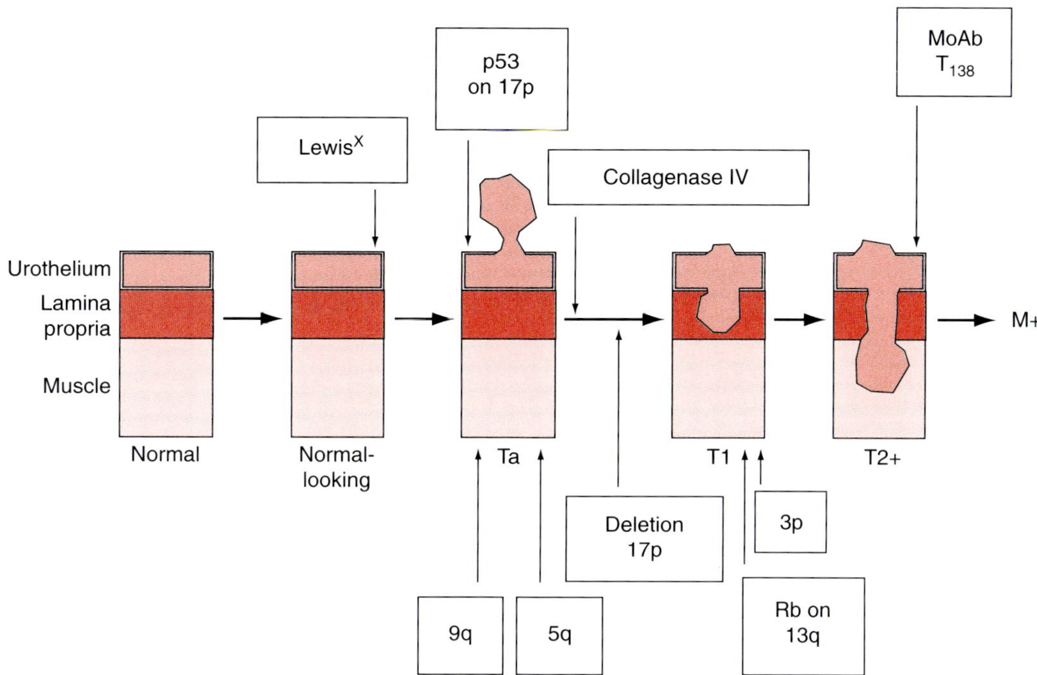

Figure 6.2. Hypothesis — bladder tumour progression.

our understanding of the molecular biology of bladder-tumour progression. Although results document the genetic changes that occur as one examines the differences between normal urothelium and muscle-invading disease, as yet, clinicians have no known way of inhibiting or augmenting the malignant process initiated by these genetic malfunctions. It is clear, however, that it is necessary to bring together basic laboratory scientists with clinicians, involved in the day-to-day care of patients with superficial bladder cancer, before any effective strategy of disease prevention and/or treatment will be forthcoming.

References

1   Dalbagni G, Presti J, Reuter V, Fair WR, Cordon-Cardo C. Genetic alterations in bladder cancer. *Lancet* 1993; **342**: 469–71.
2   Khanna OP, Son DL, Mazer H. Multicenter study of superficial bladder cancer treated with intravesical BCG or Adriamycin. *Urology* 1990; **35**: 101–8.
3   England HR, Paris AM, Blandy JP. The correlation of T1 bladder tumour history with prognosis and follow-up requirements. *Br J Urol* 1981; **53**: 593–7.
4   Cho KR, Vogelstein B. Suppressor gene alterations in the colorectal adenoma–carcinoma sequence. *J Cellular Biochem* 1992; (Suppl.) S16G 137–41.
5   Vogelstein B, Kinzler KW. The multistep nature of cancer. *Trend Genet* 1993; **9**(4): 138–41.

CHAPTER 7

Rationale and principles of intravesical therapy

P. Bassi, N. Piazza and F. Pagano

Introduction

Several intravesical agents have been proposed in the last four decades to treat superficial bladder cancer with favourable results; consequently intravesical therapy has been broadly accepted in clinical practice [1]. However, the clinical application of intravesical therapy has been based upon old habits rather than upon science. Greater knowledge in this field has lead to an attempt of rationalization of the clinical approach to intravesical therapy for superficial bladder cancer.

Rationale

The rational basis for intravesical therapy is found in the natural history of superficial bladder cancer. Superficial bladder cancer is known to eventually recur in a great proportion of patients, while a small proportion of patients progresses to a muscle-invading disease and/or more rarely to a metastatic disease. The reasons for these peculiar features of superficial bladder cancer are under study and seem to stem from the genetic alterations of the urothelial cells [2]. Moreover, the impact of intravesical therapy on recurrence and progression is clearer now [1,3].

Whatever the reasons for these events, the goals of intravesical therapy are to eradicate the existing disease, to inhibit tumour recurrence and to prevent tumour progression with the final goal being to improve survival rate. Two approaches have been applied by urologists to reach these goals: intravesical therapy (transurethral resection +/- intravesical agents) and more rarely, definitive therapy (radical cystectomy). Whatever the therapeutical approach, the indications for which are not discussed herein, the precise assessment of the status of the disease is pivotal in the identification of prognostic factors and risk categories and therefore in selecting the therapy.

Principles of intravesical therapy

Intravesical therapy has been and is generally considered effective in the eradication of an existing disease, in the inhibition of tumour recurrence and in the prevention of tumour progression. Classically, these goals are reached through 'prophylaxis' and 'therapy'. Prophylaxis implies intravesical instillation to prevent new recurrences after complete resection of all visible tumours while therapy implies intravesical instillation to treat residual unresected or unresectable disease.

When using any agent for superficial bladder-cancer therapy, several questions must be considered in order to apply the general principles of intravesical therapy scientifically.

Who is the best candidate?

Knowledge of the prognostic factors of superficial bladder cancer is used to make a selection of the patients to be treated with intravesical therapy. As a matter of fact, each individual patient must be treated according to his specific disease after a precise and complete clinical assessment including history, voided cytology, i.v. pyelography, urethocystoendoscopy with resection of all papillary tumours, cold biopsies of normal and abnormal appearing bladder mucosa and prostatic urethra, bimanual palpation under anaesthesia as well as check cytology and, when possible and worthwhile, check cystoscopy. Simplification of all of the prognostic groups is impossible due to the number of variables involved. However, the clinical evaluation paradigmatically identifies the patient's disease as treatable or untreatable with intravesical therapy as listed in Table 7.1.

What is the best drug?

The ideal agent for intravesical therapy must be active in eradicating pre-existing disease and in definitively preventing both recurrence and progression. The administration of the drug should be as simple and short as possible, while the drug itself should not cause local or systemic side-effects. It should be cost-effective as well. Unfortunately no such drug exists yet.

Several studies have tried and are trying to identify the 'best drug' but, to date, no definitive data are available due to different inclusion criteria as well as treatment regimens reported. However, a recent and elegant meta-analysis reported by D.L. Lamm *et al.* [3] claimed that intravesical chemotherapy agents are unable to

Table 7.1 *Who's the optimal candidate?*

No	Yes
Single tumour	Multiple tumours
No recurrent	Recurrent
Stage Ta	Stage T1, Tis
Low grade	High grade
No field changes	Adjacent dysplasia
Negative cytology	Positive cytology
Negative prostatic-urethra biopsy	Positive prostatic-urethra biopsy (superficial)
Small size	Large size

substantially affect the natural history of superficial bladder cancer. As a matter of fact, even though chemotherapy reduces the short-term incidence of tumour recurrences by 15–18%, the incidence of tumour recurrences within 5 years is equal to that observed in patients treated with transurethral resection (TUR) alone. More importantly, the studies published on intravesical chemotherapy failed to demonstrate a significant reduction in tumour progression or an increase in survival [1,3]. Even though conflicting data are reported about the efficacy of bacillus Calmette–Guérin (BCG) in comparison with other chemotherapeutic agents [1], a clear advantage of BCG in preventing tumour progression over TUR has been proven in three controlled studies [4–6].

The most common intravesical treatments are based upon the use of a single agent. However, experimental data demonstrated the synergistic cytotoxic effect of doxorubicin and thiotepa, as well as of doxorubicin and Mitomycin C [7]. A clinical approach using polichemotherapy with doxorubicin and Mitomycin C after TUR has been shown to prevent tumour recurrence in 70% of patients [8]. Alternating treatment with chemo- and immunotherapeutic drugs has been suggested to improve the immunotherapeutical activity by reducing the bladder barriers and enhancing the antitumoural effect [9].

The side-effects related to intravesical therapy are well known. BCG therapy cannot be used without respect for its potential for morbidity and death, since the incidence of local (cystitis) and systemic (fever, flu-like symptoms) side-effects is higher in comparison with that reported with the most common chemotherapeutic agents [10]. While chemotherapy drugs cause a lower incidence of chemical cystitis, chemical dermatitis and cutaneous allergic rashes have also been reported [11]. Significant systemic drug absorption has been observed with thiotepa causing drug-related neutropenia in about 5% of patients [11].

The cost of treatment must also be taken into account when selecting the drug for intravesical therapy. Moreover, situations vary in each country according to market and licence regulations.

What is the ideal drug preparation?

Surprisingly, very little attention has been paid to the clinical application of the most common pharmacological concepts. Several factors have been recognized as capable of altering the cytotoxic effect of chemotherapeutical drugs used for intravesical therapy such as molecular weight, lipophilicity, pH, osmolarity, concentrations and dosing volume. The main factor to be considered is the concentration as demonstrated by Walker *et al.* [12] in an experimental model; higher concentrations have been related to a higher cytotoxic effect. These findings were clinically confirmed in an escalating-dosage trial with epirubicin therapy of carcinoma *in situ* (CIS) published by Kurth *et al.* [13]. The osmotic strength of the instilled solution significantly affects the survival of the cancer cells as well [14]. Only recently, Badalament *et al.* used pharmacokinetic and pharmacodynamic knowledge in a computer simulation of Mitomycin C therapy; the optimized solution was more cytotoxic than the standard solution. These experimental data have been confirmed by an ongoing comparative randomized clinical trial [15]. In conclusion, the optimal conditions for intravesical administration of the chemotherapeutic drug have not yet been established.

On the other hand, more information is available about the optimal administration of BCG due to extensive clinical studies [16]. BCG as a lyophilized form must be diluted and reconstituted in a sterile physiological saline. No bacteriostatic agents capable of inactivating the BCG should be included in the diluent preparation. While a dose-activity relationship has been demonstrated in chemotherapeutic drugs [17], experimental and clinical evidence has demonstrated that higher doses of BCG are associated with a decrease in response rates, due mainly to an immunological breakdown as clinically stated by Ratliff and coworkers [18–20]. On the contrary, increased doses of BCG are associated with an increase in related side-effects, as shown with chemotherapy [18,20].

What is the best regimen for intravesical therapy?

Several questions arise about the optimal regimen: when to start instillations?, how many instillations?, how many courses?, does maintenance therapy make a difference?

The results of two parallel prospective comparative trials designed to compare early versus delayed instillations and short-term versus long-term treatment indicate that, with regard to recurrence rates, patients submitted to delayed and short-term treatment did worse than those submitted to early instillations or those who underwent prolonged treatment [21]. The argument for early treatment of superficial bladder cancer after TUR received further support from an EORTC trial which demonstrated that the recurrence rate was decreased by nearly half [22] after a single intravesical instillation of epirubicin, 80 mg, was administered immediately after TUR.

With regard to BCG, a South West Oncology Group (SWOG) study showed that maintenance therapy was more effective in prolonging the disease-free status than no maintenance treatment, both in patients with CIS and with papillary tumours [23]. Unfortunately and surprisingly, the definitive data on this trial have yet to be published. Concerns have been expressed regarding the potential systemic side-effects of early treatment with BCG after TUR. A waiting period of at least 15 days after resection is recommended before starting treatment [16,24]. It is clear that more intensive and prolonged regimens are associated with a higher incidence of side-effects, as well stated by Brosman [25].

The optimal number of chemotherapy instillations has not yet been defined. Solsona *et al.*'s experience with doxorubicin- and mitomycin-treated patients showed that more than 50% of the patients who failed to respond to a single 8-week course of therapy responded to a second additional 8-week course with the same drug [26]. This data underlines the fact that some early treatment failures could be caused by a sub-optimal number of instillations rather than by chemoresistance. This finding is even more evident with BCG therapy; three different experiences showed that an additional 6-week course provoked further response in 27–60% of patients, suggesting that at least 12 BCG instillations are necessary to classify a patient as a responder or non-responder [6,27,28,].

Does ideal timing exist?

Superficial bladder cancer can be considered a chronic disease. Though it is clear when to treat patients with intravesical therapy, no data are available about the best timing. However, some evidence is useful in selecting the treatment for patients with multirecurrent superficial bladder cancer. Patients who failed to respond to intravesical chemotherapy with one drug responded to a different chemotherapeutical drug in 42–62% of cases (Table 7.2) and to BCG in 38–68% of cases (Table 7.3) [29]; moreover, those who fail to respond to BCG therapy may respond to intravesical chemotherapy or to 'rescue' BCG treatment (Table 7.2–7.3) [30].

Is there a risk of a new primary malignancy after intravesical therapy?

Some concerns have been expressed about a possible increase in the risk of new primary malignancy in patients treated with intravesical therapy for superficial bladder cancer. Allen *et al.* [31] reported a 24% incidence of new malignancies in their series of MMC treated patients. No further related evidence is reported in literature about intravesical chemotherapy, though similar concerns about BCG-treated patients were reported by Khanna *et al.* [32]. Furthermore, the exhaustive work published by

Table 7.2 Second-line intravesical therapy: percentage responses.

Study	Agent	Patients (*N*)	Treatment	Resp (%)
CHEMO. after CHEMOTHERAPY				
Prout [38]	MMC after TTPA	23	Prophyl/therapy	43
Issel [39]	MMC after TTPA	57	Prophyl/therapy	42
Zincke [40]	TTPA after MMC	5	Prophylaxis	60
Milani [41]	MMC after ADM	31	Prophylaxis	62
CHEMO. after BCG				
Pinon [42]	MMC	4	Prophylaxis	100
Rintala [43]	MMC	11	Prophyl/therapy	82

Abbreviations: MMC, Mitomycin C; TTPA, Thiotepa; ADM, Adriamycin.

Table 7.3 Second-line intravesical therapy: percentage responses.

Study	Agent	Patients (*N*)	Treatment	Resp (%)
BCG after CHEMOTHERAPY				
Soloway [44]	TTPA/MMC	30	Prophyl/therapy	50
Lamm [45]	MMC/TTPA	37	Prophylaxis	38
Pagano [46]	MMC/ADM	28	Prophylaxis	68
BCG after BCG				
Bassi [47]	BCG	19	Prophyl/therapy	84

Abbreviations: TTPA, Thiotepa; MMC, Mitomycin C; ADM, Adriamycin; BCG, bacillus Calmette-Guérin.

Guinan *et al.* proved the incidence of new malignancies in BCG-treated patients to be similar to that observed in the general population [33].

Is a direct tumour-drug contact necessary?

The use of intravesical drug administration for superficial bladder cancer therapy was based upon the firm belief that high drug concentrations and direct and prolonged tumour–drug contact would lead to a better response rate without systemic effects.

However, more recent experiences stated that the oral approach is also worthwhile. High-dose vitamins, *Lactobacillus* preparation and bropirimine have proven to be active against superficial bladder cancer [34–36].

Which patients are ineligible for intravesical therapy?

There are several patients in whom intravesical therapy is unlikely to be effective. These include patients with cancer invading the muscle or extending into areas in which there is no direct contact with intravesical agents, such as the ureters and prostatic urethra. Recently, however, intravesical BCG has also been found effective in patients with transitional-cell carcinoma involvement of the prostatic urethra [37]. Intravesical therapy must be considered over treatment of single, low-grade, low-stage, non-recurrent tumours. Though no specific contraindications have been found for intravesical chemotherapy, concerns must be expressed about BCG treatment of patients with immunosuppressive diseases or status, or assuming some medications such as anticoagulants or antibiotics can render BCG inactive [16].

Major cautions must be taken in the intravesical administration of drugs to patients with small capacity bladders. No significant complications or side-effects have been noted in patients with reno-ureteral reflux submitted to intravesical chemo- or immunotherapy [17,25].

Conclusions

A survey of the literature on intravesical therapy for superficial bladder cancer substantially underlines the empirical approach to this cancer with regards to the principles applied in the clinical setting to date. However, recent efforts have been made to answer most of the impending questions regarding intravesical therapy.

As of yet, no ideal drug exists. The optimal conditions for intravesical administration are experimentally established but poorly applied in the clinical setting. The value of a single instillation, early treatment, maintenance therapy, additional treatment courses and second-line therapy has been demonstrated. The use of different administration modalities is now being experienced in clinical practice.

References

1 Lamm DL. Long term results of intravesical therapy for superficial bladder cancer. *Urol Clin N Am* 1992; **19**(3): 573–80.

2 Sandberg AA. Chromosome changes in bladder cancer clinical and other correlations. *Cancer Genet Cytogenet* 1986; **19**: 163–75.

3 Lamm DL, Riggs DR, Traynelis CL, Nseyo UO. Apparent failure of current intravesical chemotherapy prophylaxis to influence the long-term course of superficial transitional cell carcinoma of the bladder. *J Urol* 1995; **153**: 1444–50.

4 Herr HW, Laudone VP, Badalament RA. Bacillus Calmette–Guérin therapy alters the progression of superficial bladder cancer. *J Clin Oncol* 1988; **6**: 1450–5.

5 Lamm DL. Bacillus Calmette-Guérin immunotherapy for bladder cancer. *J Urol* 1985; **134**: 40–5.

6 Pagano F, Bassi P, Milani C *et al.* A low dose bacillus Calmette-Guérin regimen in superfical bladder cancer therapy: is it effective? *J Urol* 1991; **146**: 32–6.

7 Seraphim LA, Perrapato SD, Slocum HK, Rustum YM, Huben RP. *In vitro* study of the interaction of doxorubicin, thiotepa, and Mitomycin-C, agents used for intravesical chemotherapy of superficial bladder cancer. *J Urol* 1991; **145**: 613–17.

8 Ferraris V. Doxorubicin plus Mitomycin C in the prophylactic treatment of superficial bladder tumors. *Cancer* 1988; **62**: 1055–60.

9 Debruyne FMJ, van der Meijden APM, Witijes JA. Intravesical instillation therapy: alternative treatments. In: *Recent Results in Cancer Research*, Vol 126. Berlin: Springer-Verlag 1993; 119–25.

10 Lamm DL. Complications of bacillus Calmette–Guérin immunotherapy. *Urol Clin N Am* 1992; **19**(3): 565–72.

11 Thrasher JB, Crawford ED. Complications of intravesical chemotherapy. *Urol Clin N Am* 1992; **19**(3): 529–39.

12 Walker MC, Master JRW, Parris CN. Intravesical chemotherapy: *in vitro* studies on the relationship between dose and toxicity. *Urol Res* 1986; **14**: 137–44.

13 Kurth KH, Vijgh WJF, ten Kate F *et al.* Phase 1/2 study of intravesical epirubicin in patients with carcinoma *in situ* of the bladder. *J Urol* 1991; **146**: 1508–13.

14 Groos E, Masters JR. Intravesical chemotherapy: studies on the relationship between osmolarity and cytotoxicity. *J Urol* 1986; **136**: 399–402.

15 Kalns JE, Wientjes MG, Badalament RA *et al.* Pharmacokinetic interventions to improve intravesical therapy of superficial bladder cancer. *J Urol* 1995; **153**: 232A.

16 Brosman SA, Lamm DL. The preparation, handling and use of intravesical bacillus Calmette–Guérin for the management of stage Ta,T1, carcinoma *in situ* of transitional cell cancer. *J Urol* 1990; **144**: 313–16.

17 Richie JP. Intravesical chemotherapy: treatment selection, techniques, results. *Urol Clin N Am* 1992; **19**(3): 521–7.

18 Bassi P, Milani C, Meneghini A *et al.* Dose response of bacillus Calmette–Guérin in superficial bladder cancer: a phase III randomized trial low dose vs standard dose regimen. *J Urol* 1992; **147**: 273A.

19 Ratliff TL, Catalona WJ. Depressed proliferative responses in patients treated with 12 weeks of intravesical BCG. *J Urol* 1989; **141**: 230A.

20 Pagano F, Bassi P, Piazza N *et al.* Improving the efficacy of BCG immunotherapy by dose reduction. *Eur Urol* 1995; **27**(S1): 19–22.

21 Bouffioux C, Kurth KH, Bono A *et al.* Intravesical adjuvant chemotherapy for superficial transitional cell bladder carcinoma: results of 2 European Organization for Research and Treatment of Cancer randomized trials with Mitomycin C and doxorubicin comparing early versus delayed instillations and short-term versus long-term treatment. *J Urol* 1995; **153**: 1934–41.

22 Oosterlinck W, Kurth KH, Schroeder F *et al.* A prospective European Organization for Research and Treatment of Cancer Genitourinary group randomized trial comparing transurethral resection followed by a single intravesical instillation of epirubicin or water in single stage Ta,T1 papillary carcinoma of the bladder. *J Urol* 1993; **149**: 749–52.

23 Lamm DL, Crawford ED, Blumstein BA. Maintenance BCG Immunotherapy of superficial bladder cancer: a randomized prospective SWOG study. *J Urol* 1992; **147**: 274A.

24 Lamm DL. Complications of bacillus Calmette–Guérin immunotherapy. *Urol Clin N Am* 1992; **19**(3): 565–72.

25 Brosman SA. Bacillus Calmette–Guérin immunotherapy techniques and results. *Urol Clin N Am* 1992; **19**(3): 557–64.

26 Solsona E, Iborra I, Ricos JV *et al.* Carcinoma *in situ* associated with superficial bladder tumor. *Eur Urol* 1991; **19**: 93–6.

27 Catalona WJ, Hudson MLA, Gillen PA. Risks and benefits of repeated courses of intravesical bacillus Calmette-Guérin therapy for superficial bladder cancer. *J Urol* 1987; **137**: 220–6.

28 Kavoussi LR, Torrence RJ, Gillen DP. Results of 6 weekly intravesical bacillus Calmette–Guérin instillations on the treatment of superficial bladder tumors. *J Urol* 1988; **139**: 935–9.

29 Bassi P, Piazza N, Abatangelo G, Pagano F. Unresponsive superficial bladder cancer. (See chapter 16).

30 Bassi P, Milani C, Piazza N *et al*. Effectiveness of a rescue bacillus Calmette–Guérin therapy in patients who relapsed after successful response to BCG therapy of superficial bladder cancer. *J Urol* 1992; **147**: 372A.

31 Allen RJ, Johnson DE, Swanson DA. Mitomycin C for superficial bladder cancer: fate of patients 10 years later. *J Urol* 1990; **143**: 342A.

32 Khanna DP, Chou RH, Son DL *et al*. Does bacillus Calmette–Guérin immunotherapy accelerate growth and cause metastatic spread of secondary primary malignancy? *Urology* 1988; **31**: 459–68.

33 Guinan P, Brosman S, de Kernion J *et al*. Intravesical bacillus Calmette–Guérin and second primary malignancy. *Urology* 1989; **33**: 380–1.

34 Lamm DL, Riggs DR, Shriver JS *et al*. Megadose vitamins in bladder cancer: a double-blind clinical trial. *J Urol* 1994; **151**: 21–6.

35 Aso Y, Azaka H, Kotake T *et al*. Preventive effect of a *Lactobacillus casei* preparation on the recurrence of superficial bladder cancer in a double-blind trial. The BLP Study Group. *Eur Urol* 1995; **27**: 104–9.

36 Sarosdy MF, Lamm DL, Williams RD *et al*. Phase I trial of oral bropirimine in superficial bladder cancer. *J Urol* 1992; **147**: 31–3.

37 Schellhammer PF, Lagada LE, Moriarty RP. Intravesical bacillus Calmette–Guérin for the treatment of superficial transitional cell carcinoma of the prostatic urethra in association with carcinoma of the bladder. *J Urol* 1995; **153**: 53–6.

38 Prout GR Jr, Griffin PP, Nocks BN. Intravesical therapy of low stage bladder carcinoma with Mitomycin C: comparison of results in untreated and previously treated patients. *J Urol* 1982; **127**: 1096–102.

39 Issel BF, Prout GR, Soloway MS. Mitomycin C intravesical therapy in noninvasive bladder cancer after failure on thiotepa. *Cancer* 1984; **53**: 1025–30.

40 Milani C, Bassi P, Meneghini A *et al*. Mitomycin C in multiple superficial bladder cancer: short-term therapy, long-term results. *Urol Int* 1992; **48**: 154–6.

41 Zincke H, Benson RC Jr, Hilton JF. Intravesical thiotepa and Mitomycin C treatment immediately after transurethral resection and later for superficial bladder cancer: a prospective, randomized, stratified study with crossover design. *J Urol* 1985; **134**: 1110–16.

42 Pinon AA, Suarez GM, Politano VA. Experience with second and third line intravesical chemotherapy agents after initial agent failures. *J Urol* 1988; **139**: 320A.

43 Rintala E, Jauhiainen K, Alfthan O *et al*. Intravesical chemotherapy (Mitomycin C) versus immunotherapy (bacillus Calmette–Guérin) in superficial bladder cancer. *Eur Urol* 1991; **20**: 19–25.

44 Soloway MS, Perry A. Bacillus Calmette–Guérin for treatment of superficial transitional cell carcinoma of the bladder in patients who have failed thiotepa and/or Mitomycin C. *J Urol* 1987; **137**: 871–3.

45 Pagano F, Bassi P, Milani C. A low dose bacillus Calmette–Guérin regimen in superficial bladder cancer therapy: is it effective? *J Urol* 1991; **146**: 32–6.

46 Lamm DL, Grissmann J, Blumenstein B *et al*. Adriamycin versus BCG in superficial bladder cancer: a Southwest Oncology Group Study. *Prog Clin Biol Res* 1989; **310**: 263–70.

47 Bassi P, Milani C, Piazza N *et al*. Effectiveness of a rescue bacillus Calmette–Guérin (BCG) therapy in patients who relapsed after successful response to BCG therapy of superficial bladder cancer. *J Urol* 1992; **147**: 372A.

CHAPTER 8

Methodology in superficial bladder cancer trials. Objective evaluation of treatment: the need for standardization

P. Bassi

General considerations about cancer clinical trials

When a new anti-tumoural treatment becomes available for patients with cancer, a sequence of clinical studies begins [1]. The extent of the study at each stage is determined by the results obtained before that stage (Table 8.1).

The first clinical trial, usually called *Phase I*, is designed to find a dosage, schedule and route of administration that is not overly toxic and worthy of further investigation as based upon experimental evidence. The endpoint is toxicity. If a safe regimen of treatment has been determined a study, usually designated *Phase II*, can be conducted in a consecutive series of patients to obtain an estimate of the activity (the capacity of a treatment to induce modifications that will presumably induce benefits) of the proposed regimen of treatment. Since there is no aim in comparing treatments, randomized control patients are not generally needed in Phase I and II trials. If the Phase II trial proves positive, the next step is to test the relative efficacy (the capacity of a treatment to induce the benefits for which it is being administered) of the drug in a comparative Phase III study where the drug can be compared with the best available conventional treatment, either alone or in combination. A *Phase III* study is a substantial undertaking involving a protocol, a reasonable number of patients and often a long period of time; because it is also a considerable investment in time and money, it should not be undertaken unless adequate preliminary Phase I and II trials have been a carried out to rule out significant toxicity and to prove a substantial activity.

Table 8.1 Cancer clinical trials.

	Phase I (drug oriented)	Phase II (disease oriented)	Phase III (patient oriented)
Objectives	maximum tolerated dose	activity	efficacy
Endpoints	toxicity	response	survival
Type of trial	not randomized	not randomized (rarely randomized)	always randomized

Whatever the aim of a study (maximum tolerated dose, activity, efficacy), it is measured on the basis of data taken from the quantification of the relative endpoints (variables, the measures of which are used to evaluate treatment effects). Consequently, the criteria used to evaluate the response become the cardinal points on which the evaluation of the entire study is based. Moreover, the results of clinical trials have an influence on daily clinical choices making the definition of goals, endpoints and evaluation criteria important in routine practice as well as in the design of clinical studies.

Unfortunately, the information found in scientific literature does not always furnish definitive or indisputable answers to basic clinical questions such as which drug, what regime or which dose is optimal for a specific disease.

For example, there is wide disparity in reported cases of tumour response when patients with the same type of cancer are treated with similar therapy. Such a variability could suggests that it may be difficult, or impossible, to obtain a valid comparison of the rates of tumour response in clinical trials. The wide variability in reported rates of tumour response may be due to several factors. Some of these, such as differences in patient characteristics, dosage, regimen used, as well as the quality of patient care, can influence the true benefit of the therapy. Artifactual differences in the way that investigators collect and report their data are also sources of variability in reported response rates; among these factors the most important are: (1) patient selection, (2) inadequacy of the patient sample size to define the confidence intervals, (3) the frequency with which treated patients are excluded from the analysis and (4) the criteria used for the assessment of tumour response.

As far as superficial bladder cancer is concerned, a significant factor that contributes to studies reporting higher rates of response and longer median durations of response is typically the selection of patients with more favourable prognostic factors, such as focality, tumour stage, tumour grade and recurrence rate. Other factors, such as type and intensity of the treatment, differing levels of measurement error in the results assessment, will also contribute to the variability in observed response rates.

One of the most critical aspects of any trial is the choice and the precise definition of the criteria used to assess treatment results. Therefore, the quality of the criteria used in the assessment of tumour response is a factor which must be closely analysed for potential risks of misinterpretation of results. Response rate tends to be lower in reports from highly stringent response criteria. Considerable heterogeneity in the criteria used by different investigators to determine tumour response was detectable in a literature survey, despite the statement by several investigators that they had used 'standard' criteria. It is evident that 'standard' criteria are very variable among the published reports, making it difficult for readers to objectively 'understand' the reported data.

The example in Table 8.2 shows how subtle differences in response criteria may cause large changes in apparent response rates.

All authors could consider Group A patients as responders, some could record groups A and B, and some groups A, B, and C. Depending on the inclusion or exclusion of group E, the response rate could vary from 20% (i.e. A/A + B+C+D+E) to 75% (i.e. A+B+ C/A + B+C+D). Thus, subtle differences in response criteria may cause large changes in apparent tumour-response rates.

The actual evaluation of tumour response is perhaps too frequently forgotten, amidst such technical sophistry; the inherent and inevitable factor of human error is responsible for the misinterpretation and the misunderstanding of the detected effects of the therapy [2].

Table 8.2 Pitfalls in evaluating tumour response after systemic chemotherapy.

Patient groups	% of size reduction relative to the initial measurement at weeks:			
	2	4	6	8
A	> 50%	> 50%	> 50%	> 50%
B	> 50%	> 50%	~ 0%	< 50%
C	> 50%	~ 0%	< 50%	< 50%
D	~ 0%	< 50%	< 50%	< 50%
E	No follow-up			

Since at present we cannot eliminate the human error factor, it would seem advisable to make an effort to minimize such error by applying the most appropriate evaluation criteria of tumour response after a therapeutical approach. Fortunately, the new trend towards more objective and more controlled clinical trials has led to the elucidation of the many principles of proper scientific experimentation.

Superficial bladder cancer: a peculiar disease

Efforts to conduct more objective and controlled clinical investigation in cancer therapy generally also need to be made for superficial bladder cancer. Unfortunately, little attention has been paid to the matter in the past. More recently, the problem has been critically considered by the Consensus Conferences on Bladder Cancer, by the EORTC (European Organization for Research and Treatment of Cancer) Genitourinary Group and by the National Bladder Cancer Group (NBCG) [3,4].

A study of the objective evaluation criteria, after intravesical therapy, for superficial bladder cancer is reported herein.

Superficial bladder cancer is known to be associated with a high incidence of tumour recurrence and a negligible incidence of progression. Superficial bladder cancer can recur several times without progressing to invasive and/or metastatic disease, giving it a peculiar characteristic in the field of oncology, i.e. that of chronic disease.

Endoscopic resection and/or endovesical therapy are the treatment that patients with superficial bladder cancer typically undergo. Therefore, the guide pattern of the therapeutical approach consists of the ablation of the primary tumour, the prevention of recurrence and the prevention of invasive disease. The therapeutic approach is mainly directed at the prevention of progression, an occurrence which has an obvious negative effect on patient survival. Due to the relatively low incidence of progression, its significance is sometimes revaluated in favour of more rapidly appreciable endpoints which are in any case correlated, such as the ablation of a primary tumour or the prevention of recurrences. This obviously does not mean that survival is a secondary endpoint.

Ablation of primary tumour(s) = therapy

Papillary tumours
The treatment of papillary tumours is usually ablative, performed by means of transurethral resection (TUR). More rarely, in cases of non-resectable diffuse papillary disease, primary tumour ablation is accomplished with endovesical chemo- or immunotherapy.

Carcinoma in situ
Carcinoma *in situ* (CIS) can occur alone or in conjunction with papillary tumours. The latter are removed using TUR. Characteristically, CIS must be considered a multifocal disease until proven otherwise. Because the tumour may be invisible and may cover a large surface of the bladder urothelium, endoscopical treatment is not always feasible. Therefore, the use of intravesical therapy is usually necessary to eliminate the primary tumour.

Prevention of tumour recurrence(s) = prophylaxis

As far as superficial bladder cancer is concerned, *recurrence* is by definition the histologically/cytologically confirmed detection of tumour(s) at any site of the bladder during the follow-up period after the complete removal of all tumour(s) by TUR of papillary tumours. This implies that all papillary tumours are removed by means of TUR. The prevention of recurrence after TUR, or the *prophylaxis* usually consists of intravesical therapy. The prophylaxis of recurrence is directed at the destruction of coating cells which can be considered the main cause of recurrence after complete removal with TUR. The term 'recurrence' is not often used with reference to CIS. The more appropriate term used in general oncology — 'relapse' — seems to better define the reappearance of urothelial cancer after complete response to treatment (usually intravesical).

Prevention of tumour progression

Tumour progression is defined as muscle invasion ($\geq$ T2) and/or metastases (N+ and/or M+). Progression of grade is not an appropriate evaluation criterion. The inter-individual and intra-individual variabilities in the evaluation of tumour grade make it too subjective to be adopted as a criterion for response evaluation. Stage progression (upstaging, 'local' progression) among superficial bladder tumours (from Ta to T1 for example) may be used as a secondary endpoint in selected clinical trials but, in reality, offers no useful information from the practical point of view.

Superficial bladder cancer clinical trials

The stages involved in clinical trials involving superficial bladder cancer patients are summarized in Table 8.3.

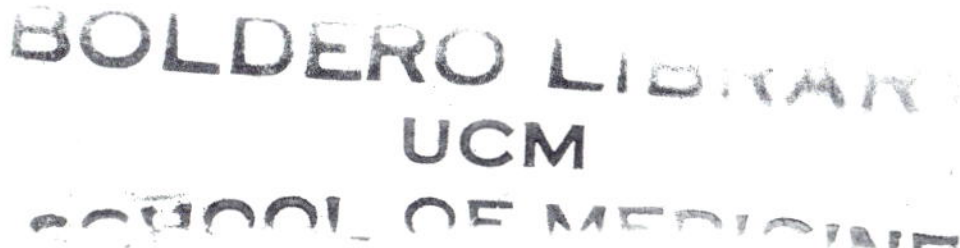

Table 8.3 Superficial bladder cancer clinical trials.

	Phase I (drug oriented)	Phase II (disease oriented)	Phase III (patient oriented)
Objectives	maximum tolerated dose	activity	efficacy
Endpoints	toxicity (local-systemic)	response (complete response, no response, progression)	time to progression, disease-free interval
Type of trial	not randomized	not randomized (rarely randomized)	randomized

Phase I trials (objective = maximum tolerated dose)

The purpose of the Phase I trial is to determine the qualitative and quantitative toxicity defining the safe dose for further studies on therapeutical activity.

Toxicity is an inherent concept of any clinical evaluation of anti-tumoural therapy. The key to the evaluation of any novel treatment is the concept of therapeutical index, that is the comparison of the benefits given to the patient with the costs in terms of treatment-related toxicity. The usefulness of any treatment for disease depends on its activity and the toxicities incurred, and also on the stage and prognosis of the specific patient population.

The assessment of treatment toxicity is a critical and challenging aspect of clinical research. The following information should be addressed in assessing toxicity: (1) which toxicity and in what percentage, (2) the severity of the toxicity, and (3) when toxicity occurs and how long it lasts. The most objective parameters possible should be used; as a consequence we should know to what extent we can or should rely on subjective information in assessing treatment toxicity. This general and complex question is important in superficial bladder-cancer trials also. Significant variations in reported toxicity of intravesical therapy result from the difficulty in defining an objective and easy standardization of grading toxicities. Due to the subjectivity of any individual interpretation of side-effects and the lack of objective parameters, the evaluation of treatment toxicity due to intravesical therapy is and will be difficult. Sometimes it is impossible to distinguish side-effects from medical complications of the cancer itself.

A simple and practical standard for the definition and grading of toxicity after intravesical therapy is proposed in Table 8.4.

Table 8.4 Grading of toxicity following intravesical therapy.

Grade 0 or absent	=	no side-effects
Grade 1 or mild	=	not requiring treatment
Grade 2 or moderate	=	requiring treatment
Grade 3 or severe	=	requiring the delay of instillations
Grade 4 or extreme	=	requiring interruption of treatment

The time of onset, the duration of a side-effect and the frequency of observation are also critical to assess whether toxicity recurs with repetitive instillations and whether or not it is cumulative in nature, as seen in patients undergoing immunotherapy.

Phase II trials (objective = activity)

The evaluation of response after treatment of superficial bladder cancer generates specific problems that make it necessary to deviate from the usual World Health Organization (WHO) guidelines for the formulation of response criteria [5].

In the past, the same considerations have been applied to Ta and T1 tumours in spite of a different prognosis. As a matter of fact, in most circumstances, the primary tumour was removed by TUR and the evaluation criteria described the prevention of tumour recurrence.

Different criteria have been applied for CIS. In reality, the recent punctualization, made by the Genitourinary Group of the EORTC, regarding the significance of the marker lesion (see chapter 9) associates the evaluation criteria for response to therapy for papillary tumours, Ta or T1 with those for carcinoma *in situ* [6]. The reliability of these criteria is totally dependent on the accuracy of the parameters in use. Sensitivity and specificity of these parameters must be taken into account. Whatever the initial treatment, TUR or intravesical therapy, the objective evaluation of the response requires an indicator lesion.

For *carcinoma in situ*, a disease that must be considered multifocal until proven otherwise, or, more rarely in cases of unresectable disease, tumour elimination (*therapy*) relies directly upon topical therapy, chemo- or immunotherapy, or other therapy.

For *papillary tumours* (Ta, T1) the only way to scientifically evaluate the activity of a treatment is to perform a Phase II study leaving a marker lesion. All but one multiple or recurrent papillary tumours must be resected before the treatment is started. This is strictly correlated to the experimental and clinical evidence that the *prophylaxis* is in part related to the destruction of the floating cells and/or residual tumour. It seems rational to correlate the prophylactic activity of a drug with its ablative ability. Authoritative studies support the principle of leaving a marker lesion. In fact prognostic factor analyses performed by the Genitourinary Group of the EORTC and the British Medical Research Council have shown that the likelihood of progression to muscle invasion in patients with multiple medium- or low-risk tumours is very low and, consequently, that treatment with unexperimental agents is feasible. Therefore, the proper selection of the patient population is mandatory for the marker lesion trials.

Ethical concerns about the risk of tumour progression have no scientific basis and can be considered unmotivated due to the negligible incidence of tumour progression reported, in trials with a marker lesion, to date. Due to proper selection of patients, tumour progression has actually been shown to be much lower than that reported in several Phase II trials in which no marker lesion was used . This approach, is the best and necessary way to objectively investigate novel agents for the treatment of Ta/T1 lesions.

Thus the response criteria for Phase II trials on superficial bladder cancer (stages Ta, T1, Tis) are the following:

Complete response (CR): Negative histology and bladder washing cytology; response should last at least 3 months.

No response (NR): Positive bladder washing cytology and/or persistence of the marker lesion regardless of the increase in size and/or number of previously described lesions. No evidence of tumour progression (stage T2 or greater, and/or N+, and/or M+).

Progression (PROG): Positive histology with muscle invasion (stage T2 or greater) of marker or new lesions, and/or nodal (N+) and/or systemic (M+) metastases, histologically proven.

Phase III trials (objective = efficacy)

Prophylactic trials (papillary tumours)

In clinical practice, TUR is used for the ablation of papillary tumours (stage Ta,T1). Adjuvant, post-operative therapies are often employed after tumour removal to prevent or limit recurrence (*prophylaxis*). Therefore, from the conceptual point of view, the evaluation of response must take into account the association of the TUR of the tumour and the adjuvant, prophylactic intravesical therapy. The radicality of TUR is a problem which is little considered in the evaluation of response. In patients undergoing early endoscopical evaluation 4 weeks after a supposedly complete TUR of their tumours, tumours which were thought to be remaining from an unwittingly incomplete resection have been found.

Because the initial treatment (TUR) of papillary tumours is considered fully ablative, the response criteria that must be employed are as follows:

Disease-Free Interval (DFI) is the time interval between the initial ablative treatment and the first recurrence, superficial or not (*time to progression*).

The *recurrence rate* (RR), considered as the number of recurrences, after an initial ablative treatment, by the time of follow-up, is less useful in evaluating the prophylactic efficacy of the combination TUR + drug under evaluation. As a matter of fact, the first recurrence (or tumour progression) proves the combination to be ineffective in the prevention of tumour recurrences and the number of recurrences, or the outcome of the patient during the subsequent follow-up, adds no substantial information with which to evaluate the prophylactic effect of the agent. Furthermore, the proportion of recurrences is strongly influenced by the duration of the follow-up period which is variable for each individual patient. From a methodological standpoint, the use of the recurrence rate in a Phase III trial implies the evaluation and comparison of the initial treatment, the prophylactic treatment and the treatment following subsequent recurrence(s). This introduces further variables which make the evaluation of the prophylactic value of the treatment under evaluation confusing and misleading.

Therapeutic trials

Therapeutic trials usually involve CIS. When potentially ablative treatment is employed as the initial ablative therapy, the evaluation criteria described for the marker-lesion trial should be used; consequently the WHO guidelines should be followed. As previously reported, the patient cannot be rendered disease-free by surgical treatments since the tumour may be invisible or may cover a large surface of the bladder. The evaluation of the response in CIS is more critical. The reliable identification of the presence or absence of the disease through cytology, histology and endoscopy is difficult. The minimal requirements for the diagnosis of CIS are still a matter of debate.

The evaluation criteria used for Phase II trials can be applied in Phase III trials: *complete response, no response, progression.* The non-responders should be followed to assess the time to progression; complete responders are followed until relapse.

Conclusion

In conclusion, the formulation of proper evaluation criteria after superficial bladder cancer therapy poses several methodological problems that are often peculiar to the disease.

The Achilles' heel of many trials is possibly found in the criteria used in the evaluation of the trial's outcome. As a consequence, total agreement regarding the criteria for response and the evaluation of response is needed. The adoption of standard response criteria should be given high priority. Uniform criteria of response should be chosen because they meet standards of reliability and statistical validity. Thus, the criteria must be reproducible and correlate with some measures of patient benefit, such as quantity and quality of survival.

References

1   Wolf H, Shipley W, Mc Lead D, Robertson C. Types, Phases of study and therapeutical approaches. In: Denis L, Niijima T, Prout G, Schröder FH (eds) *Developments in Bladder Cancer. Progress in Clinical and Biological Research* 12. New York: AR Liss 1986; 273–6.

2   Warr O, Mc Kinney S, Tannock I. Influence of measurement error on assessment of response to anticancer chemotherapy. *J Clin Oncol* 1984; **2**: 1040–6.

3   Byar D, Kailhara S, Sylvester R *et al.* Statistical analysis technique and sample size determination for clinical trials of treatments for bladder cancer. In: Denis L, Niijima T, Prout G, Schröder FH (eds) *Developments in Bladder Cancer. Progress in Clinical and Biological Research 12.* New York: AR Liss 1986; 49–64.

4   Schröder FH, Sylvester R, Gustofson H *et al.* Response criteria for phase III studies of superficial bladder cancer. In: Denis L, Niijima T, Prout G, Schröder FH (eds) *Developments in Bladder Cancer. Progress in Clinical and Biological Research 12.* New York: AR Liss 1986; 299–307.

5   World Health Organization. Who Handbook for Reporting Results of Cancer Treatment (WHO offset publication no 48). Geneva: WHO, 1979.

6   Bouffioux O, van der Maijden A, Kurth KH *et al.* Objective response of superficial bladder tumors to intravesical treatment (including review of response marker lesions). In: Schröder FH (ed) *EORTC Genitourinary Group Monograph 11: Recent Progress in Bladder and Kidney Cancer.* New York: Wiley Liss 1992; 29–42.

CHAPTER 9

Objective response criteria to intravesical therapy: the marker lesion

Ch. Bouffioux, A. van der Meijden, K. Kurth
and R. Sylvester

Introduction

The assessment of an *objective* response of a tumour to a drug requires a *measurable marker lesion.*

After completion of the treatment, changes that occur in the marker allow for definition of:

- complete response (CR): complete disappearance of the marker (proven by negative biopsy)
- partial response (PR): decrease by at least 50% of the size of the marker
- stable disease (SD): no significant change of the marker
- progressive disease (PD): increase by at least 25% of the size of the marker.

In superficial bladder cancer, these principles may be applied and adapted in the following conditions:

- In the case of *exophytic Ta, T1* superficial bladder cancer, drugs may be instilled into the bladder with an immediate *ablative purpose when transurethral resection (TUR) is not complete* either because of diffuse disease or because of anterior location. These cases have a bad prognosis and the efficacy of a treatment is difficult to appreciate, because the extension of residual disease is difficult to assess and because the delayed vanishing effect of the TUR or fulguration is not measurable and may interfere with appreciation of the results.

- In the case of carcinoma *in situ* (CIS), there is no measurable marker lesion but the disappearance of the irritative symptoms and of microscopic heamaturia, a normal aspect of the bladder at cystoscopy, negative-random biopsies (including the posterior urethra), negative urinary cytology (and probably in the near future, negative tests for markers like nuclear matrix proteins or basement membrane components) may be considered, all together, as objective parameters of response. For these reasons, CIS is probably the most appropriate material to study the objective efficacy of an intravesical therapy.

These two aspects of the objective efficacy of intravesical treatment have been covered in another paper [1] and will not be reviewed here.

- *for new drugs or for new dosages* of already known medications, it is also advocated to test them *in Phase II studies with a marker lesion* before advocating them for Phase III prophylactic studies or for clinical use.

For this purpose, the European Organization for Research and Treatment of Cancer Genitourinary Group (EORTC GU) has designed a *master Phase II protocol* (prepared by van der Meijden) that can be adapted to different intravesical or even oral medications [2].

The design of Phase II studies

The design of these Phase II studies is as follows: multiple (less than 10) primary or recurrent superficial bladder cancer (Ta, T1) patients with good or intermediate prognosis are eligible; all of the tumours but one (at least 0.5cm diameter) which is the marker, are resected.

The drug is then given following a pre-determined schedule; for intravesical treatment, it consists most often of 8 weekly instillations starting within 2–4 weeks after TUR. A control cystoscopy is performed after completion of the treatment; if the marker is still present, it is resected; if it has disappeared, a biopsy (TUR) of its previous site is performed.

If the marker disappeared (with negative histology and negative urinary cytology) without any new occurrence of tumour, it indicates a complete response; all other situations are considered as a non-response [2].

This kind of trial raises some questions

- Why multiple tumours?
- What is the risk of leaving a marker?
- Is it logical to subrogate the possible prophylactic effect of a drug to its ablative effect? In other words, is this kind of Phase II study a necessary step before embarking in Phase III prophylactic studies?

Why multiple tumours?

Because an initial deep biopsy is necessary to know the grade and the stage of the indicator lesion. Additionally, it has been postulated that such a biopsy (either with a cold cup or by TUR) can alter the blood supply of the marker which could then regress or even disappear independently of any chemical effect of the medication given later on, leading to a wrong conclusion regarding the drug's efficacy.

On the other hand, there is some risk that the grade and stage of the tumour left in place could be different from those of the removed lesions. This risk has been calculated by an EORTC referee pathologist on the material of previous EORTC studies and it is negligible [3].

Finally, the number of tumours has been arbitrarily limited to 10 because it is evident that patients with diffuse papillomatosis are at very bad risk and are not good candidates for testing new drugs.

What is the risk of leaving a marker?

Many people claim that leaving a marker is not ethically acceptable because the risk exists of progression to muscle invasion of the indicator lesion during the 8–10 weeks of treatment, before the definitive eradication, if the treatment is not efficient.

In response to these people, it may be said that in so-called complete TURs, tumours or parts of them are often forgotten [4,5] in such a way that a second look cystoscopy with biopsies has been advocated by some authors.

The EORTC GU Group and the Medical Research Council have conducted four previous studies using marker tumours [2,6,7,8]; it has been demonstrated that the risk of developing a muscle-invasive tumour is less than 1%; moreover, it is quite possible that these T2 tumours were already present at the time of initial diagnosis but that they were understaged.

The risk of superficial tumour recurrence, new tumour occurrence and progression to muscle invasion has been clarified by the multivariate analysis of patients in two previous large Phase III EORTC trials [9]. Following this analysis, patients could be classified into three risk groups (1 = good; 2 = intermediate and 3 = bad).

The theoretical risk of progression at 10 weeks was calculated. It could be shown that if the bad prognostic group is rejected, the risk of progression is extremely weak [2,10].

The true difficulty with these Phase II studies is to convince the patient to take part and to obtain his informed consent. The main objection — which is justified — is that a second TUR will be necessary; the most convincing argument is to explain that in case of recurrence, it will be known whether or not the drug may be helpful to the patient.

Are these Phase II studies a prerequisite for the evaluation of new agents or new regimens?

It has indeed been recommended by the Fourth International Bladder Cancer Consensus Conference [11].

It is clear that all the drugs exhibiting some efficacy as adjuvant treatment after TUR or in the eradication of CIS are also active on a marker in 40–70% of cases.

It is also logical to consider that these Phase II studies can give more knowledge about appropriate doses of drugs without exposing hundreds of patients in Phase III studies, for several years, to expensive drugs that may not be beneficial for superficial bladder cancer after all.

There is experimental and clinical evidence [6,12,13] that prophylaxis is partly correlated with the destruction of floating cells or residual tumour.

For these reasons, it looks logical to correlate the possible prophylactic effect of a drug with its ablative capability and thus to advocate preliminary Phase II studies for new drugs.

But we must keep in mind that some drugs (especially the immunomodulating agents) may be limited in their ablative efficacy because of the tumour volume and their inability to destroy a marker does not necessarily mean that they would be inactive on smaller numbers of cells.

In the same way, urothelial 'stabilizers' such as some vitamins may prove to be efficacious in long-term prophylaxis by way of a regulatory effect on 'urothelial instability', although they would be unable to destroy a marker.

These remarks underline the imperfection of the marker model, which, nonetheless, remains the best and necessary step to investigate new agents for the treatment or prevention of recurrence of superficial bladder cancer.

Review of some Phase II studies with a marker lesion

EORTC 30864 and 30869 protocols

These were combined Phase II–Phase III studies, one with mitomycin (MMC, protocol 30864; Coord: A. Bono), the other with epirubicin (EPI, protocol 30869; Coord; R. Hall) designed for multiple Ta, T1 transitional cell carcinoma (TCC) of the bladder [6].

Phase II Chemoresection

		R		
TUR leaving	7–15 d.	E	8 × 30 mg MMC	10 week
marker lesion		G	weekly	
	Pathol	I	8 × 50 mg EPI	Control Cysto
		S		(+ TUR)
		T		

Phase III Prophylaxis

		R	>>> No further Treat.	Endpoint:
	7–15 d.	A	(except Recur:	
	Pathol.	N	MMC/EPI wkly × 4)	First Recur.
		D		after 2 years
		O	MMC/EPI q 2 months	
		M	>>> for 2 years (if Req.	
			MMC/EPI wkly × 4)	

It was hoped that the basic question of a relationship between a therapeutic effect and a prophylactic effect could be assessed. Unfortunately, the recruitment was very poor and these studies had to be closed after 132 patients were entered (96 in 30864 and 36 in 30869) allowing an analysis of the Phase II part of the study only. (Table 9.1).

No difference could be observed between the two drugs which roughly achieved a 50% complete-response rate while 30% or the patients had no change (persistence of the marker; partial response was not considered due to difficulties in measuring tumour size) and 20% had new occurrences of tumour (there was one case of progression in stage to T2).

Table 9.1 30864–30869 protocols: Response of the marker lesion in the 10th week cystoscopy.

	30864 (MMC) (96 pts)	30869 (EPI) (36 pts)
Complete remission	48 (50%)	20 (56%)
No change	29 (30%)	9 (25%)
Progression	19 (20%)	7 (19%)

Multicentric Phase II study with epirubicin [14]

Designed for Ta/T1 primary or recurrent superficial bladder cancer, a TUR was performed, leaving a marker; epirubicin 50 mg was given intravesically, weekly for 8 weeks, and an evaluation was performed at week 12.

45 eligible patients were included in this trial. Fifteen had primary tumours and 30 had recurrent disease.

The breakdown of CR vs NC+PD in function of primary versus recurrent tumours and in consideration of pre-treatment or not is shown in Table 9.2. A 47% CR rate was noticed and the results were better in primary (67%) versus recurrent (37%) and in unpre-treated (55%) versus pre-treated (31%).

EORTC protocol 30897 [2]

Designed for intermediate risk bladder Ta, T1 multiple tumours, the study, co-ordinated by Van der Meijden [2], consisted in TUR leaving a marker followed by intravesical instillation of MMC, 30 mg weekly, for 4 weeks followed by RIVM BCG (bacillus Calmette Guerin), 6 weekly instillations, and evaluation after 12 weeks.

Thirty-two patients were eligible; 16 had a complete response documented by negative biopsies and 3 had a disappearance of the marker but refused the biopsy; 1 patient was not evaluable due to toxicity; 11 patients had no change and 1 patient progressed in stage to T2.

It must be mentioned that among these 12 NC or PD patients, 6 had very bad prognostic tumours (more than 25, already pre-treated several times) and would not be, today, eligible for the master Phase II protocol prepared by the EORTC (Table 9.3).

Table 9.2 Breakdown of CR versus NC + PD in relation to primary vs recurrent and pre-treated vs unpre-treated.

	Total	Primary	Recur.	Pre-treated*	Not pre-treated
CR	21	10	11	5	16
NC+PD	24	5	19	11	13

*pre-treated means that patients had received a previous intravesical treatment with an agent different from epirubicin.

Table 9.3 EORTC protocol 30897. Phase II sequential MMC and BCG.

Complete response	919 (59.4%)	16 pathologically (50%)
		3 cystoscopically (9%)
Not evaluable	1 (3.1%)	because of toxicity
No change	11 (34.4%)	(many bad prognostic)
Progression	1 (3.1%)	to T2 (?)
Total	32 (100%)	

MRC trial with two different strains of BCG [8]

The Medical Research Council's (MRC) subgroup on Superficial Bladder Cancer performed a trial to compare two different BCG strains in eradicating marker bladder tumours.

Ninety-nine patients with multiple recurrent Ta/T1 superficial bladder cancer were allocated at random to 6 weekly instillations of Evans BCG or Pasteur BCG after TUR of all tumours except one.

The results at 3 months (94 evaluable patients) are illustrated in Table 9.4.

Table 9.4 Response of the marker at 3 months (BCG Evans vs Pasteur).

	Pasteur	Evans	Total
No marker; no other tumour	18 (42%)	12 (24%)	30 (32%)
No marker; other tumour(s)	9 (21%)	12 (24%)	21 (22%)
Marker present; no other tumour(s)	0 (0%)	0 (0%)	0 (0%)
Marker present; other tumours	16 (37%)	27 (53%)	43 (46%)
Total	43	51	94

No significant difference was observed between the two strains regarding efficacy and toxicity.

The rate of complete response (no marker, no new occurrence) is rather low in this study as compared to other ones; this might be due to the bad prognosis of the treated tumours which could explain the unusual high incidence of new occurrences after 3 months.

At the moment, two new Phase II trials with a marker have been accepted by the EORTC GU Group. One of them has recently started: this study intends to analyse the value of BCG (1/4 dose) on a marker lesion. This Phase II study has been considered by the EORTC GU Group as a necessary step before embarking on a Phase III trial aiming to verify Pagano's trial indicating that BCG 1/2 dose is as efficient but less toxic than BCG full dose.

The other Phase II trial will study the efficacy of oral bropirimine on a marker lesion and will hopefully be activated at the beginning of 1996.

Conclusion

An objective assessment of the response of superficial transitional-cell carcinoma of the bladder to an intravesical treatment requires and indicator lesion.

In CIS, negative multiple biopsies, negative urinary cytology and negative monoclonal antibody tests, that will be available soon, may be regarded as a complete response although there is no measurable lesion. This aspect of the problem is not covered in this chapter.

For exophytic Ta, T1 lesions, the only way to objectively measure the response of an intravesical (and why not oral or systemic?) agent is to perform a Phase II study leaving a marker lesion.

This kind of trial is difficult to realize for practical and ethical reasons, even though the risk of progression of the marker during the phase of treatment is extremely weak, if bad prognostic tumours are not included.

Although the model is not perfect, a Phase II study with a marker is mandatory to evaluate new agents or regimens before testing them in Phase III prophylactic trials.

As the most common agents (mitomycin, epirubicin, BCG) achieve complete-response rates of 45–65%, an agent which would not be able to make the indicator lesion disappear in at least 40% of the cases should be considered with caution for further investigation (with the possible exception of immunomodulating agents and 'stabilizers').

References

1   Bouffioux C, van der Meijden A, Kurth KH *et al.* Objective response of superficial bladder tumors to intravesical treatment (including review of response marker lesions). In Schröder F (ed) EORTC GU Group Monograph 11. *Recent Progress in Bladder and Kidney Cancer.* Wiley–Liss; New York. 1992; 29–42.

2   van der Meijden A, Kurth KH, Brausi M *et al.* Standard Phase II Protocol for patients with intermediate risk Ta/T1 papillary carcinoma of the urinary bladder (EORTC GU Group, 1994).

3   Ten Kate F, Hall R. Personal communications 1990.

4   Oosterlinck W, Kurth KH, Schröder F *et al.* A Prospective EORTC GU Group randomized trial comparing transurethral resection followed by a single instillation of epirubicin or water in single stage Ta, T1 papillary carcinoma of the bladder. *J Urol* 1993; **149**: 749–52.

5   Bouffioux C. Intravesical adjuvant treatment in superficial bladder cancer: a review of the question after 15 years of experience with the EORTC GU group. *Scand J Urol Nephrol* (Suppl.) S138, 1991; 167–77.

6   Bono A, Hall R, Sylvester R *et al.* Topical chemotherapy in superficial bladder cancer: a chemotherapy phase II study using a marker tumour. Abstract, SIU, 22nd Congress, Sevilla, 1991.

7   Hall R. Transurethral resection for transitional cell carcinoma. *Prob Urol* 1992; **6**(3): 460–70.

8   Fellows G, Parmar M, Grigor R *et al.* Marker tumour response to Evans and Pasteur BCG in multiple recurrent pTa, pT1 bladder tumours: report from the Medical Council Subgroup on superficial bladder cancer (Urological Working Party). *Br J Urol* 1994; **73**: 639–44.

9   Kurth KH, Denis L, ten Kate F *et al.* Prognostic factors in superficial bladder tumors. *Prob Urol* 1992; **6**(3): 471–83.

10   van der Meijden A, Kurth KH, Cheuvart B *et al.* Intravesical chemotherapy for superficial bladder cancer. The EORTC GU Group experience. In: Murphy, Khoury *et al.* (eds) *Recent Advances in Urological Cancers, Diagnosis and Treatment.* 1990; 138–43.

11   Lamm D, van der Meijden A, Akaza H *et al.* Intravesical chemo- and immunotherapy: how do we assess their effectiveness and what are their limitations and uses? Proceedings of the IVth International Bladder Cancer Consensus Conference, Antwerp, 1993.

12   Soloway M, Masters S. Urothelial susceptibility to tumor cell implantation. Influence of cauterisation. *Cancer* 1980; **46**: 1158–63.

13   Bouffioux C, Kirth KH, Bono A *et al.* Intravescial adjuvant chemotherapy: results of 2 EORTC randomized trials with MMC and doxorubicin comparing early vs delayed instillation and short-term vs long-term treatment. *J Urol* 1995; **153**(3/2): 934–41.

14   Calais da Silva F, Denis L, Bono C, Bollack C, Bouffioux C. Intravesical chemo-resection with 4′-epi-doxorubicin in patients with superficial bladder tumors. *Eur Urol* 1988; **14**: 207–9.

CHAPTER 10

Doxorubicin and epirubicin

T.M. de Reijke and K. Kurth

Introduction

Since the early 1970s adjuvant (Ta, T1) and therapeutic (Tis) intravesical chemotherapy has become a common practice for the treatment of superficial bladder cancer [1,2]. Differences in treatment results when transurethral resection (TUR) alone is compared with adjuvant treatment are defined as net benefit. This net benefit averages from 17–31%, with ranges from 0–42% for the different drugs depending on the treatment schedule applied and prognostic factors [3,4]. There is up to now no evidence for the superiority of one cytostatic agent compared to others.

In the following the place of the anthracyclines, doxorubicin and epirubicin in patients with superficial bladder cancer is discussed.

Pharmacology and experimental studies

Doxorubicin hydrochloride (Adriamycin®) was isolated in 1963 by aerobic fermentation of *Streptomyces peucetius*, a variant of *S. caesius*, as an anti-neoplastic antibiotic agent [5]. Chemically it is an anthracycline, exerting its cytostatic activity through binding specifically with DNA by intercalation between adjacent base pairs of the double helix, interrupting the DNA synthesis and the protein synthesis [6].

Epirubicin differs from doxorubicin by the epimerization of the hydroxyl group at the 4′ position of the amino acid [7]. It was developed with a view to enhancing the therapeutic activity and decreasing the incidence of adverse events observed using doxorubicin when given parenterally. Both compounds have been used as well locally, for superficial bladder cancer, as parenterally for muscle invasive bladder cancer. If applied intravesically, systemic toxicity is not to be expected for either of the anthracyclines, due to their high molecular weight of 579.9 kD. It has also been shown, both experimentally and clinically, that the resorption of these agents through the bladder wall is low and only at the detection level, even in case of bladder damage [8–11]. This explains the low incidence of haematologic side-effects like thrombocytopenia and/or leucopenia.

However, local toxicity has been reported for both drugs. In a mouse study, bladder damage after doxorubicin instillation was significantly less pronounced compared with Mitomycin C [12]. Chemical cystitis, frequency of voiding or haematuria have been reported in 4–26% of patients receiving doxorubicin [13,14] and in 3–26% of patients receiving epirubicin [10,15], depending on the doses used and the number of instillations. Cessation of further instillations due to toxicity has been reported in 0.7–20% of patients [10,16,17]. In comparative studies the local toxicity did not significantly differ for the two agents [18].

Doxorubicin, being the first isolated anthracycline, has been investigated experimentally most extensively. Usansky *et al.* [19] found a rapid uptake of doxorubicin in a human bladder cancer-cell line (UM-UC-6) and an even faster uptake in a multidrug-resistant cell line (UM-UC-6DOX). The anthracycline molecule uptake was mainly restricted to the urothelium and papillary formations, the basement membrane acted like a barrier for doxorubicin [9].

Several experimental reports describe methods to enhance the anti-tumour activity of doxorubicin, these include combination with (2″R)-4′-O-tetrahydropyranyl (THP), [20], Tween 80 [21] or lonidamine [22], influence of osmolality [23], concentration–time curve and pH [24]. Ueda *et al.* [25] added a mucous adhesive agent to doxorubicin (hydroxypropylcellulose-doxorubicin [HPC-Dox]). Three days after instillation of HPC-Dox higher levels could be detected in the bladder mucosa as well as in the tumour tissue compared with the aequous solution of doxorubicin. Synergistic effects of a combination of cytostatic agents was investigated by Seraphim *et al.* [26], using a well-differentiated human bladder tumour-cell line (RT-4). The combination of doxorubicin with thiotepa or Mitomycin C yielded the most synergistic effect.

Although all of the above-mentioned combinations showed some enhanced activity, none of them has been introduced into routine clinical practice.

The question of possible tumour induction by anthracycline application intravesically has been investigated by Deutz *et al.* [27], who could not demonstrate epithelial proliferations in dogs in contrast to earlier observations made in mice [28].

Results from Phase II and Phase III studies

Marker lesions
In order to investigate the efficacy of a new drug for the treatment of superficial bladder cancer the responsiveness of a marker lesion can be used [29]. Only one small study with doxorubicin and three studies with epirubicin have been published (Table 10.1). Overall complete-response rates ranging from 12–67% were achieved, with various instillation schemes in patients with different tumour characteristics. A single instillation of HPC-Dox, 20mg/20ml, resulted in a complete response of 37.5% (6/16) [33]. Ueda *et al.* [34] also compared the effect of HPC-Dox as a single treatment or combined with local hyperthermia. The combination resulted in a higher complete response of the marker lesion, 35% (7/20) and 54.5% (6/11), respectively.

Carcinoma in situ *(CIS)*
Overall complete-response rates with anthracyclines in the treatment of CIS ranged from 29 to 70% (Table 10.2). However, only scarce data are available about the long-term follow-up of these patients, thus the percentage of patients relapsing and/or developing muscle-invasive disease after long-term follow-up (>36 months) is

Table 10.1 Anthracyclines and marker lesions.

Study	Treatment	Patients (*N*)	T-stage	Response
Khanna *et al.* [30]	ADM 50 mg/50 ml weekly × 6 2 weeks after TUR	13	Ta/T1/Tis	CR: 38%
Matsumura *et al.* [15]	EPI 50–80 mg/ 30 ml 3 consec. days × 2 (4 days rest)	35 (33 eval.)	Ta/T1 G1–3	CR: 12%
da Silva *et al.* [31]	EPI 48 hr after TUR 50 mg/50 ml weekly × 8	46 (1 lost)	Ta/T1 G1–3 prim/ recur.	CR total: 47% CR prim: 67% CR recur: 37% CR pretr: 31% CR non-pretr: 55%
Popert *et al.* [32]	EPI 50–100 mg/ 50 ml × 1 10–21d. after TUR	81	Ta/T1 G1–3 prim/ recur.	Cr total: 46% CR prim: 56% CR recur: 39%

Abbreviations: ADM, Adriamycin; TUR, transurethral resection; CR, complete response; EPI, epirubicin; consec, consecutive; eval, evaluable; prim, primary; recur, recurrent; pretr, pretreated; non-pretr, non-pretreated.

Table 10.2 Anthracyclines and carcinoma *in situ*.

Study	Treatment	Patients (*N*)	Response
Jakse *et al.* [35]	ADM 40 mg/ 20 ml biweekly	9	CR total : 66%
	ADM 80 mg/40 ml monthly, thereafter 1 or 2 × monthly, 1 year therapy	6	FU (mean): 12, 3 mos
Edsmyr *et al.* [36]	ADM 300 μgr/ml/hr, monthly, 13 courses average	19 (prim) 23 (sec)	CR prim : 29% CR sec : 48% FU : > 1 year
Kurth *et al.* [10]	EPI 30, 50, 80 mg/50 ml weekly × 8	34 (22 evaluable)	CR 30 mg : 43% CR 50 mg : 60% CR 80 mg : 70% FU (mean) : 35.3 mos

Abbreviations: ADM, Adriamycin; CR, complete response; FU, follow-up; mos, months; prim, primary; sec, secondary; EPI, epirubicin.

unknown. At this moment an European Organization for Research and Treatment of Cancer-Genitourinary (EORTC-GU) Group randomized study (protocol 30906) is in progress comparing bacillus Calmette–Guérin (BCG) and epirubicin in patients with CIS of the bladder. Results of this study have to be awaited.

Phase III studies

The net benefit of adjuvant treatment of superficial bladder cancer with anthracyclines ranged between 5 and 39% compared to transurethral resection (TUR) alone [3]. Comparing the prophylactic activity of doxorubicin and epirubicin, no difference was found [37]. Anthracycline instillations did not result in lower recurrences compared with any of the cytostatic drugs tested (Table 10.3). Based on prognostic factors instillation regimens can be adapted [4] and Oosterlinck *et al.* [42] found that the recurrence rate was decreased by nearly 50% after a single instillation of 80 mg epirubicin within 24 hours of TUR, in patients with a single, primary or recurrent Ta/T1 tumour, compared with water instillation.

Long-term therapy (12 months) was found to be advantageous as far as recurrence rate is concerned for those patients who received delayed instillations (7–15 days after TUR) [43], but short-term (6 months) therapy was equivalent when given early after TUR (< 7 days). Melekos *et al.* [44] observed that maintenance therapy with epirubicin was especially beneficial for patients with multiple recurrent tumours. Bono *et al.* [45] reported a series of 128 consecutive patients with primary T1G3 tumours who received doxorubicin (50 mg/50 ml; weekly × 4 and monthly × 11). They found a recurrence rate of 56.3% and a progression in 23.4%. They concluded that adjuvant therapy in T1G3 tumours is appropriate, but on first recurrence cystectomy should be considered.

Since the introduction of BCG treatment in 1976 by Morales *et al.* [46] the place of cytostatics has been questioned by some authors. Randomized studies comparing BCG with doxorubicin or epirubicin have been reported (Table 10.4) [47–50]. From the presently available data it can be concluded that, for patients with low to intermediate risk for recurrence, cytostatic treatment is as good as BCG. In high-risk groups BCG is superior, although additional comparative studies are still underway and definitive data have to be awaited.

Combination therapy of two cytostatic agents (doxorubicin plus Mitomycin C) has been applied for Ta/T1 tumours, this resulted in more pronounced side-effects and only marginally improved results [51]. In CIS of the bladder complete response after sequential cytostatic therapy was comparable to BCG therapy alone [52].

Combination therapy using a cytostatic agent and an immunomodulating agent has been reported by various authors. Chemoimmunotherapy using epirubicin and BCG resulted in a high percentage of local toxicity and in 35.7% (5/14 patients) side-effects necessitated discontinuation of further therapy [53]. With the immunomodulator, interferon alpha (IFNα), the results achieved were comparable to those with cytostatic agents, however, the high percentage of local toxicity observed with BCG was not evident [54]. The anti-tumoural action of IFNα given intravesically is explained by the induction of infiltration of natural killer cells and T lymphocytes into the bladder wall and the increased concentration of the urinary cytokines interleukin 2 and 4 [55]. The theoretical advantage of combining cytostatic and immunomodulating therapy is the possible promotion of necrosis and inflammatory action of the cytostatic agent, resulting in lymphocytic infiltration. Sequential therapy with IFNα could activate the local immune response through the T lymphocytes, eventually resulting in enhanced tumour destruction. The hypothesis of an enhanced response is not yet proven beyond any doubt but it is supported by the observation of some authors.

Ferrari *et al.* [56] reported that the combined treatment of epirubicin and IFN in patients with superficial bladder cancer tended to reduce the percentage of relapses and to extend the disease-free interval. Raitanen and Lukkarinen [57] randomized 81

Table 10.3 Anthracyclines in randomized Phase III studies.

Study	Treatment	Patients (N)	T-stage	Recurrences
Zincke *et al.* [38]	Water : 60 ml	28	Ta: 26; T1: 2	71%
	TTP: 60 mg/60 ml	30	Ta: 28; T1: 2	30%
	DX : 50 mg/60 ml	31	Ta: 30; T1: 1	32%
	one instillation immediately		G1–3, concom. Tis prim/rec	TTP/DX vs Water p <.01
				Endpoint: 4 mos
Kurth *et al.* [39]	TUR only	69	Ta: 41; T1: 28	68%
	DX : 50 mg/50 ml	151	Ta: 80; T1: 71	47%
	Epodyl : 1.13 gm/100 ml	159	Ta: 84; T1: 75	49%
	weekly × 4		G1–3, concom. Tis prim/recur	Epodyl/DX vs TUR p <.001
	monthly × 11			FU (mean) : 29 mos
Bouffioux *et al.* [40]	TTP : 30 mg/50 ml	97	Ta: 58; T1: 51	61%
	DX : 50 mg/50 ml	88	Ta: 55; T1: 57	65%
	CP : 50 mg/50 ml	81	Ta: 50; T1: 42	64%
	weekly × 4		G1–3	p: n.s.
	monthly × 11		recur	FU (mean) : 20 mos
da Silva *et al.* [41]	EPI : 50 mg/50 ml	32	Ta: 6; T1: 26	62.5%
	MMC : 30 mg/30 ml	28	Ta: 3; T1: 25	64.2%
	weekly × 4		G1–3	p: n.s.
	monthly × 11		prim/recur	FU (mean) : 17 mos

Abbreviations: TTP, thiotepa; DX, doxorubicin; concom, concomitant; prim, primary; recur, recurrent; mos, months; TUR, transurethral resection; FU, follow-up; CP, cisplatin; EPI, epirubicin; MMC, Mitomycin-C.

Table 10.4 Randomized studies comparing anthracyclines with BCG.

Study	Treatment	Patients (*N*)	T-stage	Response
Martinez Piñeiro *et al.* [47]	TTP: 50 mg/50 ml	56	Ta: 23; T1: 33	Rec: 35.7%; PD: 3.6%
	DX : 50 mg/50 ml	53	Ta: 21; T1: 32	Rec: 43.3%; PD: 7.5%
	BCG: 150 mg/50 ml	67	Ta: 18; T1: 49	Rec: 13.4%; PD: 1.5%
	weekly × 4		G1–3, concom. Tis	TTP vs DX: n.s.
	monthly × 11		prim/recur	TTP vs BCG: p = 0.003
				DX vs BCG: p = 0.002
				FU (mean): 3 yr
Lamm *et al.* [48]	BCG: 120 mg/50 ml+sc	127	Ta–1: 63; Tis: 64	CR Tis : 70%
	weekly × 6, maint.			Rec Ta–1: 65.1%
	DX: 50 mg/50 ml	135	Ta–1: 68; Tis: 67	CR Tis : 34%
	weekly × 4			Rec Ta–1: 80.9%
	monthly × 11			Tis: DX vs BCG: p = 0.001
				Ta–1: DX vs BCG: p = 0.015
				FU (median) : 65 mos
Melekos *et al.* [49]	TUR alone	32	Ta: 21; T1: 11	Rec: 59.4%, PD: 12.5%
	EPI: 50 mg/50 ml	67	Ta: 42; T1: 25	Rec: 40.3%, PD: 4.5%
	BCG: 150 mg/50 ml	62	Ta: 41; T1: 21	Rec: 32.2%, PD: 3.2%
	weekly × 6, 1		G1–3, concom. Tis	EPI vs BCG: n.s.
	instil 3-monthly for 2 yr,		prim/recur	FU (mean): 25.6 mos
	6-monthly thereafter			
Bassi and Pagano [50]	EPI : 80 mg/50 ml	95	Ta/T1	DFS: 40.8%, PD: 1%
	BCG: 75 mg/50ml	89	G1–3	DFS: 38.4%, PD: 13%
			prim/recur	EPI vs BCG: n.s.
				FU (mean): 36 mos

Abbreviations: TTP, thiotepa; DX, doxorubicin; BCG, bacillus Calmette–Guérin; concom, concomitant; prim, primary; recur, recurrent; rec, recurrence; PD, progressive disease; FU, follow-up; sc, subcutaneous; maint, maintenance; CR, complete response; TUR, transurethral resection; EPI, epirubicin; concom, concomitant; DFS, disease-free survival.

patients between TUR only, epirubicin 50 mg/50 ml and epirubicin 50 mg/50 ml immediately followed by IFN-α-2b 10 MU/50 ml. Patients received one instillation a week during the first month, followed by one instillation a month over the next 11 months. With a mean follow-up of 20 months recurrences were lower in the chemo-immunoprophylaxis group (EPI + IFN: 50%, EPI: 75%; Control: 89%) and progression was seen in 7%, 9% and 11% of patients, respectively.

Conclusion

From Phase II studies anti-tumour activity has clinically been proven for both anthracyclines. Compared with control patients they significantly reduce the recurrence rate per year and prolong the disease-free interval. Because in comparative studies no cytostatic was found to be superior, other factors become important for decision making regarding which agent should be used (e.g. cost, toxicity, pharmaceutical properties). Systemic toxicity (dizziness, nausea, fever, hypotension) is observed in only a small percentage of patients (3–5.8%) after intravesical instillation of either doxorubicin or epirubicin, local toxicity is comparable with that of other cytostatic agents (9–34%) depending on dosage, number and interval of instillations given. Based on prognostic factors an individualized instillation scheme can be instituted. Whenever possible a short interval between TUR and the first instillation is preferable. In patients with a single tumour a single instillation early after TUR should be considered. In the low- and intermediate-risk group for recurrence comparable results have been reported of the anthracyclines (long-term treatment) and BCG. For the high-risk group BCG is superior, but randomized studies should be awaited for CIS of the bladder. Chemo-immunoprophylaxis seems theoretically a rational approach and the first clinical reports are encouraging.

However, recent evaluation of the EORTC-GU group data [58] showed that, in randomized trials, intravesically applied cytostatics did not increase the duration of survival compared to TUR alone.

References

1   Torti FM, Lum BL. Superficial bladder cancer: risk of recurrence and potential role for interferon therapy. *Cancer* 1987; **59**: 613–16.
2   Heney NM, Nocks BN, Daly JJ *et al.* Ta and T1 bladder cancer: location, recurrence and progression. *Br J Urol* 1982; **54**: 152–7.
3   Lamm DL. Long term results of intravesical therapy for superficial bladder cancer. *Urol Clin N Am* 1992; **19**: 573–80.
4   Kurth KH. Intravesical chemotherapy for superficial bladder tumors category Ta/T1: who should be treated and how? *Semin in Urol* 1996; **14**: 30–5.
5   Carter SK. Adriamycin — A review. *J Nat Cancer Inst* 1975; **55**: 1265–7.
6   Di Marco A, Zunino F, Silvestrini R *et al.* Interaction of some daunomycin derivatives with deoxyribonucleic acid and their biological activity. *Biochem Pharmacol* 1971; **20**: 1323–8.
7   Cersosimo RJ, Hong WK. Epirubicin: a review of the pharmacology, clinical activity, and adverse events of an Adriamycin analogue. *J Clin Oncol* 1986; **4**: 425–39.
8   Engelmann U, Bürger RA, Rumpelt JH, Jacobi GH. Adriamycin permeability of the rat bladder under different conditions. *J Urol* 1983; **129**: 862–4.
9   Jacobi GH, Kirth KH. Studies on the intravesical action of topically administered G3H-doxorubicin hydrochloride in men: plasma uptake and tumor penetration. *J Urol* 1980; **124**: 34–7.

10 Kurth KH, van der Vijgh WJF, ten Kate F *et al.* Phase 1/2 study of intravesical epirubicin in patients with carcinoma *in situ* of the bladder. *J Urol* 1991; **146**: 1508–13.

11 Mross K, Maessen P, van der Vijgh WJF *et al.* Absorption of epi-doxorubicin after intravesical administration in patients with *in situ* transitional cell carcinoma of the bladder. *Eur J Cancer Clin Oncol* 1987; **23**: 505–8.

12 Post JG, te Poele JA, Oussoren Y, Stewart FA. Bladder damage in mice after single and repeated intravesical instillations of Mitomycin C or doxorubicin. *J Urol* 1993; **150**: 1965–9.

13 Kurth KH, Schröder FH, Tunn U *et al.* Adjuvant chemotherapy of superficial transitional cell bladder carcinoma: preliminary results of a European Organization for Research and Treatment of Cancer randomized trial comparing doxorubicin hydrochloride, ethoglucid and transurethral resection alone. *J Urol* 1984; **132**: 258–62.

14 Schulman CC, Denis LJ, Oosterlinck W *et al.* Early adjuvant Adriamycin in superficial bladder carcinoma. *World J Urol* 1983; **1**: 86–8.

15 Matsumura Y, Tsushima T, Ozaki Y *et al.* Intravesical chemotherapy with 4′-epi-Adriamycin in patients with superficial bladder tumors. *Cancer Chemother Pharmacol* 1986; **16**: 176–7.

16 Burk K, Schultze-Seeman W, Rodeck G, Jonas D. Der Einfluss von Adriamycin auf das Progressionsverhalten von oberflächlichen Harnblasenkarzinomen (pp. 55–60.) In: *Proceedings Tenth International Symposium Chemotherapeutics of Bladder Cancer.* Vienna: Medical Academy Press, 1987.

17 Lundbeck F, Mogensen P, Jeppesen N. Intravesical therapy of noninvasive bladder tumors (stage Ta) with doxorubicin and urokinase. *J Urol* 1983; **130**: 1087–9.

18 Shuin T, Kubota Y, Noguchi S *et al.* A Phase II study of prophylactic intravesical chemotherapy with 4′-epirubicin in recurrent superficial bladder cancer: comparison of 4′-epirubicin and Adriamycin. *Cancer Chemother Pharmacol* 1994; **35**: 52–6.

19 Usansky JI, Liebert M, Wedemeyer G, Grossman HB, Wagner JG. The uptake and efflux of doxorubicin by a sensitive human bladder cancer cell line and its doxorubicin-resistant subline. *Selective Cancer Ther* 1991; **7**: 139–50.

20 Akaza H, Niijima T, Hisamatsu T, Fujigaki M. Comparative investigation on use of (2″R)-4′-O-tetrahydropyranyl-Adriamycin and Adriamycin as intravesical chemotherapy for superficial bladder tumors. *Urology* 1988; **32**: 141–5.

21 Parris CN, Masters JRW, Walker MC *et al.* Intravesical chemotherapy: combination with Tween 80 increases cytotoxicity *in vitro. Urological Res* 1987; **15**: 17–20.

22 Popert RJ, Masters JR, Coptcoat M, Zupi G. Relative cytotoxicities of Adriamycin and epirubicin in combination with lonidamine against human bladder cancer cell lines. *Urological Res* 1995; **22**: 367–72.

23 Groos E, Masters JRW. Intravesical chemotherapy: studies on the relationship between osmolality and cytotoxicity. *J Urol* 1986; **136**: 399–402.

24 Eksborg S, Nilsson S-O, Edsmyr F. Intravesical instillation of Adriamycin. A model for standardization of the chemotherapy. *Eur Urol* 1980; **6**: 213–15.

25 Ueda K, Sakagami H, Ohtaguro K, Masui Y. Studies on the retention of the mucous-membrane-adhesive anticancer agent hydroxypropylcellulose-doxorubicin. *Eur Urol* 1992; **21**: 250–2.

26 Seraphim LA, Perrapato SD, Slocum HK, Rustum YM, Huben RP. *In vitro* study of the interaction of doxorubicin, thiotepa, and Mitomycin-C, agents used for intravesical chemotherapy of superficial bladder cancer. *J Urol* 1991; **145**: 613–17.

27 Duetz F-J, Moll F, Friedrichs R *et al.* Long-term experimental study of intravesical chemotherapy: effect on the normal urothelium in dogs. In: Jacobi GH, Rübben H, Harzmann R (eds) *Invest Urol* 2. Berlin: Springer Verlag, 1985: 47–55.

28 Rübben H. Thesis: Die intravesikale Chemotherapie des Blasenkarzinoms. Experiment und Klinik. Habilitationsschrift vor der Medizinischen Fakultät der RWTH Aachen, 1983.

29 Lamm DL, vd Meijden APM, Akaza H *et al.* Intravesical chemotherapy and immunotherapy: how do we assess their effectiveness and what are their limitations and uses? *Int J Urol* 1995; **2**: 23–35.

30 Khanna OP, Son DL, Mazer H *et al.* Superficial bladder cancer treated by intravesical bacillus Calmette–Guérin or Adriamycin: multicenter study interim report. *Urology* 1987; **30**: 520–8.

31 Calais da Silva F, Denis L, Bono A *et al.* Intravesical chemoresection with 4′-epi-doxorubicin in patients with superficial bladder tumors. *Eur Urol* 1988; **14**: 207–9.

32 Popert RJM, Goodall J, Coptcoat MJ *et al.* Superficial bladder cancer: the response of a marker tumour to a single intravesical instillation of epirubicin. *Br J Urol* 1994; **74**: 195–9.

33 Ueda K, Sakagami H, Masui Y, Okamura T, Ohtaguro K. One-shot intravesical instillation of the mucous adhesive anticancer agent hydoxypropylcellulose-doxorubicin for the treatment of superficial bladder carcinoma is sufficient to determine antitumor effects. *Eur Urol* 1993; **24**: 62–5.

34 Ueda K, Sakagami H, Masui Y, Okamura T. Single instillation of hydroxypropyl cellulose-doxorubicin as treatment for superficial bladder carcinoma. *Cancer Chemother Pharmacol* 1994; **35**: 81–3.

35 Jakse G, Hofstädter F, Marberger H. Intracavitary doxorubicin hydrochloride therapy for carcinoma *in situ* of the bladder. *J Urol* 1981; **125**: 185–90.

36 Edsmyr F, Andersson L, Esposti P-L. Intravesical chemotherapy of carcinoma *in situ. Urology* 1984; **23**(Suppl): S37–9.

37 Shinohara N, Nonomura K, Tanaka M *et al.* Prophylactic chemotherapy with anthracyclines (Adriamycin, epirubicin, and pirarubicin) for primary superficial bladder cancer. *Cancer Chemother Pharmacol* 1994; **35**: 41–5.

38 Zincke H, Utz DC, Taylor WF, Myers RP, Leary FJ. Influence of thiotepa and doxorubicin instillation at time of transurethral surgical treatment of bladder cancer on tumor recurrence: a prospective, randomized, double-blind, controlled trial. *J Urol* 1983; **129**: 505–9.

39 Kurth KH, Schröder FH, DeBruyne F *et al.* Long-term follow-up in superficial transitional cell carcinoma of the bladder: prognostic factors for time to first recurrence, recurrence rate and survival. *Prog Clin Biol Res* 1989; **303**: 481–90.

40 Bouffioux C, Denis L, Oosterlinck W *et al.* Adjuvant chemotherapy of recurrent superficial transitional cell carcinoma: results of a European Organization for Research and Treatment of Cancer randomized trial comparing intravesical instillation of thiotepa, doxorubicin and cisplatin. *J Urol* 1992; **148**: 297–301.

41 da Silva FC, Ferrito F, Brandao T, Santos A. 4′-epidoxorubicin versus Mitomycin C chemoprophylaxis of superficial bladder cancer. *Eur Urol* 1992; **21**: 42–4.

42 Oosterlinck W, Kurth KH, Schröder F *et al.* A prospective European Organization for Research and Treatment of Cancer Genitourinary Group randomized trial comparing transurethral resection followed by a single intravesical instillation of epirubicin or water in single stage Ta, T1 papillary carcinoma of the bladder. *J Urol* 1993; **149**: 749–52.

43 Bouffioux C, Kurth KH, Bono A *et al.* Intravesical adjuvant chemotherapy for superficial transitional cell bladder carcinoma: results of 2 European Organization for Research and Treatment of Cancer randomized trials with Mitomycin C and doxorubicin comparing early versus delayed instillations and short-term versus long-term treatment. *J Urol* 1995; **153**: 934–41.

44 Melekos MD, Dauaher H, Fokaefs E, Barbalias G. Intravesical instillations of 4-epi-doxorubicin (epirubicin) in the prophylactic treatment of superficial bladder cancer: results of a controlled prospective study. *J Urol* 1992; **147**: 371–5.

45 Bono AV, Benvenutti C, Damiano G, Lovisolo J. Results of transurethral resection and intravesical doxorubicin prophylaxis in patients with T1G3 bladder cancer. *Urology* 1994; **44**: 334–5.

46 Morales A, Eidinger D, Bruce AW. Intracavitary bacillus Calmette–Guérin in the treatment of superficial bladder tumors. *J Urol* 1976; **116**: 180–3.

47 Martínez-Piñeiro JA, León JJ, Martínez-Piñeiro Jr L *et al.* Bacillus Calmette–Guérin versus doxorubicin versus thiotepa: a randomized prospective study in 202 patients with superficial bladder cancer. *J Urol* 1990; **143**: 502–6.

48 Lamm DL, Blumenstein BA, Crawford ED *et al.* A randomized trial of intravesical doxorubicin and immunotherapy with bacille Calmette–Guérin for transitional cell carcinoma of the bladder. *N Engl J Med* 1991; **325**: 1205–9.

49 Melekos MD, Chionis HS, Paranychianakis GS, Dauaher HH. Intravesical 4′-epi-doxorubicin (epirubicin) versus bacillus Calmette–Guérin: a controlled prospective study on the prophylaxis of superficial bladder cancer. *Cancer* 1993; **72**: 1749–55.

50 Bassi P, Pagano F. Epirubicin vs BCG as prophylaxis in superficial bladder cancer: a prospective randomized multicenter Phase III trial. Presented at DUA IV, Nijmegen 1995.

51 Fukui I, Kihara K, Sekine H *et al.* Intravesical combination chemotherapy with Mitomycin C and doxorubicin for superficial bladder cancer: a randomized trial of maintenance versus no maintenance following a complete response. *Cancer Chemother Pharmacol* 1992; **30**(Suppl): S37–40.

52 Sekine H, Fukui I, Yamada T *et al.* Intravesical Mitomycin C and doxorubicin sequential therapy for carcinoma *in situ* of the bladder: a longer follow-up result. *J Urol* 1994; **151**: 27–30.

53 Erol A, Ozgur S, Basar M, Cetin S. Trial with bacillus Calmette-Guérin and epirubicin combination in the prophylaxis of superficial bladder cancer. *Urol Int* 1994; **52**: 69–72.

54 Höltl W, Hasun R, Albrecht W. Prospective, randomized trial to evaluate high versus low-dose interferon-alpha-2b versus conventional chemotherapy in prevention of the recurrence of superficial transitional cell carcinoma of the urinary bladder. *Anti-Cancer Drugs* 1992; **3**(Suppl): S29–32.

55 Serretta V, Corselli G, Piazza B *et al.* Correlation between clinical response and urinary interleukin levels using different doses and intravesical administration schedules of interferon-alpha-2b combined with epirubicin: a pilot study. *Urological Res* 1993; **21**: 353–7.

56 Ferrari P, Castagnetti G, Pollastri CA *et al.* Chemoimmunotherapy for prophylaxis of recurrence in superficial bladder cancer: interferon-alpha-2b versus interferon-alpha-2b with epirubicin. *Anti-Cancer Drugs* 1992; **3**(Suppl): S25–27.

57 Raitanen M-P, Lukkarinen O. A controlled study of intravesical epirubicin with or without alpha-2b-interferon as prophylaxis for recurrent superficial transitional cell carcinoma of the bladder. *Br J Urol* 1995; **76**: 697–701.

58 Pawinski A, Sylvester R, Bouffioux C *et al*. A combined analysis of EORTC/MRC randomized clinical trials for the prophylactic treatment of TaT1 bladder cancer. *J Urol* (in press).

CHAPTER 11

Overview on Mitomycin C

A.P.M. van der Meijden

Introduction

Mitomycin C (MMC) is approved for use in treating various malignant tumours and has been used extensively in the treatment of superficial bladder cancer over the past 30 years. Its molecular weight of 329 leads to minimal absorption from the bladder into the circulation. Mitomycin C is relatively non-toxic. Chemical cystitis may occur but represents no real clinical problem. A systemic contact dermatitis is observed in up to 9% of cases. This entity is more common than one would expect but only a few reports in the urological literature exist. The results of several Phase II studies, in which MMC has been used as an ablative agent against existing tumours, have been reported. In this chapter European Organization for Research and Treatment of Cancer (EORTC) results of the sequential combination of intravesical therapy with MMC and bacillus Calmette–Guérin (BCG) on a marker tumour are presented. Response rates of different studies comparing MMC to BCG after transurethral resection (TUR) in patients with pTa, pT1 and carcinoma *in situ* (CIS) bladder tumours suggest that BCG is superior to MMC. However, several studies are quoted in which the superiority of BCG over Mitomycin C could not be demonstrated by us. Finally the frequency of side-effects and the nature of cutaneous reactions to the intravesical instillation of MMC are discussed.

Mitomycin C in Phase I and II trials

In 1975 Mishina *et al.* [1] reported the results of a 7-year Phase II trial using intravesical MMC for the treatment of superficial bladder cancer. It was one of the first reports in the literature on MMC. Fifty patients received 20 mg Mitomycin C in 20 ml sterile water, which they held in the bladder as long as possible (average 3 hours). The instillations were repeated three times weekly and maintained for 7 weeks. Complete response was achieved in 22 of 50 patients (44%), partial response occurred in 16 patients (32%). Mishina demonstrated in this trial the ablative effect of mitomycin in 76% of the treated patients. A strong correlation was found with tumour size, stage and grade. The investigators suggested that the therapy was most effective in small tumours (less than 1 cm) and in low-stage and low-grade tumours. In 1980 the results of another multi-institutional Phase I–II study of MMC therapy was reported by De Furia *et al.* [2]. Complete remission was defined in this study as the disappearance of all visible tumour while partial remission was considered to be a greater than 50% reduction of tumour load. Different doses of MMC were used but the final concentration was in most cases 1 mg/ml, achieved by dissolving the 20- and 40-mg doses with 20 and 40 ml of sterile water respectively.

Twenty-one patients (45%) achieved a complete response and 13 (22%) had a partial response. The investigators reported no clear dose–response relationship although there was a trend for higher response rate when 60 mg of MMC was used.

Similar results were reported by Bracken *et al.* [3]. They treated 43 patients whose tumours were not amenable to TUR, mostly due to bulky disease.

Complete response was observed in 49% and partial response in 30% of patients respectively.

Harrison *et al.* treated 23 patients in a Phase II study. Of these 4 patients had CIS, 2 had CIS and papillary tumours and 17 had only papillary tumours, mostly T1.

After administration of instillations of 20 mg MMC in 20 ml sterile water, three times weekly, for 7 weeks a complete-response rate of 77% was achieved; a partial-response rate of 18% was recorded [4].

It is known that BCG immunotherapy is one of the most active intravesical therapies for Ta, T1 papillary tumours and for CIS. The EORTC Genitourinary group has addressed the issue of combined treatment with MMC and BCG on a marker tumour. The ablative activity of intravesical MMC followed by intravesical BCG on a papillary marker tumour and the incidence and severity of side-effects were determined [5]. Thirty-five patients with multiple Ta or T1 bladder tumours underwent complete TUR with the exception of one marker tumour measuring 0.5–1 cm. MMC, 40 mg in 50 ml of saline, was administered weekly for four consecutive weeks, followed by BCG (RIVM strain), 5×10^8 colony-forming units in 50 ml of saline, weekly for six consecutive weeks. Thus the total regimen consisted of 10 consecutive weekly instillations. Cystoscopy was performed at 12 weeks (2 weeks after the last instillation). All visible lesions were resected including the marker lesion, if not destroyed. In the case of complete destruction of the marker tumour a biopsy was taken at the site of the previous tumour.

Complete response was defined as the complete destruction of the marker lesion, confirmed by negative cytology and negative biopsy at the site of the marker tumour, and the appearance of no new tumours elsewhere. No change was either the destruction of the marker lesion with positive cytology and/or stabilization of the marker lesion with a stage less than or equal to T1 and/or appearance of new tumour(s) with a stage less than or equal to T1. Progressive disease was defined as the occurrence of a tumour with a stage greater than T1, either at the marker or new lesion(s). Partial response, e.g. a decrease in the size of the marker tumour was not taken into account in this trial because it was difficult to measure the diameter of a bladder tumour with sufficient accuracy.

Thirty-two patients entered by 10 different centres were evaluable for response or adverse effects. Of the patients, 27 were males and 5 females. The age of the patients varied from 45 to 85 years, median 70 years. Five patients had multiple primary tumours and 27 had multiple recurrent tumours. The number of tumours at entry varied in general between 2 and 10, but three patients had 16, 19 and 60 tumours, respectively. The stage and grade of the tumours are depicted in Table 11.1. Thirty-one patients

Table 11.1 Tumour stage (Ta–T1) and tumour grade (G1–3) in 32 evaluable patients.

Tumour stage (WHO)	Tumour grade			Total number of events
	G1	G2	G3	
Ta	12	8	0	20
T1	3	8	1	12
Total	15	16	1	32

received the full dose of MMC plus BCG. One patient had to stop instillation therapy after the second MMC instillation due to chemical cystitis (grade 3). This patient was inevaluable for response. Toxicity of the sequential regimen is reported in Table 11.2. Apart from the patient with severe chemical cystitis, no patient had to stop instillations, although postponement for 1 week was necessary in the case of three patients.

None of the patients had CIS or severe dysplasia in any of the randomly taken biopsies, or in biopsies that were taken from areas suspected of CIS.

The overall response in 32 eligible patients is shown in Table 11.3. Complete response (CR) (no tumour, negative cytology) was seen in 16 (50%) of the patients. Another three patients (9.4%) had a tumour-free bladder and negative cytology, but they refused biopsy. No change (NC) (CR of marker lesion, appearance of new lesion) was noted in three (9.4%) patients, and NC (stable marker tumour, no new tumours) was observed in eight (25%) of the patients. Progressive disease (PD) to muscle invasive tumour (T2) was seen in one (3.1%) patient.

Table 11.2 Side-effects reported during treatment using WHO standards.

	Toxicity, WHO grade					Grade 1–2 %	Grade 3–4 %
	0	1	2	3	unknown	%	%
Nausea/vomiting	30	1	0	0	0	3.23	0
Drug fever	29	2	0	0	0	6.45	0
Allergy	31	0	0	0	0	0	0
Local reaction (a,c)	15	11	3	2	0	15.61	6.45
Cutaneous reaction	30	1	0	0	0	3.23	0
Haemorrhage (b)	29	2	0	0	0	6.45	0
Flu-like syndrome	30	1	0	0	0	3.23	0
Other toxicity	30	0	1	0	0	3.23	0

a. Chemical or bacterial cystitis, dysuria, bladder irritation.
b. Mild haematuria.
c. Bacterial cystitis in two cases.

Table 11.3 Best overall response (32 eligible patients).

Response	Observations	Frequency
Complete response	16	50.00
No change (CR in marker lesion + new lesion)	3	9.37
No change (stable marker lesion)	8	25.00
Progression	1	3.12
Inevaluable: not confirmed CR	3	9.38
Inevaluable: toxicity	1	3.12
Total patients	32	= 100%

The rate of CR appeared to be associated with the number of tumours upon entry. Of the 18 patients who had 2–5 tumours, 11 (66%) achieved CR. Three of nine patients with $\geq$ 10 tumours showed CR and none of the patients with $\geq$ 15 tumours was completely free of tumour after 3 months. In December 1993 (cut-off follow-up period) all patients were alive. The median disease-free interval among responders was 19.8 months (range 7–38 months). Three of 16 responders had one recurrence, and 5 of 12 non-responders had one recurrence (Ta or T1). In one patient the marker tumour progressed to T2.

Mitomycin C for carcinoma *in situ*

Mitomycin C has been used successfully for the treatment of CIS. A compilation of results in the literature [6] is presented in Table 11.4.

Data have to be interpreted with caution due to small series, different doses of MMC used, different instillation schedules and duration of follow-up. In 147 patients treated with MMC the complete response was 53%. For doxorubicin and thiotepa these results are respectively 48% and 38%.

However, for patients treated with BCG results appear to be superior over chemotherapeutic agents including MMC. Lamm *et al.* [6] reported a complete response in 500 of 718 BCG-treated patients (70%).

Because of these data there is a consensus that the treatment of choice for CIS is BCG despite the high toxicity of BCG.

Table 11.4 Response in carcinoma *in situ* treated with Mitomycin C.

Study*	Mitomycin C	Complete response
Fluchter	6	6 (100%)
Harrison	6	4 (67%)
Issel	14	4 (29%)
Bouffioux	5	3 (60%)
Powell	5	3 (60%)
Soloway	12	5 (42%)
Koontz	20	9 (45%)
Jauhainen	11	9 (82%)
Cant	12	5 (42%)
Lucero	5	4 (80%)
Hetherinton	4	4 (100%)
Stricker	19	15 (79%)
Stanisic	7	0 (0%)
Soloway	21	7 (33%)
Mitomycin C sub-totals	147	78 (53%)
Chemotherapy total response	448	213 (48%)

*This data is taken from ref. 5 and all the studies mentioned are detailed therein.

Mitomycin and BCG in Phase III trials

Presently many investigators consider BCG to be the most effective intravesical agent known for the prevention of recurrence of superficial bladder tumours [7].

Multiple studies have established that BCG prophylaxis following complete TUR significantly reduces recurrences and prolongs the disease-free interval in Ta, T1 bladder cancer in comparison to TUR alone and in comparison to chemotherapeutic agents such as thiotepa, doxorubicin and MMC. In contrast randomized controlled studies have failed to show the superiority of one chemotherapeutic drug over another cytotoxic agent.

As illustrated in Table 11.5 the comparison of BCG with chemotherapeutic agents in prospective randomized trials shows that BCG is superior to thiotepa and to doxorubicin [6].

However, with MMC the advantages of BCG have not been clearly apparent [6]. There are two studies indicating that BCG is superior over MMC [8,9]. The Finnbladder study [8] reports a recurrence rate of 35% for BCG-treated patients and 62% for MMC-treated patients.

The SWOG study [9] comparing 50 mg of Tice BCG with 20 mg of MMC in 469 patients using the same 6-weekly and then monthly-treatment schedule had to be stopped at the first interim analysis due to a highly significant ($p < 0.006$) advantage of BCG over MMC. The overall recurrence was reduced from 32.6% with MMC, to 19.5% with BCG and the median time to recurrence was prolonged from 20 months to more than 36 months.

Table 11.5 Recurrence rate with BCG versus chemotherapy.

Study	BCG	Thiotepa	Doxorubicin	Mitomycin	TUR	p-value
Brosman	0%	47%				< 0.01
Netto	7%	43%				< 0.01
Martinez	13%	36%	43%			< 0.01
SWOG	63%		83%			< 0.02
Debruyne	30%			25%		N.S.
Finnblad	35%			62%		< 0.01
Rübben	28%			35%	42%	N.S.
Witjes	29% (RIVM)			26%		N.S.
	24% (Tice)					

However, there are three studies in the literature suggesting that MMC was equal to BCG in terms of efficacy but superior with regards to adverse effects.

Rübben using maintenance therapy could not find a significant difference between TUR alone versus TUR plus BCG versus TUR plus MMC [10].

The EORTC-GU Group conducted a randomized prospective two-arm study in which the treatment with BCG (RIVM strain) was compared to MMC in patients with primary or recurrent superficial bladder tumours, including CIS [11].

BCG (5×10^8 colony-forming units) was instilled once a week for six consecutive weeks. No maintenance was given. MMC (30 mg in 50 ml saline) was instilled once a week for 1 month (weeks 1–4) and thereafter once a month for a total of 6 months. The total number of MMC instillations was nine versus six for BCG.

The tumour recurrence rate in 325 patients was reported after 21 months of follow-up. Of the patients treated with BCG (n = 158), tumour(s) recurred in 66 (42%), whereas of those patients who received MMC (n = 167), 60 (36%) had recurrences. The recurrence rate is 0.28 for BCG and 0.24 for MMC respectively (p = 0.40, not significant).

The tumour stage at entry, the tumour grade, the number of tumours and the number of primary versus recurrent tumours are shown in Tables 11.6–11.9.

Table 11.6 Tumour category at study entry.

Therapy	Tumour pathology (stage)*			Total (%)
	pTis	pTa	pT1	
BCG-RIVM	5	107	60	172 (50)
Mitomycin	5	109	58	172 (50)
Totals	10	216	118	344 (100)

*Number of patients.

Table 11.7 Tumour grade in patients at study entry.

Therapy	Tumour grade (Gx = G unknown)				
	G1	G2	G3	Gx	Total (%)
BCG-RIVM	48	90	29	5	172 (50)
Mitomycin	61	82	24	5	172 (50)
Totals	109	172	53	10	344 (100)

Table 11.8 Number of tumours in patients at study entry.

Therapy	Number of tumours				
	Unknown	1	2–3	4–10	Total (%)
BCG-RIVM	0	90	45	37	172 (50)
Mitomycin	1	92	43	36	172 (50)
Totals	1	182	88	73	344 (100)

Table 11.9 Primary/recurrent bladder cancer in patients at study entry.

Therapy	Bladder cancer		Total (%)
	Primary	Recurrent	
BCG-RIVM	120	52	172 (50)
Mitomycin	120	52	172 (50)
Totals	240	104	344 (100)

Because of the lack of superiority of BCG over MMC, the efficacy of BCG-RIVM strain was questioned. BCG is a biological product consisting of living bacteria, subcellular debris and adjuvant compounds.

Considerable differences in the various strains and even lots of the same strain can be present [12].

Therefore another trial was designed in which two BCG strains were used: BCG-RIVM and BCG-Tice. As a third arm MMC was again chosen [13]. The doses and instillation schedules were exactly the same as in the previous trial where BCG-RIVM was compared to MMC.

Tumour characteristics of evaluable patients are shown in Table 11.10.

For stages pTa and pT1 papillary tumours the time to first recurrence was recorded. In patients treated with MMC a recurrence was observed in 58 of 136 patients (43%), 75 of 117 patients (64%) treated with BCG-Tice had a recurrent tumour while 62 of 134 patients (46%) treated with BCG-RIVM had a recurrence. The estimated percentages of disease-free patients in the three treatment arms are shown in Table 11.11. The analysis of efficacy in the patients with papillary tumours shows a

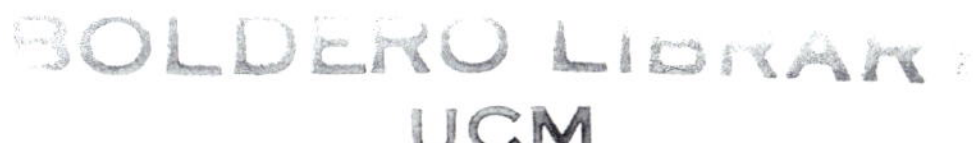

Table 11.10 Tumour characteristics of evaluable patients and allocation to treatment.

	Mitomycin C	Tice-BCG	RIVM-BCG	Total no. (%)
Stage pTa				
Grade 1	24	28	32	84
Grade 2	55	48	54	157
Grade 3	4	5	4	13
Total				254 (65.6)
Stage pT1				
Grade 1	–	–	–	–
Grade 2	31	18	23	72
Grade 3	22	18	21	61
Total				133 (34.4)
Primary	104	87	108	299
Recurrent	32	30	26	88
Total papillary tumours	136	117	134	387
CIS	12	23	15	50
Totals	148	140	149	437

Table 11.11 Treatment efficacy defined as percentage of patients free of tumour at 5 years of follow-up.

Yrs	Mitomycin C	Tice-BCG	RIVM-BCG
1	73 ± 4	66 ± 5	70 ± 4
2	61 ± 5	53 ± 5	61 ± 5
3	59 ± 5	42 ± 5	55 ± 5
4	57 ± 5	36 ± 5	54 ± 5
5	57 ± 5	36 ± 5	54 ± 5

Percent disease-free with standard error and all papillary tumours.
*No failures seen after 4 years.

borderline statistically significant difference among the treatment arms ($p = 0.04$). The MMC and BCG-RIVM treatments were equally effective ($p = 0.53$), but MMC was more effective than BGC-Tice ($p = 0.01$).

For CIS the number of patients investigated was too small to permit solid conclusions. Progression in stage (pT2 or higher) was observed in eight (6%) of the MMC group, seven (5%) of the BCG-Tice group and eight (6%) treated with BCG-RIVM.

Side-effects of Mitomycin C

Local toxicity, expressed as the occurrence of bacterial cystitis, drug-induced cystitis and other local side-effects [13] was analysed (Table 11.12). The severity of local side-

Table 11.12 Side-effects during instillation period.

	Mitomycin C	Tice-BCG	RIVM-BCG	Total (%)
Bacterial cystitis ($p = 0.20$)				
No	121	102	115	338
Yes, without delay	25	26	24	75
Yes, with delay	1	11	10	22
Stop treatment	1	1	–·	2
Total number yes (%)	27 (18.2)	38 (27.1)	34 (22.8)	99 (22.7)
Drug-induced cystitis ($p = 0.009$)				
No	122	98	101	321
Yes, without delay	25	40	45	110
Yes, with delay	1	1	2	4
Stop treatment	–	1	1	2
Total number yes (%)	26 (17.6)	42 (30.0)	48 (32.2)	116 (26.5)
Allergic reaction ($p = 0.30$)				
No	141	137	146	424
Yes, without delay	4	2	2	8
Yes, with delay	1	1	1	3
Stop treatment	2	–	–	2
Total number yes (%)	7 (4.7)	3 (2.1)	3 (2.0)	13 (3.0)
Other local side-effects ($p = 0.004$)				
No	141	117	127	385
Yes, without delay	7	3	20	50
Yes, with delay	–	–	2	2
Total number yes (%)	7 (4.7)	23 (16.4)	22 (14.8)	52 (11.9)
Systemic side-effects ($p < 0.001$)				
No	142	102	122	366
Yes, without delay	6	32	24	62
Yes, with delay	–	3	1	4
Stop treatment	–	3	2	5
Total number yes (%)	6 (4.1)	38 (27.1)	27 (18.1)	71 (16.3)

effects was classified in three categories: (1) not requiring delay of instillations, (2) requiring delay of instillations, and (3) requiring a definitive cessation of instillation therapy. Bacterial cystitis (not caused by BCG) was observed in 18.2% of MMC-treated patients, 27.1% of BCG-Tice-treated patients and 22.8% of BCG-RIVM patients. The differences are not significant ($p = 0.20$). Drug-induced cystitis was encountered in 17.6% for the MMC group, 30.0% for the BCG-Tice group and 32.2% for the BCG-RIVM patients respectively ($p = 0.009$). Other local side-effects, such as haematuria, pain, etc. were observed in 4.7%, 16.4% and 14.8% for the three groups respectively

($p = 0.004$). Again, MMC-treated patients suffered less side-effects than BCG-treated patients. Systemic side-effects [13], such as fever, malaise and flu-like symptoms, were seen in 4.1% of the MMC patients, in 27.1% of the BCG-Tice-treated patients and in 18.1% of the BCG-RIVM-treated patients respectively ($p < 0.001$).

In conclusion MMC-treated patients showed significantly fewer side-effects than BCG-treated patients with the exception of bacterial cystitis. There was no difference in adverse effects between BCG-Tice and BCG-RIVM.

Frequency of cutaneous reactions caused by Mitomycin C

To assess the frequency of mitomycin-related cutaneous reactions, we reviewed 35 clinical reports of mitomycin-instillation therapy. Side-effects were not mentioned or specified in eight reports [14]. The relevant data on side-effects from 27 reports are therefore summarized in Table 11.13. Cutaneous reactions to mitomycin therapy were specified in 23 reports (85%). Overall, of 1450 patients treated in the 27 studies reviewed, 126 (8.7%) had dermatological reactions.

Although skin rashes from mitomycin use occur frequently, adequate dermatological descriptions of these reactions in the urological literature are lacking, as shown in Table 11.13. Relatively few patients taking mitomycin have been evaluated by dermatologists. Furthermore, the descriptions in these studies do not allow conclusions as to the morphology of mitomycin-related skin reactions. On review of the data, two types of cutaneous reactions can be distinguished. The most common reaction is found on the hands and/or genitals and sometimes on the feet. The skin reaction on the palms and soles is either desquamation or vesicular dermatitis. The other type is a more diffuse reaction, also involving the trunk. Skin rashes never develop after the first treatment, but usually do so after five to eight instillations. In many cases, especially when only the hands are involved, mitigation of the local reaction can be accomplished using topical corticosteroids and therapy with intravesical mitomycin instillations can be continued, although each subsequent treatment will reproduce the symptoms. However, in our review of the literature, of 126 patients in whom cutaneous reactions developed, 37 (29%) had to interrupt treatment.

We recently investigated seven patients who had cutaneous reactions during intravesical mitomycin therapy. They were patch-tested with either water- or petrolatum-based concentrations of mitomycin ranging from 0.06% to 0.6%. Positive patch-test reactions were observed in six patients, indicating delayed hypersensitivity. The only patient not reacting had suffered from generalized exanthem with fever. He had used many other drugs, of which one may have been responsible. Thus, there is evidence that most, if not all, cases of cutaneous side-effects from mitomycin are caused by delayed hypersensitivity reactions. (1) The cutaneous reaction first develops after repeated instillation treatments, never after the first administration. (2) After the first skin reaction, renewed treatment with mitomycin generally reproduces the symptoms. (3) After intravenous administration of mitomycin, exanthems are rare. If such reactions were non-immunological in nature, the low plasma concentrations that occur after intravesical mitomycin administration would be highly unlikely to cause cutaneous problems. (4) Contact allergy to mitomycin has been demonstrated in several patients with mitomycin-related skin reactions.

Table 11.13 Type and frequency of cutaneous side-effects: literature review*

Series	Patients treated (n)	Type/frequency of cutaneous reaction
Mishina *et al.*	50	No dermatological side-effects mentioned
Van Helsdingen *et al.*	31	Contact eczema 3 (10%); generalized exanthem 3 (10%)
Huland and Otto	54	Allergy 1; dermatitis 2 (6%)
Issel *et al.*	58	Skin reactions on hands or genitals 7 (12%)
Harrison *et al.*	23	Rash 4 (17%)
Stricker *et al.*	19	Rash on hands or genitals 3 (16%)
Zincke *et al.*	42	Rash and contact dermatitis 2 (5%)
Heney *et al.*	76	Rash 14 (18%)
DeBruyne *et al.*	87	Allergic reactions 6 (7%)
Huland *et al.*	329	Allergy and other side-effects 33 (10%)
Soloway, 1985	70	Penile rash 3 (4%); palmar erythema and/or dermatitis 4 (6%)
MacFarlane and Tolley	25	Rash 1 (4%)
Prout *et al.*	28	Rash 1 (4%)
Soloway *et al.*	16	Palmar rash 3 (19%)
Bracken *et al.*	43	Desquamation of palmar skin 2 (5%)
Nissenkorn *et al.*	29	Desquamation of palmar skin 4 (14%), and also erythema of perianal region and penile oedema in 2 (6%); generalized rash 1 (3%)
Hetherington *et al.*	43	Palmar rash 5 (12%)
Jauhiainen *et al.*	17	No dermatological side-effects mentioned
Ausfeld *et al.*	57	Cutaneous reactions 10 (18%): desquamation of hands and genitals 3, extremities or face 3, extremities and trunk 4
Devonec *et al.*	26	Palmar surface desquamation 3 (12%)
DeFuria *et al.*	57	Rash on hands 3 (5%)
Koontz *et al.*	117	Rash on hands or feet 19 (16%)
Flanigan *et al.*	25	Generalized or severe palmar rash 8 (32%)
Fukui *et al.*	30	No dermatological side-effects mentioned
Maier and Baumgartner	56	Skin rash 2 (4%)
Jurincic *et al.*	23	No dermatological side-effects mentioned
Stricker *et al.*	19	Generalized or localized rash on hands or genitalia 3 (16%)
TOTAL	1,450	Dermatologic side-effects 126 (8.7%)

*Adapted from data in ref. 14. All the studies listed are detailed therein.

From our own experiences and the literature, we conclude that up to 9% of patients treated with intravesical instillations of mitomycin will develop cutaneous side-effects. Most, if not all, of these reactions are caused by contact allergy. The dermatitis is usually localized in the palms of the hands, on the feet, and in the area of the genitals and anus; widespread reactions occur less frequently. This distribution pattern is the result of systemic-contact dermatitis caused by absorption of mitomycin from the bladder mucosa.

Conclusion

Intravesical therapy with MMC delays the time to first recurrence. For a long time it was unknown whether intravesical chemotherapy influences progression and survival. A recent meta-analysis of four EORTC and two Medical Research Council (MRC) studies, comprising 2535 patients treated either with TUR alone versus TUR plus intravesical chemotherapy, suggests that chemotherapy does not influence progression and survival [15].

Intravesical immunotherapy with BCG may prolong the time to progression but more data and longer follow-up are needed to confirm early data [6].

How can our favourable results of MMC versus BCG be explained? In the two Phase III trials mentioned before obviously the number of patients with high-risk superficial bladder cancer was significantly lower than in the SWOG 8795 study [9]. In this study at least three major differences can be noted compared to our two trials [11,13].

In study 8795 only patients with rapidly recurring tumours (high risk) were enrolled; they were treated with a relatively low dose of MMC (20 mg) and they received maintenance therapy. In our studies a relatively large number of patients with intermediate risk, according to prognostic factors, were treated. They had predominantly primary tumours, solitary tumours or pTa tumours. Few patients with CIS were treated.

Obviously BCG is the agent of preference in patients with high-risk papillary tumours and CIS [6]. However, nearly a third of all patients belong to the intermediate-risk group and half of the patients to the low-risk group [16]. It is questionable as to whether low-risk tumours need any instillation therapy and if so a single instillation may be sufficient [17]. Patients with intermediate risk will be at an advantage with intravesical therapy, mainly with regard to recurrence. The risk of progression in this category is fairly low. This group of patients, especially, may benefit from intravesical MMC and suffer fewer side-effects than caused by BCG. Therefore, MMC is an agent which still has an important role in the treatment of patients with low- or intermediate-risk superficial bladder cancer.

References

1   Mishina T, Oda K, Murata S *et al.* Mitomycin C bladder instillation therapy for bladder tumours. *J Urol* 1975; **114**: 217–19.

2   De Furia M, Bracken B, Johnson DE *et al.* Phase I–II study of Mitomycin C topical therapy for low-grade, low stage transitional cell carcinoma of the bladder: an interim report. *Cancer Treat Rep* 1980; **64**(2–3): 225–30.

3   Bracken B, Johnson DE, van Eschenbach AC *et al*. Role of intravesical Mitomycin C in management of superficial bladder tumours. *Urology* 1980; **16**(1): 11–15.

4   Harrison GSM, Green DF, Newling DWW *et al*. A phase II study of intravesical Mitomycin C in the treatment of superficial bladder cancer. *Br J Urol* 1983; **55**: 676–9.

5   Van der Meijden APM, Hall RR, Pavone-Macaluso M *et al*. Marker tumour response to the sequential combination of intravesical therapy with mitomycin C and BCG-RIVM in multiple superficial bladder tumours. Report from the European Organisation for Research and Treatment on Cancer-Genitourinary Group (EORTC 30897). *Eur Urol* 1996; **29**: 199–203.

6   Lamm DL, Van der Meijden APM, Akaza H *et al*. Intravesical chemotherapy and immunotherapy: how do we assess their effectiveness and what are their limitations and uses? *Int J Urol* 1995; **2**(Suppl2): S23–35.

7   Herr HW, Laudone VP, Whitmore WF. An overview of intravesical therapy for superficial bladder tumors. *J Urol* 1987; **138**: 1363–8.

8   Jauhiainen K, Rintala E, Alfthan O, the Finnbladder Group. Immunotherapy (BCG) versus chemotherapy (MMC) in intravesical treatment of superficial urinary bladder cancer. In: deKernion JB (ed) *Immunotherapy of Urological Tumors*. Edinburgh: Churchill-Livingstone, 1990; 13–26.

9   Lamm DL, Crawford ED, Blumenstein B *et al*. SWOG 8795: a randomized comparison of bacillus Calmette–Guérin and Mitomycin C prophylaxis in stage Ta and T1 transitional cell carcinoma of the bladder. *J Urol* 1993; **149**(2): 275A–82A.

10 Krege S, Otto T, Rübben H *et al*. Final report on a randomized multi-centre trial on adjuvant therapy in superficial bladder cancer: TUR only versus TUR and mitomycin versus TUR and bacillus Calmette–Guérin. *J Urol* 1996; **155**: 494A, Abstract 734.

11 Debruyne FMJ, Van der Meijden APM, Geboers AD, Franssen MP, Van Leeuwen MJ, Steerenberg PA, De Jong WH, Ruitenberg JJ. BCG-RIVM versus Mitomycin C intravesical therapy superficial bladder cancer. *Urology* 1988; **31**(Suppl3): S20–5.

12 Kelley DR, Ratliff TL, Catalona WJ *et al*. Intravesical bacillus Calmette–Guérin therapy for superficial bladder cancer: effect of bacillus Calmette–Guérin viability on treatment results. *J Urol* 1985; **134**: 48–53.

13 Vegt PDJ, Witjes JA, Witjes WPJ *et al*. A randomized study of intravesical Mitomycin C, bacillus Calmette–Guérin Tice and bacillus Calmette–Guérin RIVM treatment in pTa–pT1 papillary carcinoma and carcinoma *in situ* of the bladder. *J Urol* 1995; **153**: 929–33.

14 De Groot AC, Van der Meijden APM, Conemans JMH and Maibach HI. Frequency and nature of cutaneous reactions to intravesical instillation of mitomycin for superficial bladder cancer. *Urology* 1992; **31**: (Suppl) S40: 16–19.

15 Pawinski A, Sylvester R, Kurth K *et al*. A combined analysis of European Organization for Research and Treatment of Cancer and Medical Research Council randomized clinical trials for the prophylactic treatment of stage Ta,T1 bladder cancer. *J Urol* 1996; **155**: 1934–41.

16 Van der Meijden APM. New approaches to intravesical chemo- and immunotherapy in superficial bladder cancer. In: EORTC Genitourinary Monograph: *Recent Progress in Bladder and Kidney Cancer*. New York: Wiley–Liss 1992; 95–101.

17 Oosterlinck W, Kurth KH, Schröder F *et al*. A prospective European Organization for Research and Treatment of Cancer Genitourinary Group randomized trial comparing transurethral resection followed by a single intravesicular instillation of epirubicin or water in single stage Ta, T1 papillary carcinoma of the bladder. *J Urol* 1992; **149**: 749–52.

CHAPTER 12

Overview on bacillus Calmette–Guérin

D.L. Lamm

Introduction

The live attenuated tuberculosis vaccine, bacillus Calmette–Guérin (BCG), was noted to have potential anti-neoplastic effects by Pearl in 1929. However, it was not until 1976 that Morales *et al.* [1] first reported the use of intravesical BCG in the management of early stage bladder cancer. Many studies have since shown the efficacy of intravesical BCG in the treatment of superficial bladder cancer, and currently BCG remains the standard by which treatments of aggressive superficial bladder cancer must be compared. Immunotherapy with BCG heralds a new era in the management of bladder cancer.

Mechanisms of action

BCG is recognized as a non-specific immune stimulant. Intravesical BCG induces inflammation of the bladder with infiltration of a broad range of cell types. BCG may activate macrophages, T lymphocytes, B lymphocytes, natural killer cells and killer cells [2]. BCG stimulates cytokine production, and this in turn enhances natural killer cell activity, which increases after BCG immunotherapy [3–5]. BCG produces a T-cell mediated immune response that has been linked to anti-tumour activity in both humans and mice [6]. The anti-neoplastic effect of BCG is most likely the result of a combination of enhanced activity of various arms of the immune system. The mechanism of BCG–tumour cell interaction is not completely understood. After intravesical instillation live mycobacteria attach to the urothelial lining, facilitated by fibronectin, a component of the extracellular matrix [7]. Integrin is required for the direct attachment and internalization of BCG by bladder tumour cells [7,8,9]. This process leaves bacterial cell-surface glycoproteins attached to epithelial cell membranes, and this antigen is thought to mediate the immune response [10]. Tumour-cell motility is also thought to be inhibited by BCG through a mechanism involving the BCG–fibronectin–tumour cell interaction [11]. Intravesical BCG immunotherapy results in cytokine production including interleukins 1, 2, and 6, interferon-γ and tumour necrosis factor-α [12], which can be measured in the urine for many hours after instillation. Bladder biopsies following BCG administration show increased expression of HLA DR antigens on tumour cells and infiltration of tumour and stroma with lymphocytes, predominantly T-helper cells, and macrophages. The helper/suppressor ratio in infiltrating lymphocytes is increased. Changes in peripheral blood are also seen, including heightened immunoproliferative response to BCG antigen and production of specific antibody [13,14].

Principles of immunotherapy

To use immunotherapy effectively in the management of bladder cancer or other malignancy it is important to consider basic principles and understand the differences between immunotherapy and chemotherapy. Currently, chemotherapy is limited in specificity and basically inhibits or destroys rapidly dividing cells. Generally, tumour cell destruction is proportional to drug concentration so treatments are pushed to the limit of tolerance. In contrast, immunotherapy may be either non-specific or specific. More often than not optimal responses to immunotherapy are seen at less than the maximum tolerated dose because high-dose treatment invokes complex immune regulatory mechanisms. The typical dose–response curve with biological-response modifiers, such as BCG, is therefore bell-shaped, with optimal responses occurring at intermediate doses [15].

The failure of BCG immunotherapy in many previous trials in other malignancies is probably in part a result of ignoring the principles of optimal BCG immunotherapy previously defined by animal studies. These principles, as reviewed by Bast *et al* [16], include juxtaposition of BCG and tumour cells, minimization of tumour burden, and use of an adequate number of viable bacteria. Clinically, ensuring direct contact of BCG with tumour may require resection of the prostate or instillation of BCG in the upper tract for disease outside the bladder. BCG has a complete response rate of 60% or more when used to treat residual stage Ta or T1 bladder cancer, but based on animal studies I prefer to resect all visible tumour when possible prior to beginning treatment. The optimal dose of BCG remains to be defined, and may, like the optimal treatment schedule, vary from patient to patient. Current data suggest that intravesical doses of between one hundred million (1×10^8) and one billion (1×10^{10}) colony-forming units (CFU) are effective, but responses have been reported with doses as low as 10 million CFU or 1 mg BCG [17]. The wide variation in effective clinical doses probably relates to the mode of administration. With intravesical instillation only those organisms that attach to the bladder wall stimulate an immune response. Consideration must therefore also be given to avoid administration of medications that can limit the effectiveness of the dose given. Agents that inhibit clot formation reduce fibronectin expression and can reduce BCG attachment, immune stimulation, and anti-tumour activity [18–20]. Similarly, concern has been raised that administration of anti-tubercular antibiotics such as isoniazid, which inhibits intravesical BCG attachment and immune stimulation in the guinea pig model [21], may also reduce the efficacy of BCG therapy. For this reason I avoid the prophylactic use of isoniazid, trimethoprim/sulfamethoxazole, and quinolone antibiotics in patients receiving BCG, but do not hesitate using such antibiotics to treat the side-effects of BCG or intercurrent infection.

Efficacy

BCG is most effective in the treatment of carcinoma *in situ* (CIS) of the bladder, as discussed in chapter 20, and is highly effective in the treatment of residual superficial transitional-cell carcinoma. While complete responses have been observed in patients with muscle-invasive disease, more aggressive treatments are recommended for these patients. By far the most frequent use of BCG is the prevention of tumour recurrence. The relative efficacy of BCG and intravesical chemotherapy in the prevention of tumour recurrence is reviewed in chapter 7, but a discussion of the possible reasons for the high efficacy of BCG is appropriate here.

In CIS the world-wide experience of a more than 70% complete response rate to BCG immunotherapy is unparalleled. The flat, non-invasive nature of CIS facilitates direct contact, so it is not surprising that CIS is exquisitely sensitive to BCG, but the configuration of CIS does not explain the superiority of BCG over chemotherapy, which is even more dependent on direct contact. Surprisingly, evidence suggests that low-grade tumours may be more sensitive to chemotherapy than high-grade tumours, so CIS may be relatively resistant to chemotherapy by virtue of its high grade. In contrast, high grade, more undifferentiated tumours may be more antigenic and therefore more susceptible to immunotherapy. Patients with CIS are presumed to be at high risk for new tumour formation, even if all existing carcinoma is eradicated. Chemotherapy is effective only at the time of administration, but the immune stimulation induced by BCG is known to persist for many months. This continued effect of BCG may contribute to the superior long-term results observed.

Persistent immune stimulation may also explain the superior results that are seen with BCG prophylaxis. Intravesical chemotherapy is used following tumour resection to eradicate residual microscopic disease, and maintenance chemotherapy is used to prevent microscopic carcinomas from becoming clinically evident, but chemotherapy acts only at the time of administration. The concept of 'prophylactic chemotherapy' is therefore a misnomer, because chemotherapy can only treat existing disease. Immunotherapy, on the other hand, has the potential to correct weakness in the defence system against cancer, so that future tumours may be avoided.

Perhaps the greatest disappointment in the development of intravesical therapy for superficial bladder cancer is the inability to demonstrate that chemotherapy reduces the risk of disease progression. While this limitation may be partly related to the difficulty in following large groups of patients for long periods of time, it is clear that if chemotherapy has any effect on progression, it must be very small. Considering the mechanism of action of intravesical chemotherapy, this limitation might be anticipated. Since chemotherapy diffuses into the bladder wall and tumour primarily by a concentration gradient, the deepest portions of the tumour receive the lowest drug concentration, and hence the least effective treatment. These tumour cells, at the depth of the tumour, have the greatest propensity to invade the detrusor muscle and are least subject to eradication by chemotherapy.

Evidence continues to mount suggesting that BCG immunotherapy can significantly reduce disease progression. In most studies progression is reduced by about one half. This advantage of BCG may relate to the observation that BCG is relatively more effective against higher grade tumours or to the ability of BCG to penetrate deep within the bladder wall. BCG attaches to the bladder wall by means of fibronectin receptors and to tumour cells by means of integrin receptors. BCG organisms and granuloma can be found deep within the detrusor muscle, within regional nodes, and even beyond. The ability of BCG to penetrate the bladder and persist long after termination of treatment may explain the long-term beneficial results in stage T1 and even an infrequent stage T2 bladder tumour. Unfortunately, as discussed in the next section, these propensities may also result in adverse reactions.

Safety

The benefit of BCG immunotherapy far exceeds the risk of treatment for patients with aggressive bladder tumours, but serious and even lethal adverse reactions can occur. Because patients who are at risk for serious reactions cannot be reliably identified, BCG immunotherapy is restricted to patients who are at risk for stage progression or multiple, intractable recurrences. Such patients include those with CIS, grade 3, or stage-T1 disease. Patients with multiple grade-1 or -2, stage Ta tumours may be treated with intravesical chemotherapy or immunotherapy. I certainly believe that BCG is appropriate for these patients if they continue to have recurrence after having received intravesical chemotherapy. Patients with a solitary grade-1, stage Ta tumour do not require intravesical therapy, but a single post-operative chemotherapy instillation is safe, effective, and reasonably inexpensive.

The potential toxicity of BCG treatment should be respected but not feared. On one hand, much of the reported toxicity of BCG is merely the expected consequence of effective immune stimulation, and should be regarded as a beneficial sign. On the other hand, serious toxicity from BCG can come unexpectedly, and both patients and treating urologists should beware of untoward reactions. The incidence of complications are listed in Table 12.1, but rather than explore each complication in detail, I will discuss the prevention, diagnosis and treatment of BCG reactions in general and emphasize the principles involved.

The most common reactions to BCG are urinary frequency, mild dysuria, low-grade fever, and mild malaise. These symptoms are a reflection of the immune stimulation resulting from BCG and should be considered a favourable sign. Such symptoms typically begin after the third instillation and last for up to 2 days. If necessary, they can be treated symptomatically with acetaminophen, phenazopyridine, anticholinergics, or antihistamines. Patients who fail to respond or develop fever above 38.8°C are treated with isoniazid, 300 mg, daily. Treatment is continued for several days after symptoms resolve and can be reinstituted 1 day before subsequent BCG instillations and again continued for several days after symptoms resolve or for 3 days if significant symptoms are prevented. It is important to withhold BCG treatment until all symptoms from previous administrations have resolved.

Serious reactions to BCG fortunately occur in less than 1% of patients. The risk for systemic BCG reaction can be significantly reduced by appropriately treating local BCG infection and avoiding conditions that increase the risk of intravenous administration such as traumatic catheterization or administration in the presence of cystitis or after surgery or cystoscopy. Both patients and physicians should be aware that serious BCG reactions can be delayed for months and even years after termination of treatment. Most delayed reactions occur in patients who have had increased symptoms during treatment, inadequate treatment of BCG

Table 12.1 Complications in 2,602 patients according to sub-strains of BCG.

	Total no. (%) (2,602 pts)	% Armand Frappier (718 pts)	% Tice (726 pts)	% Connaught (353 pts)	% Pasteur (325 pts)	% RIVM (129 pts)
Fever	75 (2.9)	3.8	4.7	4.7	0.6	2.1
Granulomatous prostatitis	23 (0.9)	1.8	1.0	0.2	0.6	0.0
Pneumonitis/ hepatitis	18 (0.7)	0.4	0.8	0.6	1.2	0.8
Arthralgia	12 (0.5)	0.7	0.1	0.6	1.8	0.0
Haematuria	24 (1.0)	0.3	0.6	2.4	1.0	0.4
Rash	8 (0.3)	0.4	0.0	0.9	0.0	0.0
Urethral obstruction	8 (0.3)	0.6	0.4	0.2	0.0	0.0
Epididymitis	10 (0.4)	0.4	0.0	0.2	1.2	0.8
Contracted bladder	6 (0.2)	0.0	0.3	0.2	0.6	0.0
Renal abscess	2 (0.1)	0.0	0.0	0.4	0.0	0.0
Sepsis	10 (0.4)	0.1	0.4	0.9	0.2	0.0
Cytopenia	2 (0.1)	0.0	0.3	0.0	0.0	0.0

Table source: Copyright: reproduced with permission of Lamm DL *et al.*: Incidence and treatment of complications of bacillus Calmette–Guérin intravesical therapy in superficial bladder cancer. *J Urol* 1992; **147**: 596–600.

reaction, inappropriate BCG administration, resulting in intravenous absorption, or immunosuppression. However, delayed progressive BCG infection can occur without these predisposing features and can even occur despite the use of isoniazid. Fortunately, BCG remains very sensitive to anti-tubercular antibiotics, so once the diagnosis is made treatment, generally with isoniazid and rifampin, is quite successful. The signs and symptoms of BCG infection are extremely varied because BCG can infect nearly any organ, but patients will typically have intermittent fever, malaise, and weight loss. Common sites of infection are liver, typically with elevation of liver-function tests, bone, lung, epididymis and prostate, and choroiditis, renal and retroperitoneal abscess, mycotic aneurysm and infection of artificial joints have been reported. A high index of suspicion in patients who have received BCG is important, because treatment is highly effective but diagnostic tests may be negative.

The most dangerous and dramatic complication of BCG therapy is the septic reaction. Current estimates are that sepsis occurs in 1 of 50,000 patients now that the importance of prevention of intravenous BCG absorption is recognized. Studies [22,23] now confirm that hypersensitivity is a major component of the BCG-septic reaction, and treatment with isoniazid, 300 mg, rifampin, 600 mg, and most importantly prednisolone, 40 mg, daily is highly effective.

Conclusions

BCG is an archaic vaccine that profoundly and diffusely stimulates the immune system. Prior to the advent of modern chemotherapy astute clinicians observed that BCG could have a beneficial effect in cancer patients, an effect that was later confirmed in animal studies. Despite numerous clinical attempts, the use of BCG in the treatment of human cancer was largely unsuccessful until Morales applied the knowledge gained by animal studies to the successful use of BCG in the treatment of bladder cancer. Today BCG is the standard by which all treatments for superficial bladder cancer must be compared. Research in the use of BCG, as discussed in this text, has further improved the safety and efficacy of treatment.

References

1   Morales A, Eidinger D, Bruce AW. Intracavitary bacillus Calmette–Guérin in the treatment of superficial bladder tumors. *J Urol* 1976; **116**: 180–3.
2   Davies M. Bacillus Calmette–Guérin as an antitumor agent. The interaction with cells of the mammalian immune system. *Biochim Biophys Acta* 1982; **651**: 143–74.
3   Sosnowski JT, Lamm DL. Immunotherapy for bladder cancer. In: Rous SN (ed) *Urology Annual*. East Norwalk, Connecticut: Appleton & Lange, 1990; **4**: 123–56.
4   Haaff EO, Catalona WJ, Ratliff TL. Detection of interleukin 2 in the urine of patients with superficial bladder tumors after treatment with intravesical BCG. *J Urol* 1986; **136**: 970–2.
5   Morales A, Ottenhof PC. Clinical application of a whole blood assay for human natural killer (NK) cell activity. *Cancer* 1983; **52**: 667–70.
6   Ratliff TL, Gillen D, Catalona WJ. Requirement of a thymus dependent immune response for BCG-mediated antitumor activity. *J Urol* 1987; **137**: 155–8.
7   Ratliff TL, Hudson MA, Catalona WJ. Strategy for improving therapy of superficial bladder cancer. *World J Urol* 1991; **9**: 95–7.
8   Becich MJ, Carroll S, Ratliff TL. Internalization of bacille Calmette–Guérin by bladder tumor cells. *J Urol* 1991; **145**: 1316–24.
9   Kuroda K, Brown EJ, Telle WB, Ratliff TL. Characterization of the internalization of bacillus Calmette–Guérin by human bladder tumor cells. *J Clin Invest* 1993; **91**: 69–76.
10 Morales A, Nickel JC. Immunotherapy of superficial bladder cancer with BCG. *World J Urol* 1986; **3**: 209.
11 Garden RJ, Liu BCS, Redwood SM *et al.* Bacillus Calmette–Guérin abrogates *in vitro* invasion and motility of human bladder tumor cells via fibronectin interaction. *J Urol* 1992; **148**: 900–5.
12 De Boer EC, De Jong WH, Steerenberg PA *et al.* Induction of urinary interleukin-1 (IL-1), IL-2, IL-6, and tumor necrosis factor during intravesical immunotherapy with bacillus Calmette–Guérin in superficial bladder cancer. *Cancer Immunol Immunother* 1992; **34**: 306–12.
13 Schmidt AC, Bouic PJ, Heyns CF, De Kock ML. Peripheral blood lymphocyte response in patients with superficial transitional cell carcinoma of the bladder treated with intravesical bacillus Calmette–Guérin: a useful marker of response? *Br J Urol* 1993; **71**: 179–82.
14 Winters WD, Lamm DL. Antibody responses to bacillus Calmette–Guérin during immunotherapy in bladder cancer patients. *Cancer Res* 1981; **41**(7): 2672–76.
15 Lamm DL, Reichert FD, Harris SC, Lucio RM. Immunotherapy of murine transitional cell carcinoma. *J Urol* 1982; **128**(5): 1104–8.
16 Bast RC Jr, Zbar B, Borsos T *et al.* BCG and cancer 1. *N Engl J Med* 1974; **290**: 1413–15.
17 Corti Ortiz D, Rivera Garay P, Aviles Jasse J *et al.* Prophylaxis del cancer vesical superficial con 1 mg de BCG: comparación con otras dosis. *Actas Urol Esp* 1993; **17**: 239–42.
18 Ratliff TL, Kavoussi LR, Catlona WJ. Role of fibronectin in intravesical BCG therapy for superficial bladder cancer. *J Urol* 1988; **139**: 410–14.
19 Hudson MA, Yvan JJ, Catalona WJ *et al.* Adverse effect of fibrin clot inhibitors on intravesical bacillus Calmette–Guérin therapy for superficial bladder tumors. *J Urol* 1990; **144**: 1362–4.
20 Rogerson JW. Intravesical bacillus Calmette–Guérin in the treatment of superficial transitional cell carcinoma of the bladder. *Br J Urol* 1994; **73**: 655–8.

21 De Boer LC, Steerenberg PA, Van der Meijden PM *et al.* Impaired immune response by isoniazid treatment during intravesical BCG treatment in the guinea pig. *J Urol* 1992; **148**: 1577–82.

22 DeHaven JI, Traynelis CT, Riggs DR, Lamm DL. Antibiotic and steroid therapy of massive bacillus Calmette–Guérin (BCG) toxicity. *J Urol* 1992; **147**: 738–42.

23 Koukol SC, DeHaven JI, Riggs DR, Lamm DL. Drug therapy of systemic BCG sepsis. *Urol Res* 1995; **22**: 373–6.

CHAPTER 13

The use of biological modifiers in the treatment of superficial bladder cancer

J.M. Harris and M.F. Sarosdy

Introduction

The normal control of cell growth, differentiation, division, and death is dependent on a complex balance of production of growth factors, growth-factor receptors, inhibitors of growth (tumour suppressors), and regulators of programmed cell death (apoptosis). Increased production of growth factors or their receptors by gene amplification or transfection with their viral ancestors (oncogenes) results in uncontrolled cell proliferation and tumour formation, while loss of tumour suppressors produces the same result. Recently it has become clear that loss of apoptosis may play an important role in oncogenesis as well.

The causes of such alterations in gene production are multiple and include viral transfection, hereditary DNA deletion or translocation, and DNA mutations. Oncogenesis often follows an autosomal dominant pattern in that loss of both alleles is required for tumour formation. Knudsen first proposed the 'two hit hypothesis' in which the first hit can be an inherited defect, and the second hit is a post-gestational mutation. Post-gestational mutations are caused by radiation or chemicals known as carcinogens which damage DNA and result in loss of expression, or more frequently, expression of products which have lost normal function. Once an imbalance occurs and abnormal proliferation begins, growth may be held in check by elimination of the abnormal cells by the immune system. Natural killer cells and cytokines are produced in response to the abnormal cells and normally are helpful in causing cell death. Cancers can cause a relative immune deficiency and reduce the effectiveness of this system.

Early attempts to eradicate cancers used chemicals which target and kill rapidly dividing cells. Since this was non-specific, rapidly dividing normal cells were targetted as well, and resulting toxicity frequently limited doses and therefore their efficacy. A better understanding of the molecular mechanisms of tumour formation and elimination has allowed us to attack the biological systems at the molecular level to eradicate tumours. Biological modification can be directed at the restoration of the balance of gene expression of growth factors and tumour suppressors through gene therapy. Carcinogens can be eliminated or neutralized by anti-oxidants. And finally, immunostimulants can be employed to intensify the immune response to tumours and improve its ability to kill cancer cells. All of these techniques are being employed in the treatment of recurrent superficial bladder cancer, and will likely become the mainstay in the treatment of this common malignancy.

Immunotherapy

Since the initial report of Morales *et al.* [1], the primary means of immunotherapy for the last 20 years has been the use of intracavitary bacillus Calmette–Guérin (BCG). The principles of immunomodulation of BCG deserve mention, as they may serve as a template for other immunological agents. Ratliff *et al.* [2] showed that direct contact of the bacillus with binding to the fibronectin receptor is required to evoke the immune response. It was further shown that heat-killed bacilli were just as effective as live bacilli, and that bacilli bind selectively to tumour cells [3]. An intact T-cell system has also been shown to be required with subtypes CD3, CD4, CD8, and CD56 being involved [4–7]. A multitude of cytokines including interleukin-2 (IL-2), interleukin-6 (IL-6), interleukin-8 (IL-8), tumour necrosis factor (TNF), and interferon-gamma (INF-γ) have been implicated in the tumoricidal response illicited by BCG [8–13].

Bropirimine

Bropirimine (2-amino-5-bromo-6-phenyl-4-(3H)-pyrimidinone) is an orally active immunomodulator which increases endogenous interferon-alpha (IFN-α) and other cytokines. It also activates several cell-mediated immunological defence mechanisms, producing a wide array of antitumour, antiviral, and immunomodulatory effects [14–17]. Cell-mediated cytotoxicity has been demonstrated by blocking studies to involve both natural killer cells as well as macrophages. Since it is active when given orally, it has the potential to treat upper tract as well as metastatic tumours. Initial animal studies revealed limited activity as a single agent in murine tumours [18,19], but it appeared to have synergistic activity when combined with BCG [20]. As a result of this activity, a Phase I trial was performed in patients with either marker papillary tumours or residual carcinoma *in situ* (CIS) [21]. Five of 11 patients with CIS experienced a complete response, including four of six patients receiving a dose of at least 3 g a day for three consecutive days repeated weekly for 12 weeks. There was less activity against papillary tumours, with only one showing complete regression and this was at the highest dose used (5.25 g).

A confirmatory Phase II trial was then performed in patients having CIS, with positive cytology still present after biopsy, initially using 4.5 g a day for three consecutive days and repeated weekly [22]. This study was closed well before meeting its accrual goal due to toxicity. Forty-two patients with biopsy- and cytology-proven CIS were then enrolled at a dose of 3.0 g/day. At this lower dose, toxicity was acceptable, with only 2 of 42 patients (4%) having Grade 3 or higher toxicity, and 15 of 42 (36%) having no toxicity at all. Only 1 of 42 patients (2%) dropped because of toxicity. Twenty of 33 evaluable patients (61%) converted bladder-wash cytology and biopsies to negative, including 6 of 12 (50%) who failed previous BCG and 14 of 21 (67%) who had not received prior BCG. No large difference was seen between patients with multifocal (13 of 25 or 52% responded) versus unifocal (6 of 8 or 75% responded). However, a large difference that approached but did not achieve statistical significance was seen with responses in 12 of 15 (80%) patients with primary CIS compared to 8 of 18 (44%) with secondary CIS ($p = 0.08$, Chi-square).

A possible advantage of bropirimine as an oral systemic agent is potential activity in the upper tracts. This was evaluated in a recently completed multi-centre trial [23]. To be eligible, patients were required to have positive upper-tract cytologies and negative retrograde pyeloureterograms. Twenty-four patients were enrolled and 21 were evaluable for efficacy. Among the 21, 10 demonstrated conversion of positive cytology to negative. Five did so after 12 weeks of treatment, and five more after an additional 12 weeks of treatment. Among the non-responders, six stopped the drug after 12 weeks, and five continued for between 6 and 12 months without response. Of the responders, only two reverted back to positive cytology, one after 24 weeks, and the other after 48 weeks, with the median duration of response not yet reached but in excess of 9 months.

Other trials underway include a Phase II trial in patients with BCG-failed CIS and a Phase III trial comparing oral bropirimine to intravesical BCG in newly diagnosed CIS. A Phase II trial combining oral bropirimine with intravesical BCG is also in progress in the Southwest Oncology Group. It is anticipated that future trials evaluating bropirimine in tumour-recurrence prophylaxis and in patients with metastatic disease will open soon [24].

Keyhole limpet haemocyanin

Keyhole limpet haemocyanin (KLH) is a protein of the mollusk *Megathura crenulata*, and as a highly immunogenic protein, has been used for many years as an experimental antigen in the study of delayed-type hypersensitivity. It has been known to possess anti-tumour activity in superficial bladder cancer for years, yet it has not been submitted to a multicentre trial and only recently has been studied in animal models. Olsson first noted a marked reduction in papillary tumour recurrence among patients that were immunized with subcutaneous KLH to test immunological responsiveness [25]. A small prospective trial was then performed and confirmed this apparent anti-tumour effect of KLH, with minimal adverse effects [26]. In a later study, Jurincic *et al.* [27] compared combination intradermal and intravesical KLH (1 mg and 10 mg) to 20 mg of intravesical Mitomycin C for tumour prophylaxis [27]. Superficial tumours recurred in only 3 of 21 patients (14%) in the KLH arm, compared to 9 of 23 patients (39%) who received Mitomycin C ($p < 0.07$).

KLH efficacy in animal bladder-cancer models has been studied recently. Lamm *et al.* showed that both crude KLH and Immucothel, a KLH antigen modified for clinical use, had good activity when injected into MBT2 tumour implants [28,29]. The crude KLH required immunization prior to tumour implantation. Swerdlow *et al.*, using the murine intravesical model MB-49, showed that a KLH preparation (KLH Immune Activator) resulted in decreased tumour growth [30]. Dosages of 10 μg and 100 μg were given intravesically on days 1, 4, 7, 14, and 21, and a prior immunization was required before activity was seen. A simultaneous toxicity study was performed using 4 mg/kg and 40 mg/kg and no toxicity was noted.

More recently, KLH has been shown to have activity in the prevention of recurrent tumours associated with schistosomal infestation [31]. KLH has antigens similar to schistosomal antigens, and thus was chosen as a candidate to treat these unique bladder tumours. KLH immunotherapy reduced the recurrence rate of superficial bladder tumours, in patients with Ta, Tis, T1 tumours, to 15.4% compared to 76.9% before therapy. A prospective randomized trial comparing intracavitary KLH versus intracavitary ethoglucide was performed to test the efficacy of prevention of tumour recurrence [32]. The KLH patients received a subcutaneous, 1 mg, dose of KLH and were then given KLH, 30 mg, intracavitary weekly for 6 weeks and then monthly for a year. There was no difference between the two groups in time to recurrence, number of recurrences, or progression of disease.

It is clear that KLH possesses activity against superficial bladder tumours with very minimal toxicity. The optimal dosage and route of delivery are not known and need to be determined in a dose–response study. The efficacy of KLH also needs to be determined through large multi-centre trials. These studies are not currently underway. Also, relative lack of availability of KLH has been cited as one problem.

Interferon

Interferons are naturally occurring glycoproteins with anti-viral and anti-proliferative properties, and have proven to be very safe in the treatment of superficial bladder cancers. Toxicities have been limited to mild flu-like symptoms which resolve with cessation of therapy. The IFN which has the most activity in bladder cancer is IFN-α, which acts primarily through the stimulation of natural killer cells. IFN-β and IFN-γ have been used in small Phase I trials but have shown only limited activity [33,34]. Christophersen *et al.* first reported on the successful treatment of superficial bladder cancer using intramuscular injections of recombinant IFN-α2b [35] (Table 13.1). Ikic *et al.* then reported that direct injections of recombinant IFN-α2b into tumours daily for 3 weeks resulted in complete regression of tumour in four of eight patients [36].

Table 13.1 *Phase I–II* studies of interferon-alpha (IFN-α).

Principal investigator	IFN & source	Regimen	Number of patients (tumour)	Response
Christophersen *et al.* [35]	Leukocyte IFN-α	4.0×10^6 U IM qd × 2 months, then TIW	3	3/3 PR
Ikic *et al.* [36]	Leukocyte IFN-α	4.0×10^6 U intralesional qd × 21 days	8	4/8 CR
Oliver *et al.* [38]	Lymphoblastoid IFN-α	50×10^6 U intravesical q week 8	8 (Ta) 8 (Tis)	3/8 PR 3/8 CR 0/8
Torti *et al.* [39]	Recombinant IFN-α	$50–1000 \times 10^6$ U intravesical q week × 8	16 (Ta, T1) 19 (Tis)	4/16 CR 6/17 CR
Glashan [40]	Recombinant IFN-α	10 MU or 100 MU intravesical q week × 12 then q month × 12	38 (Tis) low dose 47 (Tis) high dose	2/38 CR 20/43 CR

Table 13.2 Properties of cytokines stimulated by BCG.

Cytokine	Source	Effect
Interleukin-2	Activated TH1 cells	Activates NK cells
		Activates LAK cells
Interleukin-6	Activated TH2 cells	T-cell stimulant
Interleukin-8	Macrophages	Chemoattractant
TNF	Macrophages	Tumour necrosis
		Vascular thrombosis
Interferon-α	NK cells	Antiviral
		Anti-tumour

Abbreviations: LAK, lymphokine-activated killer; NK, natural killer; TNF, tumour necrosis factor.

Intralesional injection is not practical, and is not even feasible for CIS or multiple tumours, so the efficacy of intravesical therapy was assessed by Shortliffe *et al.* [37]. They reported resolution of CIS in four of eight patients who received doses ranging from 50–200 million units of IFN-α weekly for 8 weeks. Oliver *et al.* used intravesical lymphoblastoid IFN-α to treat eight patients with CIS and eight patients with papillary tumours [38]. There were no responses in the CIS group, but there were three complete regressions and three partial regressions in the papillary group. Torti *et al.* reported a Phase I/II trial of the Northern California Oncology Group using intravesical recombinant IFN-α-2b at dosages ranging from 50 million to 1 billion units weekly for 8 weeks [39]. Complete resolution of CIS was seen in 6 of 17 patients (32%) and resolution of marker papillary tumours occurred in 4 of 16 patients.

As a result of this recognized activity, a large multi-centre Phase III trial was undertaken comparing intravesical administration of 10 million units of recombinant IFN-α-2b to 100 million units in patients with biopsy-proven CIS and positive cytologies [40]. Complete resolution was seen in 20 of 47 (47%) patients at the higher dose, compared to only 2 of 38 (5%) patients at the lower dose. In addition, five of the patients receiving the higher dose had previously failed BCG, and two of these had complete responses.

Preliminary studies of IFN-α-2b for prophylaxis of recurrent papillary tumours have also been reported. In a European study, Boccardo *et al.* compared intracavitary recombinant IFN-α-2b to Mitomycin C for tumour-recurrence prophylaxis [41]. Patients were randomized to receive either 50 million units of recombinant IFN-α-2b or 40 mg of mitomycin weekly for 8 weeks. Mitomycin proved to be more effective in terms of time to first recurrence and recurrence rate. Whether this was because the IFN dose was inadequate cannot be known. Da Silva *et al.* reported a Phase II study of intravesical IFN-α-2b in the treatment of patients with recurrent superficial papillary tumours, comparing a 60 million-unit dose to a 100 million-unit dose [42]. Each was given weekly for 8 weeks, and then twice a month for 4 months, and then monthly for 6 months. Toxicity was minimal, and there was no difference in recurrence rates between the two groups; 26 of 64 (40%) had recurrence in the low-dose group compared to 21 of 63 (33%) in the high-dose group. However, since there was no control group, nor a group given BCG, the efficacy of the therapy is not clearly known.

The exact role for recombinant IFN-α-2b is not clear. It is now commercially available (Intron), and is reimbursed by Medicare in many states, but it is very expensive. It is also unknown if a dosage lower than 100 million units (but higher than 10 million units) would have similar efficacy, and studies to determine this are needed. For now, it seems reasonable to use Intron in the treatment of BCG-failed CIS, as a potential alternative to cystectomy in selected patients.

Miscellaneous immunomodulators

Several small studies have evaluated IL-2 in the treatment of superficial bladder cancer. IL-2 is a T-cell growth factor produced by certain T cells and it induces the proliferation of a variety of subsets of T cells with tumoricidal activity. Early studies utilized cumbersome intralesional injections [43]. Gomella *et al.* reported a pilot study in which 14 patients with Ta, T1, or Tis tumours were given weekly intravesical treatment of 12 million units of recombinant IL-2 (rIL-2) for 8 weeks [44]. Three of 14 patients (21%) had complete responses with durations of 3 to greater than 9 months. All of these patients had failed prior intravesical therapy, and toxicity was minimal. Schwaibold *et al.* gave continuous infusion and intermittent high-dose IL-2 to patients with advanced local disease, not eligible for standard therapy, to assess toxicity and found it to be minimal [45]. This suggests that systemic IL-2 may be a safe regimen for evaluation in prevention of papillary recurrence, but efficacy reports have not been published.

Intravesical recombinant TNF (rTNF) has recently been evaluated in a small, single institution, Phase I trial by Grampsas *et al.* involving patients with refractory superficial bladder cancer [46]. Sixteen patients were given intravesical rTNF twice a week for 4 weeks at doses ranging from 10 to 500 $\mu g/m^2$. Only minimal toxicities were noted and no maximum dose was determined as toxicities were not increased even at the maximum dosage. There were two complete responders and nine partial responders, and only one patient had progressive disease.

Numerous combinations of immunomodulators have been anecdotally reported in the management of superficial bladder cancer. Sosnowski *et al.* evaluated the anti-tumour effects of rIL-2 alone and in combination with rIFN-γ and found them both to be effective [47]. Ikemoto *et al.* evaluated IL-2 and BCG in the treatment of TCC using the MBT2 murine model and found that IL-2 and BCG in combination were superior to either therapy alone [48]. However, Phase II trials of adequate size have not been

Table 13.3 Types of interferons (IFNs).

Name	Other terms	Cell source	Effects
IFN-α	Leukocyte interferon	Macrophage	Antiviral, activates
	Type-1 IFN	D-cells	NK cells
IFN-β	Leukocyte interferon	Somatic cells	Antiviral, activates
	Type-1 IFN		NK cells
IFN-γ	Immune interferon	TH1 cells	Antiviral, activates
	Type-II IFN	NK cells	NK cells

Abbreviations: NK, natural killer.

reported, nor have any Phase III trials comparing combinations to single-agent therapy been attempted. Thus, there is currently no justification for use of combination immunotherapies in patients unless it is part of a clinical trial.

Modifiers of carcinogens

Although more useful in prevention of carcinoma, anti-oxidants deserve mention as they are in essence a form of biological modifier. Specifically, certain vitamins have been shown to reduce the levels of carcinogens in urine as a result of free oxygen radical scavenging [49]. Lamm *et al.* evaluated a preparation which contains high doses of vitamin A, C, E, B6, and zinc in combination with BCG compared to BCG and recommended daily allowances (RDA) of the same vitamins [50]. They found a marked reduction in tumour recurrence in the megadose group. A valid criticism of the report was the failure to explain a very high recurrence rate in the BCG plus RDA controls compared to historical controls with BCG alone. Further study of chemoprevention of tumours in patients with first-time tumours is warranted, but is thus far not underway.

Gene therapy and other new agents

A new era of biological therapy is emerging and includes genetically engineered proteins, genetically engineered BCG, and gene-replacement therapy. Most of these have not been applied in clinical trials, but this is not very far away.

Gene-replacement therapy holds great promise for the treatment of all malignancies, but the bladder stands poised as the first to benefit because of its ease of accessibility and large surface area for prolonged contact with gene vectors. The feasibility of gene therapy has been documented in studies by Morris *et al.* [51], using an adenovirus as a vector. Transfection and gene expression was confirmed in their rat model. Abnormalities in the *p53* and *Rb* tumour-suppressor genes have been identified in bladder cancer, and gene replacement of these defective genes will be a part of clinical trials soon [52]. Epidermal growth factor (EGF) receptors have been shown to be increased in bladder cancer [53,54] and can perhaps be a target for gene-'knockout' therapy. Hiura *et al.* [55] recently transfected the IFN-γ gene into MBT-2 murine cell line and rendered it non-tumourogenic.

Genetically engineered proteins have already been tested in a Phase I clinical trial. The engineered protein TP-40 is the receptor binding fragment of transforming growth factor-α (TGF-α) fused to the *Pseudomonas* exotoxin PE-40 [56]. The protein binds to EGF receptors which are much more dense on malignant transitional cells, and the toxin is then internalized, leaving normal cells unharmed. This fusion protein was found to be highly effective *in vitro* [57], so TP-40 was used in a Phase I trial [58]. The protein was given in escalating doses to a total of 43 patients. Although it had no apparent tumoricidal activity in papillary tumours, it converted cytologies to negative in two and produced partial responses in six of nine evaluable patients with CIS. No dose-related toxicities were noted, with all toxicities related to vesical irritability.

Genetic manipulation of BCG is a novel approach recently attempted by O'Donnell *et al.* [59]. The gene coding for murine IL-2 was transfected into BCG under the control of the BCG HSP60 promoter and was found to secrete the murine IL-2. The genetically engineered BCG was found to increase production of IFN-γ when exposed to mouse splenocytes. Obviously, other cytokine genes can be transfected using this technique, providing a novel means of delivering cytokines to superficial bladder cancers.

Conclusions

Biological modifiers now play a key role in the management of patients with superficial bladder cancer. With the explosion of molecular biological research, the use of biological modifiers will only increase. Future modifiers may not only have better efficacy, but perhaps more importantly, will be less toxic to patients. The continued willingness of all urologists to enrol patients into statistically valid clinical trials, as these new agents arrive on the scene, is critical to improve our management of superficial bladder cancer.

References

1   Morales A, Eidinger D, Bruce AW. Intracavitary bacillus Calmette–Guérin in the treatment of superficial bladder tumors. *J Urol* 1976; **116**: 180–3.
2   Ratliff TL, Kavoussi LR, Catalona WJ. Role of fibronectin in intravesical BCG therapy for superficial bladder cancer. *J Urol* 1988; **139**: 410–14.
3   Schneider B, Thanhauser A, Jocham D *et al.* Specific binding of bacillus Calmette–Guérin to urothelial tumor cells *in vitro. World J Urol* 1994; **12**(6): 337–44.
4   Ratliff TL, Gillen D, Catalona WJ. Requirement of a thymus dependent immune response for BCG-mediated antitumor activity. *J Urol* 1987; **137**: 155–8.
5   Prescott S, James K, Hargreave TB *et al.* Intravesical Evans Strain BCG therapy: quantitative immunohistochemical analysis of the immune response within the bladder wall. *J Urol* 1992; **147**: 1636–42.
6   Ratliff TL, Ritchey JK, Yuan JJJ *et al.* T-cell subsets required for intravesical BCG immunotherapy for bladder cancer. *J Urol* 1993; **150**: 1018–23.
7   Bohle A, Thanhauser A, Ulmer AJ *et al.* On the mode of action of intravesical bacillus Calmette–Guérin: *in vitro* characterization of BCG-activated killer cells. *Urol Res* 1994; **22**(3): 185–90.
8   Stassar MJ, Vegt PD, Steerenberg PA *et al.* Effects of isoniazid (INH) on the BCG-induced local immune response after intravesical BCG therapy for superficial bladder cancer. *Urol Res* 1994; **22**(3): 177–84.
9   Thanhauser A, Reiling N, Bohle A *et al.* Pentoxifylline: a potent inhibitor of IL-2 and IFN-gamma biosynthesis and BCG-induced cytotoxicity. *Immunology* 1993; **80**(1): 151–6.
10 Huygen K, Vandenbussche P and Heremans H. Interleukin-6 production in *Mycobacterium bovis* BCG-infected mice. *Cell Immunol* 1991; **137**(1): 224–31.
11 Kurisu H, Matsuyama H, Ohmoto Y, Shimabukuro T, Naito K. Cytokine-mediated antitumor effect of bacillus Calmette–Guérin on tumor cells *in vitro. Cancer Immunol Immunother* 1994; **39**: 249–53.
12 Saito F, Takashima T, Sonchoru O, Fukushi M, Suzuki T. A study of the mechanism of action of BCG against transitional cell carcinoma of the bladder — the change of TNF-alpha and IL-2 in the serum and urine. *Nippon Hinyokika Gakkai Zasshi* 1994; **85**(3): 466–72.
13 Esuvaranathan K, Alexandroff AB, McIntyre M *et al.* Interleukin-6 production by bladder tumors is upregulated by BCG immunotherapy. *J Urol* 1995; **154**: 572–5.
14 Wierenga W. Antiviral and other bioactivities of pyrimidinones. *Pharmacol Ther* 1985; **30**: 67–89.
15 Lotzova E, Savary CA, Stringfellow DA. 5-Halo-6-phenyl-pyrimidinones: New molecules with cancer chemotherapeutic potential and interferon-inducing capacity are strong inducers of murine natural killer cells. *J Immunol* 1983; **130**: 965–9.
16 Lotzova E, Savary CA, Khan A, Stringfellow DA. Stimulation of natural killer cells in two random-bred strains of athymic rats by interferon-inducing pyrimidinone. *J Immunol* 1984; **132**: 2566–70.

17 Tracey DE, Richard KA. Mechanisms of immunostimulation by pyrimidinones. In: *Immunopharmacology of infectious diseases: vaccine adjuvants and modulators of nonspecific resistance*. New York: Alan R. Liss, Inc., 1987, pp. 279–89.

18 Simmons WB, Reichert DF, Lucion RM *et al*. Pyrimidinone interferon inducers in the treatment of murine transitional cell carcinoma. *J Urol* 1983; **129**: 169A.

19 Sidky YA, Borden EC, Wierenga W *et al*. Inhibitory effects of interferon-inducing pyrimidinones on the growth of transplantable mouse bladder tumors. *Cancer Res* 1986; **46**: 3798–802.

20 Sarosdy MF, Kierum CA. Combination immunotherapy of murine transitional cell carcinoma using BCG and an interferon-inducing pyrimidinone. *J Urol* 1989; **142**: 1376–9.

21 Sarosdy MF, Lamm DL, Williams RD *et al*. Phase I trial of oral bropirimine in superficial bladder cancer. *J Urol* 1992; **147**: 31–3.

22 Sarosdy MF, Lowe BA, Schellhammer PF *et al*. Oral bropirimine immunotherapy is active in carcinoma *in situ* of the bladder: results of a Phase II trial. *Urol* 1996; **48**: 21–7.

23 Sarosdy MF, Pisters LL, Carroll PR *et al*. Bropirimine immunotherapy of upper urinary tract carcinoma *in situ*. *Urol* 1996; **48**: 28–32.

24 Sarosdy MF. Immunotherapy of superficial bladder carcinoma, AUA Update Series, Lesson 29 1995; **XIV**: 234–9.

25 Olsson C, Rao C, Menzoian J *et al*. Immunologic unreactivity in bladder cancer patients. *J Urol* 1972; **107**: 607.

26 Olsson C, Chute R, Rao C. Immunologic reduction of bladder cancer recurrence rate. *J Urol* 1974; **111**: 173.

27 Jurincic CD, Engelman V, Gasch J *et al*. Immunotherapy in bladder cancer with keyhole-limpet hemocyanin: a randomized study. *J Urol* 1988; **139**: 723.

28 Lamm DL, DeHaven JI, Riggs DR, Delgra C, Burrell R. Keyhole limpet hemocyanin immunotherapy of murine bladder cancer. *Urol Res* 1993; **21**(1): 33–7.

29 Lamm DL, DeHaven JI, Riggs DR, Ebert RF. Immunotherapy of murine bladder cancer with keyhole-limpet hemocyanin (KLH). *J Urol* 1993; **149**(3): 648–52.

30 Swerdlow RD, Ratliff TL, La Regina M, Ritchey JK, Ebert RF. Immunotherapy with keyhole limpet hemocyanin: Efficacy and safety in the MB-49 intravesical murine bladder tumor model. *J Urol* 1994; **151**(6): 1718–22.

31 Wishahi MM, Ismail IM, Ruebben H, Otto T. Keyhole-limpet hemocyanin immunotherapy in the bilharzial bladder: a new treatment modality? Phase II trial: superficial bladder cancer. *J Urol* 1995; **153**: 926–8.

32 Flamm J, Donner G, Bucher A *et al*. Topical immunotherapy (KLH) vs. chemotherapy (Ethoglucid) in prevention of recurrence of superficial bladder cancer. A prospective randomized study. *Urologe A* 1994; **33**(2): 138–43.

33 Forni G, Giovarelli M, Jemma C *et al*. Perilymphatic injections of cytokines: a new tool in active cancer immunotherapy: experimental rationale and clinical findings. *Ann First Super Sanita* 1990; **26**: 3–4.

34 Niijima T. Intravesical treatment of bladder cancer with recombinant human interferon-β. *Cancer Immunol Immunother* 1989; **30**: 81–5.

35 Christophersen IS *et al*. Interferon therapy in neoplastic disease. *Acta Med Scand* 1978; **204**: 471–6.

36 Ikic D *et al*. Application of human leukocyte interferon in patients with urinary bladder papillomatosis, breast cancer, and melanoma. *Lancet* 1981; **1**: 1022–4.

37 Shortliffe LC *et al*. Intravesical interferon therapy for carcinoma *in situ* and transitional cell carcinoma of the bladder. *J Urol* 1984; **131**: 171.

38 Oliver R, Waxman J, Kwok H *et al*. Alpha lymphoblastoid interferon for non-invasive bladder cancer. *Br J Cancer* 1986; **53**: 432.

39 Torti FM *et al*. Alpha-interferon in superficial bladder cancer: a northern California oncology group study. *J Clin Oncol* 1988; **6**: 475.

40 Glashan R. A randomized controlled study of intravesical α-2b-interferon in carcinoma *in situ* of the bladder. *J Urol* 1990; **144**: 658–61.

41 Boccardo F, Cannata D, Rubagotti A *et al*. Prophylaxis of superficial bladder cancer with mitomycin or interferon alfa-2b: results of a multicentric Italian study. *J Clin Oncol* 1994; **12**(1): 7–13.

42 Da Silva FC. Interferon alpha 2b 60 Millions vs 100 Millions in intravesical prophylaxis of superficial bladder cancer. *J Urol* 1993; **149**: 282A.

43 Pizza G, Severini G, Menniti D *et al*. Tumour regression after intralesional injection of interleukin 2 (IL-2) in bladder cancer: preliminary report. *Int J Cancer* 1984; **34**: 359–67.

44 Gomella LG, McGinnis DE, Lattime EC *et al*. Treatment of transitional cell carcinoma of the bladder with intravesical interleukin-2: a pilot study. *Cancer Biother* 1993; **8**(3): 223–7.

45 Schwaibold H, Huland E, Heinzer H *et al.* Toxicity of local, continuous and cyclic, high-dose bladder perfusion with recombinant and natural interleukin-2 in advanced cancer of the urinary bladder. *J Cancer Res Clin Oncol* 1995; **121**(4): 239–46.

46 Grampsas SA, Kahm K, Crawford ED. Intravesical RTNF therapy of superficial bladder cancer. A phase I study of recombinant tumor necrosis factor administered intravesically to patients with superficial bladder cancer. *J Curr Clin Trials* 1994; **3**:

47 Sosnowski J, DeHaven J, Riggs D *et al.* Treatment of murine transitional cell carcinoma with intralesional interleukin 2 and murine interferon gamma. *J Urol* 1991; **146**: 1164–7.

48 Ikemoto S, Kamizuru M, Wada S *et al.* Combined effect of interleukin-2 and bacillus Calmette–Guérin in the therapy of mice with transitional cell carcinoma. *Urol Int* 1991; **47**(4): 250–4.

49 Mirvish SS, Wallcave L, Eagen M, Shubik P. Ascorbate–nitrate reaction: possible means of blocking the formation of carcinogenic N-nitroso compounds. *Science* 1972; **177**: 65–8.

50 Lamm DL, Riggs DR, Shriver JS *et al.* Megadose vitamins in bladder cancer: a double-blind clinical trial. *J Urol* 1994; **151**(1): 21–6.

51 Morris Jr, BD, Drazan KE, Csete ME *et al.* Adenoviral-mediated gene transfer to bladder *in vivo. J Urol* 1994; **152**: 506–9.

52 Griffin KP, Segura L, Kan N *et al.* The effects on proliferation, metabolism and tumorigenicity of MBT-2 using a retroviral vector human wild type *p53* gene. *J Urol* 1988; **139**: 723.

53 Neal D, Bennet M, Hall R *et al.* Epidermal-growth-factor receptors in human bladder cancer: Comparison of invasive and superficial tumors. *Lancet* 1985; **1**: 366–8.

54 Messing EM. Clinical implications of the expression of epidermal growth factor receptors in human transitional cell carcinoma. *Cancer Res* 1990; **50**: 2530–7.

55 Hiura M, Hashimura T, Watanabe Y, Kuribayashi K, Yoshida O. Induction of specific anti-tumor immunity by interferon-gamma gene-transferred murine bladder carcinoma MBT-2. *Folia Biol* 1994; **40**: 49–61.

56 Siegall CB, Xu Y, Chaudhary V *et al.* Cytotoxic activities of a fusion protein compromised of TGF-α *Pseudomonas* exotoxin. *FASEB* 1989; **3**: 2647–52.

57 Sarosdy MF, Hutzler DH, Yee D *et al. In vitro* sensitivity testing of human bladder cancers and cell lines to TP40: a hybrid protein with selective targeting and cytotoxicity. *J Urol* 1993; **150**: 1950–5.

58 Goldberg MR, Heimbrook DC, Russo P *et al.* Phase I clinical study of the recombinant oncotoxin TP40 in superficial bladder cancer. *Clin Cancer Res* 1995; **1**: 57–61.

59 O'Donnell MA, Aldovini A, Duda RB *et al.* Recombinant *Mycobacterium bovis* BCG secreting functional interleukin-2 enhances gamma interferon production by splenocytes. *Infect Immun* 1994; **62**(6): 2508–14.

CHAPTER 14

Intravesical chemotherapy versus immunotherapy

D.L. Lamm

Introduction

The goals of intravesical therapy, eradication of carcinoma *in situ* (CIS) or residual stage Ta or T1 transitional-cell carcinoma, prevention of tumour recurrence, disease progression and patient mortality, are generally the same whether we select chemotherapy or immunotherapy. The mechanisms of action of these treatments and the expected results are in some instances quite different. Consideration of the differences in chemotherapy and bacillus Calmette–Guérin (BCG) immunotherapy will facilitate selection of the best treatment for individual patients.

Mechanisms of action

Most of the commonly used intravesical chemotherapies, such as mitomycin, thiotepa, and epodyl, are alkylating agents. Doxorubicin and epirubicin are intercalating agents and inhibitors of topoisomerase II [1]. When a patient fails one intravesical chemotherapy it would seem reasonable to select an alternative treatment with a different mechanism of action to reduce the chance of shared resistance, but this principle has not been demonstrated in intravesical chemotherapy trials. Resistance to one intravesical chemotherapy does increase resistance to others. Fortunately, the mechanism of action of BCG immunotherapy is completely different from that of intravesical chemotherapy and cross resistance has not been demonstrated.

The mechanism of action of BCG is complex, as might be expected considering BCG is a living organism rather than a defined molecule. Stimulation of cellular immunity or the TH1 type response is thought to be the most important aspect of BCG's action. Following intravesical BCG instillation an increase in urinary IL-1, IL-2, IL-6, IL-8, IL-10, IL-12, tumour necrosis factor-alpha (INF-α), interferon-alpha (IFN-α), and interferon-gamma (IFN-γ) is seen. BCG stimulates natural killer cells, helper and cytotoxic T cells and lymphokine-activated killer (LAK) cells as a newly described cytotoxic cell termed the 'BCG activated killer' (BAK) cell [2]. Biopsy of bladders after BCG shows increased cellular infiltration with granuloma and lymphocytes and an increase in helper/suppressor ratio, CD25 positive cells, and expression of HLA DR antigen. Functionally, BCG stimulates phagocytosis by macrophages, urothelial cells and tumour cells, and decreases tumour-cell motility.

The differing mechanisms of action of chemotherapy and BCG immunotherapy result in contrasting results and expectations of treatment. Cytotoxic chemotherapy kills tumour cells directly within a short period of time. A single instillation of chemotherapy may be sufficient to prevent attachment and growth of malignant cells following tumour resection. Tumour destruction by BCG depends on the induction of an immune response in the host, and several weekly BCG treatments, generally six initially and three subsequently, are required to induce the maximal response. Therefore, a single early post-operative instillation of chemotherapy would be expected to produce an excellent and prompt response in patients with microscopic residual disease. In contrast, early post-operative BCG administration is found to greatly increase treatment toxicity without increasing efficacy.

Early post-operative BCG treatment should be strictly avoided. Complete response to BCG treatment often does not occur until the sixth week after completion of instillations and in patients with CIS complete response has been observed to take up to 6 months to occur.

Side-effects

Intravesical chemotherapy is generally associated with relatively few side-effects, especially when single instillations or short courses are used. Irritative bladder symptoms are common, particularly with doxorubicin, but with high molecular weight compounds such as doxorubicin, systemic absorption and side-effects are rare. Myelosuppression, which can occur with thiotepa or mitomycin, can be avoided by checking a blood count prior to administration. Serious and even fatal reactions to intravesical alkylating agents have been reported, but should be preventable by such monitoring and limiting dose.

BCG immunotherapy produces local irritative bladder symptoms more frequently than most chemotherapies. Mild to moderate dysuria, for example, was found in 52% of patients given 50 mg of BCG monthly compared with 36% of patients given 20 mg of mitomycin monthly in the Southwest Oncology Group randomized comparison [3]. Systemic symptoms, as exemplified by fever, occur much more frequently with BCG (17% versus 3.6% for mitomycin in the SWOG study). Minor symptoms such as dysuria and low-grade fever are related to the immune stimulation induced by BCG, and are actually correlated with an improved anti-tumour response. Serious side-effects are fortunately rare. The most serious side-effect, systemic BCG sepsis/hypersensitivity, is thought to result from intravenous absorption. About 10 fatalities are temporally related to BCG administration, most from the early years when the importance of avoiding intravasation of BCG was not appreciated. The side-effects of BCG have been overemphasized in many instances, but the remote potential for serious toxicity is real. BCG is therefore generally limited to patients at risk for disease progression and those with lower risk tumours who have failed chemotherapy prophylaxis.

Carcinoma *in situ* (CIS)

In the United States, BCG immunotherapy is the only Food and Drug Administration-approved intravesical treatment for CIS. Response rates reported with other treatments are generally lower, and the Southwest Oncology Group (SWOG) randomized comparison revealed complete-response rates of 70% for BCG and 34% for doxorubicin ($p < 0.001$), with overall 5-year estimates of remaining disease-free of 45% and 18%, respectively ($p = 0.015$) [4]. Reported complete-response rates for commonly used intravesical treatments for CIS are listed in Table 14.1 and average 34% for thiotepa, 48% for doxorubicin, 53% for mitomycin and 72% for BCG. Mitomycin was found to have a statistically significant increased response relative to thiotepa, but not doxorubicin. IFN-2b had a complete-response rate of 47% in patients who received doses of 50 million units or more. The efficacy of interferon immunotherapy in CIS compares favourably with chemotherapy, but appears to be less than that of BCG. BCG complete-response rates are significantly higher than all other reported intravesical therapies [5].

Table 14.1 Complete response in CIS.

	Series	CR/total	% CR
Chemotherapy			
Thiotepa	4	34/89	38
Doxorubicin	8	101/212	48
Mitomycin	14	78/147	53
Immunotherapy			
Interferon-α	2	29/62	47
BCG	34	975/1354	72

Abbreviations: CR, complete response.
Reference: Lamm DL, Torti FM. Bladder cancer 1996. *CA Cancer J Clin* 1996; **46**: 93–112.

Superficial bladder cancer prophylaxis

Intravesical therapy is much more commonly used to prevent tumour recurrence than treat CIS because only 10% of patients with bladder cancer have CIS. Comparison of the results of intravesical chemotherapy and BCG immunotherapy versus surgery alone reveals that thiotepa, doxorubicin, mitomycin, epodyl, and epirubicin clearly reduce tumour recurrence, but not to the extent reported with BCG [6]. Results of controlled prophylaxis trials are illustrated in Table 14.2 and 14.3. Average reduction in tumour recurrence is 12% for thiotepa, 15% for doxorubicin, 9% for mitomycin, 31% for epodyl, 12% for epirubicin, and 42% for BCG. Studies of the long-term effect of intravesical prophylaxis suggest that the benefit of intravesical therapy is of 2–3 years duration, while the benefit of BCG persists for 5 or more years. Unfortunately, attempts to prolong the benefit of chemotherapy with maintenance treatments have been unsuccessful.

Table 14.2 Effect of intravesical chemotherapy on recurrence in controlled studies.

| Source | Total number | Control (TURBT) | | Chemotherapy | | | |
		Control (N)	Recurred (N) (%)	Treated (N)	Recurred (N) (%)	Difference % recurred	p value
Thiotepa							
Burnand	51	32	31 (97%)	19	11 (58%)	39	0.001
Byar & Blackar	86	48	29 (60%)	38	18 (47%)	13	0.016
Nocks	42	22	14 (64%)	20	13 (65%)	−1	n.s.
Asahi	134	56	23 (41%)	78	31 (40%)	1	n.s.
Schulman	209	104	72 (69%)	105	62 (59%)	10	n.s.
Koontz	93	47	31 (66%)	46	18 (39%)	27	0.02
Zincke	58	28	20 (71%)	30	9 (30%)	41	0.002
Prout	90	45	43 (76%)	45	29 (64%)	12	0.05
MRC	367	123	46 (37%)	244	97 (40%)	−3	n.s.
Total	1130	505	309 (61%)	625	288 (49%)	12	
Mitomycin C							
Huland & Otto	58	30	15 (50%)	28	2 (7%)	43	0.01
Niijima	278	139	86 (62%)	139	79 (57%)	5	n.s.
Kim & Lee	43	22	18 (82%)	21	17 (81%)	1	n.s.
Tolley	397	130	85 (65%)	267	137 (51%)	14	0.001
Rübben	83	40	17 (42%)	43	15 (35%)	5	n.s.
Akaza	298	148	49 (33%)	150	36 (24%)	9	n.s.
Total	1157	509	270 (53%)	648	286 (44%)	9	
Doxorubicin							
Niijima	436	139	86 (62%)	297	135 (45%)	17	0.05
Zincke	59	28	20 (71%)	31	10 (32%)	39	0.01
Kurth	217	70	41 (59%)	147	52 (35%)	24	0.006
Rübben	220	82	50 (61%)	138	77 (56%)	5	n.s.
Akaza	457	148	49 (33%)	309	77 (25%)	8	n.s.
Total	1389	467	246 (53%)	922	351 (38%)	15	
Ethoglucid							
Kurth	209	70	41 (59%)	139	39 (28%)	31	0.0004
Epirubicin							
Oosterlinck	399	205	84 (41%)	194	56 (29%)	12	0.0152
Cumulative result	3899	1756	950 (54%)	2528	1020 (40%)	14	

TURBT: Transurethral resection of bladder tumour.

p value as reported by the authors.

n.s. = not significant.

Adv = advantage. Advantage is defined as the total percent recurrence following transurethral resection alone minus percent recurrence following surgery plus intravesical chemotherapy. Lengths of follow-up and risk factors vary from study to study, therefore, statistical comparisons, other than those reported by original authors, are not appropriate and therefore are not reported. Averages are presented for interest only.

Reference: Lamm DL. Long term results of intravesical therapy for superficial bladder cancer. *Urol Clin N Am* 1992; **19**: 573–80.

Table 14.3 Effect of intravesical BCG on recurrence in controlled studies.

| Source | Total number (N) | Control (TURBT) | | Bacillus Calmette–Guérin | | | |
		Control (N)	Recurred (N) (%)	Treated (N)	Recurred (N) (%)	Difference % recurred	p value
Lamm	57	27	14 (52%)	30	6 (20%)	32	< 0.001
Herr	86	43	41 (95%)	43	18 (42%)	53	< 0.001
Herr	49	26	26 (100%)	23	8 (35%)	65	< 0.001
Pagano	133	63	52 (83%)	70	18 (26%)	57	< 0.001
Melekos	94	32	19 (59%)	62	20 (32%)	27	< 0.02
Rübben	77	40	17 (42%)	37	13 (35%)	7	n.s.
Total	496	231	169 (73%)	265	83 (31%)	42	

Reference: Lamm DL, Rigg DR, Traynelis CL, Nseyo UO. Apparent failure of current intravesical chemotherapy prophylaxis to influence the long-term course of superficial transitional cell carcinoma of the bladder. *J Urol* 1995; **153**: 1444–50.
Abbreviations: TURBT, transurethral resection of bladder tumour.

Direct randomized comparisons of prophylactic BCG therapy with thiotepa, doxorubicin and mitomycin chemotherapy, as illustrated in Table 14.4, have demonstrated BCG to provide superior protection from tumour recurrence. Statistically significant reduction in recurrence with BCG has been consistently reported in comparisons with thiotepa and doxorubicin, but the advantage of BCG over mitomycin has been inconsistent [7]. These findings would suggest that

Table 14.4 Recurrence in controlled comparison trials.

Source	BCG	Thiotepa	Doxorubicin	Mitomycin C	p value
Brosman	0	47%			< 0.01
Netto	7%	43%			< 0.01
Martinez	13%	36%	43%		< 0.01
BCG/Thiotepa avg	7%	42%			
SWOG	63%		83%		< 0.02
BCG/Doxorubicin avg	38%		63%		
Debruyne	30%			25%	n.s.
Juahianen	288%			62%	< 0.01
Rübben	35%			35%	n.s.
Witjes	29% (RIVM)			26%	n.s.
	34% (Tice)				n.s.
SWOG	20%			33%	< 0.01
BCG/Mitomycin avg	29%			36%	
BCG avg	25%				
Chemotherapy avg	43%				

mitomycin may be superior to other intravesical chemotherapies, but direct randomized-comparison studies have shown no advantage of mitomycin therapy.

The studies showing BCG to provide superior protection from tumour recurrence have used what we now know to be sub-optimal BCG treatment schedules. Using 1 instillation weekly for 3 weeks at 3 months, 6 months, and every 6 months to 3 years the complete-response rate in CIS is significantly increased and the long-term benefit of BCG in preventing tumour recurrence in patients with high-risk stage Ta, T1 TCC nearly doubled.

Tumour progression

Intravesical chemotherapy has not achieved the goal of reducing disease progression. No individual controlled chemotherapy trial has resulted in statistically significant reduction of stage progression, and analysis of the combined experience shows no evidence that chemotherapy reduces progression (Table 14.5). The inability to demonstrate reduction of progression with chemotherapy may be due to the high percentage of low-risk patients entered into chemotherapy trials, the consequent low incidence of progression, the duration of follow-up, or intercurrent treatment. Nonetheless, with over 4000 patients entered into controlled chemotherapy trials it is disappointing that no evidence of reduction in progression is found, and if any reduction in progression exists it must be quite small.

Table 14.5 Effect of intravesical chemotherapy on progression in controlled studies.

Source	Treatment		Control	
	N	Progression (%)	N	Progression (%)
Thiotepa				
Green *et al.*	25	1 (4)	31	6 (19)
Prout *et al.*	45	6 (13.3)	45	4 (8.9)
MRC	244	7 (2.8)	123	2 (1.6)
Mitomycin				
Huland & Otto	28	1 (4)	30	6 (20)
Tolley *et al.*	267	6 (2.2)	130	2 (1.5)
Total ($N = 455$)	295	7 (2.4)	160	8 (5.0)
Doxorubicin				
Rübben *et al.*	138	19 (14)	82	10 (12)
Kurth *et al.*	165	20 (12)	70	7 (10)
Total ($N = 455$)	303	39 (12.9)	152	17 (11.2)
Totals	912	60 (6.6)	511	37 (7.2)

Reference: Lamm DL. Long term results of intravesical therapy for superficial bladder cancer. *Urol Clin N Am* 1992; **19**: 573–80.

Patients entered into randomized, controlled, BCG trials have generally been at higher risk for recurrence and progression than those entered into chemotherapy trials. Demonstration of reduction in progression is therefore less difficult. As illustrated in Table 14.6, controlled trials suggest a statistically significant and consistent reduction in progression, but in some of the listed studies, definitions other than stage progression above T2 have been included.

Table 14.6 Effect of BCG on progression in controlled studies.

Source	BCG N (%)	Control N (%)	p value
Herr (43)	12 (28%)	15 (35%)	< 0.01
Lamm (53)	8 (15%)	21 (37%)	< 0.01
Pagano (165)	7 (4%)	28 (17%)	< 0.01
Totals (261)	27 (10%)	64 (24%)	< 0.001

Reference: Lamm DL. Long term results of intravesical therapy for superficial bladder cancer. *Urol Clin N Am* 1992; **19**: 573–80.

Conclusions

Intravesical chemotherapy has been demonstrated to reduce tumour recurrence by about 14% in controlled randomized trials, but unfortunately has no effect on the subsequent incidence of stage progression. BCG immunotherapy reduces tumour recurrence by approximately 42% and controlled comparison studies have confirmed this improved protection from recurrence when compared with thiotepa, doxorubicin and mitomycin. Unlike chemotherapy, the reduction in tumour recurrence afforded by BCG is associated with a reduction in the incidence of tumour progression. The superior efficacy of BCG is associated with an increase in side-effects, but the vast majority of side-effects are minor and reflect the desired immune stimulation that is the mechanism of action of the treatment. To date all of the comparison studies have used BCG-treatment schedules that are now known to be sub-optimal. Even better results should be obtained with the 3-weekly maintenance BCG schedule.

References

1   Traynelis CL, Lamm DL. Current status of intravesical therapy for bladder cancer. In: Rous SN (ed) *Urology Annual* Vol 8. W.W. New York: Norton & Company, 1994; 113–43.
2   Bohle A, Thanhauser A, Ulmer AJ *et al.* Dissecting the immunobiological effects of bacillus Calmette–Guérin (BCG) *in vitro*: evidence of a distinct BCG-activated killer (BAK) cell phenomenon. *J Urol* 1993; **150**: 1932–7.
3   Lamm DL, Blumenstein BA, Crawford ED *et al.* Randomized intergroup comparison of bacillus Calmette–Guérin immunotherapy and Mitomycin C chemotherapy prophylaxis in superficial transitional cell carcinoma of the bladder, a Southwest Oncology Group study. *Urol Oncol* 1995; **1**: 119–26.
4   Lamm DL, Blumenstein BA, Crawford ED *et al.* A randomized trial of intravesical doxorubicin and immunotherapy with bacille Calmette–Guérin for transitional-cell carcinoma of the bladder. *NEJM* 1991; **325**: 1205–9.

5   Lamm DL. Carcinoma *in situ*. In: Lamm DL (ed) *The Urologic Clinics of North America*. Philadelphia, PA: W.B. Saunders Co., 1992; **19**: 499–508.

6   Lamm DL, Riggs DR, Traynelis CL, Nseyo UO. Apparent failure of current intravesical chemotherapy prophylaxis to influence the long-term course of superficial transitional cell carcinoma of the bladder. *J Urol* 1995; **153**: 1444–50.

7   Lamm DL, Torti FM. Bladder cancer 1996. *CA Cancer J Clin* 1995; **46**: 93–112.

8   Lamm DL. Long term results of intravesical therapy for superficial bladder cancer. *Urol Clin N Am* 1992; **19**: 573–80.

CHAPTER 15

Photodynamic therapy of bladder carcinoma

D. Jocham

Introduction

Phototherapy is the use of visible or near-visible light as a therapeutic agent in clinical medicine. Photodynamic therapy (PDT) falls into two categories: *direct*, without an administered photosensitizer (e.g. treatment of neonatal jaundice with blue/white light) and *indirect*, where the effect is achieved via an administered photosensitizer which is the effective light absorber. Of course, light must be absorbed in either case, but it is useful, nonetheless, to distinguish between both categories, as the administration of both the sensitizing drug and light dosage in the *indirect* category means that consideration must be given to additional parameters (e.g. chemical structure of the photosensitizer and length of drug–light interval). At the present time, one of the most active areas of research in the field of phototherapy is tumour phototherapy. This subject has become known as photodynamic therapy, which arises from the term 'photodynamische Wirkung' (photodynamic effect) coined by German physiologists in order to describe the destruction of living tissue by a combination of photosensitizer, visible light, and oxygen.

In the case of bladder tumours, PDT combines the use of a modern, up to date, usually systemically applied photosensitizer with laser irradiation, primarily aiming at the destruction of rapidly proliferating tissue, as for example, tumour tissue. The production of photodynamic-active photoproducts (in the main singlet oxygen) is activated by light in the photosensitized tissue, thus effectively destroying tumour tissue [1,2,3,4].

As a result of the increased accumulation of the photosensitizer in tumour tissue, a specific tumour therapy is possible, even in the case of a multifocal tumour, providing that all tumour areas are exposed to irradiation.

At the present time, in the clinical application of, exclusively, photosensitizers of the so-called 'first generation' (porphyrins), it is only possible to obtain a curatively successful treatment in superficial tumours. This is due to the limited intensity of photodynamic therapy. Therefore, currently, the treatment of tumours at an early stage appears to be the domain of PDT. The clinical application of PDT in the region of permitted trials, however, is also being undertaken with a palliative aim, e.g. in the recanalization of the bronchial tree in the case of an obstructing bronchial carcinoma or to open an oesophagus closed by a tumour.

The question of the future role of the topically applicable fluorescent marker — delta-aminolevulinic acid (ALA) (e.g. bladder instillation) — which acts as a precursor in intracellular protoporphyrin IX is unclear, on account of suitability to treatment [5,6,7].

On account of the contact-free application of PDT treatment, without the occurrence of thermical processes, this procedure is predestined to be utilized in other clinical disciplines, dealing especially with cosmetic aspects (skin), or to protect tissue structures immediately in the operation area (central nervous system).

A particular advantage of this procedure is the fact that treatment can be undertaken, in the main, without anaesthesia being necessary; also, treatment can be repeated, as in comparison to most other forms of therapy (nuclear-orientated), different cellular mechanisms are activated (PDT-dependent destruction of cell membrane, e.g. mitochondria). Thus, the possibility of the utilization of PDT in other forms of therapy-resistant tumours exists. A disadvantage of the procedure, however, is the hypersensitivity of the skin to light, on account of the current utilization of porphyrins, which subsequent to intravenous application of the photosensitizer (Photofrin®, manufactured by QLT, Vancouver, Photosan®, Seelab or the Russian Photog(h)em) result in a clinically relevant hypersensitivity of the skin to light for a primary median period of 30 days [5,8,9–11,13,16,19–21,33].

PDT in bladder tumours

In 1976, Kelly and Snell reported on the first clinical endoscopic utilization of PDT in humans. They were able to destroy papillary tumours of the bladder by means of focally applied irradiation, following a systematic application of a haematoporphyrin derivative, administered 48 hours prior to treatment [20].

Benson, D'Hallewin, Dugan, Harty, Hisazumi, Kriegmair, Manyak, Naito, Nseyo, Prout, Schumaker and Jocham have all reported on the clinical application of PDT in carcinoma of the bladder; however, in all cases different dosages of photosensitizers were administered, i.e. haematoporphyrin derivative, Photofrin or Photosan-3, as well as different irradiation modalities (Table 15.1) [5,8,11,13,16–19,26,27,30,31,33, 35,36].

At the present time, taking into account a background of experimental and clinical data, PDT therapy, with a curative aim, can only be performed in the case of superficial tumours, stages Tis, Ta and T1. Prior to PDT, exophytic areas of tumour tissue should have been mechanically extracted by means of transurethral resection (TUR), or in the case of papillomatosis, subsequent to an adequate histological expert opinion and treatment with Nd:YAG laser (1064 nm). In order to validate treatment with PDT in tumours of the bladder, controlled, prospective randomized clinical trials are essential. The well-known clinical side-effects of PDT (pollacisuria, contraction of the bladder, retention of urine in the bladder), during the course of clinical trials, and in tumour stages where a high risk of a local process or metastatic spread exists, should be taken into consideration. Consequently, this means that in tumours known to have a low rate of malignancy (TaG1), as well as in tumours with a very high rate of malignancy where complete destruction is unclear (T1G3; $T \geq 2,\text{G1–G3}$), treatment with PDT should not be performed. This classification can also be applied to the administration of porphyrin mixtures in the form of photosensitizers, which are known to have a limited-depth effect. By the utilization of

Table 15.1 Photodynamic therapy of carcinoma of the bladder.

Main author/ year	N. of patients N. of tumours	Type of tumour	Photosensitizer dosage mg/kg/bw	PDT output/ dosage	Irradiation modalities	Therapy success CR	PR	NR	Rec.	Follow-up (months)
Benson [4] 1985	27/31	15 focal CIS	HpD 2.5	150 J/cm^2	smooth fibre microlens	15	0	0	8	6–32
		12 diffuse CIS		25–45 J/cm^2 (3 or	spherical scattered light	12	0	0	2	(median 7)
		2 Ta	HpD 4–5	48 h after HpD i.v.)	150–250 ml saline	0	0	2	0	
		2 T2								
Dugan [10] 1991	24	21 Ta	Photofrin 2 after TUR	12 patients	spherical scattered light	median time to recurrence in				
				15 J/cm^2 integral		control arm was 93 days in				
				12 patients control period		PDT arm not achieved				
Ha 1983	6	Urothel-Ca., T	HpD 5	?	?	3	1	0	?	1
Harty [33] 1989	7	2 CIS	Photofrin 2	100 J/cm^2 focal	spherical scattered light	1	0	1	0	?
		3 Ta		+25 J/cm^2 integral	microlens	3	0	0	1	
		2 Ta				1	0	1	0	
Hisazumi 1983	9/48	Ta, T1	HpD 2–3.2	150–300 mW/cm^2	smooth fibre					
				100–200 J/cm^2	200 ml saline					
	< 1 cm					22	6	5	–	1
	1–2 cm					4	2	3	–	
	2–3 cm					0	1	2	–	
	> 3 cm					0	0	1	–	
Jocham [19] 1990	20/28	CIS	10 × HpD 3	15–75 J/cm^2	special catheter	23	–	5	14	12–60
		therapy refractory	8 × Photofrin 2		intralipid scattering media					(median 33)
			2 × Photofrin 1.5							
Kriegmair 1992	11	3 CIS	Photofrin 2	15 J/cm^2	spherical scattered light	3	0	0	0	5–15
		7 Ta G1/2				5	0	2	4	3–14
		1 T2				1	0	0	0	15 (+MVECI)
Manyak 1991	11	Urothel-Ca.	Photofrin 1.5	15–20 J/cm^2	scattered media	3	?	?	?	18+
Naito [30] 1991	35	Urothel-Ca.	22 × HpD 3	10–30 J/cm^2	spherical scattered light	24	0	11	14	5–60
			13 × Photofrin 2							(median ?)
Nseyo [32] 1987	23	6 CIS	Photofrin 2	16–200 J/cm^2	spherical scattered light	4	1	1	?	2–12
		8 Ta			microlens	3	3	2	?	
		8 T1			cylindrical light	2	5	1	?	
		3 T2				0	1	2	?	
		1 T3				0	0	1	?	
Prout [35] 1987	20/50	3 CIS	Photofrin 2	5.5–10 J/cm^2	spherical scattered light	3	0	0	?	3
		50 Ta/T1		100–200 J/cm^2	microlens	12	25	13	2	
Shumaker [36] 1987	16	12 CIS	Photofrin 2	< 20 J/cm^2	150 ml saline	7	2	?	3	6–36
		4 Ta				2	0	2	0	6–15
Tsuchiya 1983	8	Ta-T2	HpD 2.5	120–260 J/cm^2	smooth fibre	8	0	0	2	6–18

Table 15.2. Dosimetry test: table of values. (This table shows the permissible area of values for the fluence rate [mW/cm^2] in relation to the laser light output L [W] on the detector fibre and volume of the bladder V [cm^3].)

V [cm^2] L [W]	100	120	140	160	180	200	220	240	260	280	300	320	340	360	380	400	420	440	460	480
1.20	29–88	26–78	23–70	21–64	20–60	19–56	17–52	16–49	16–47	15–44	14–42	14–41	13–39	13–38	12–36	12–35	11–34	11–33	11–32	10–31
1.30	32–95	28–85	25–76	23–70	22–65	20–60	19–56	19–53	17–50	16–48	15–46	15–44	14–42	14–41	13–39	13–38	12–37	12–36	12–35	11–34
1.40	34–103	30–91	27–82	25–75	23–69	22–65	20–61	19–57	18–54	17–52	16–49	16–47	15–45	15–44	14–42	14–41	13–39	13–38	12–37	12–36
1.50	37–110	33–98	29–88	27–81	25–74	23–69	22–65	20–61	19–58	18–55	18–53	17–51	16–49	16–47	15–45	15–44	14–42	14–41	13–40	13–39
1.60	39–117	35–104	31–94	29–86	26–79	25–74	23–69	22–66	21–62	20–59	19–56	18–54	17–52	17–50	16–48	16–47	15–45	15–44	14–42	14–41
1.70	42–125	37–111	33–100	30–91	28–84	26–79	25–74	23–70	22–66	21–63	20–60	19–57	18–55	18–53	17–51	17–50	16–48	15–46	15–45	15–44
1.80	44–132	39–117	35–106	32–97	30–89	28–83	26–78	25–74	23–70	22–67	21–64	20–61	19–58	19–56	18–54	17–52	17–51	16–49	16–48	15–46
1.90	47–140	41–124	37–111	34–102	31–94	29–88	27–82	26–78	25–74	23–70	22–67	21–64	21–62	20–59	19–57	18–55	18–54	17–52	17–50	16–49
2.00	49–147	43–130	39–117	36–107	33–99	31–93	29–87	27–82	26–78	25–74	24–71	23–68	22–65	21–63	20–60	19–58	19–56	18–55	18–53	17–52
2.10	51–154	46–137	41–123	38–113	35–104	32–97	30–91	29–86	27–82	26–78	25–74	24–71	23–68	22–66	21–63	20–61	20–59	19–57	19–56	18–54
2.20	54–162	48–143	43–129	39–118	36–109	34–102	32–95	30–90	28–85	27–81	26–78	25–74	24–71	23–69	22–66	21–64	21–62	20–60	19–58	19–57
2.30	56–169	50–150	45–135	41–123	38–114	35–106	33–100	31–94	30–89	28–85	27–81	26–78	25–75	24–72	23–69	22–67	22–65	21–63	20–61	20–59
2.40	59–176	52–156	47–141	43–129	40–119	37–111	35–104	33–98	31–93	30–89	28–85	27–81	26–78	25–75	24–72	23–70	23–68	22–66	21–64	21–62
2.50	61–184	54–163	49–147	45–134	41–124	39–116	36–109	34–102	32–97	31–92	29–88	28–85	27–81	26–78	25–75	24–73	24–71	23–68	22–66	22–65
2.60	64–191	56–169	51–153	47–140	43–129	40–120	38–113	35–106	34–101	32–96	31–92	29–88	28–84	27–81	26–78	25–76	24–73	24–71	23–69	22–67
2.70	66–198	59–176	53–158	48–145	45–134	42–125	39–117	37–111	35–105	33–100	32–95	30–91	29–88	28–84	27–81	26–79	25–76	25–74	24–72	23–70
2.80	69–206	61–182	55–164	50–150	46–139	43–130	41–122	38–115	36–109	34–103	33–99	32–95	30–91	29–88	28–84	27–82	26–79	26–77	25–74	24–72
2.90	71–213	63–189	57–170	52–156	48–144	45–134	42–126	40–119	38–113	36–107	34–102	33–98	31–94	30–91	29–87	28–85	27–82	26–79	26–77	25–75
3.00	73–220	65–195	59–176	54–161	50–149	46–139	43–130	41–123	39–116	37–111	35–106	34–101	32–97	31–94	30–90	29–87	28–85	27–82	27–80	26–77
3.10	76–228	67–202	61–182	55–166	51–154	48–143	45–135	42–127	40–120	38–115	36–109	35–105	34–101	32–97	31–93	30–90	29–87	28–85	27–82	27–80
3.20	78–235	69–208	63–188	57–172	53–159	49–148	46–139	44–131	41–124	39–118	38–113	36–108	35–104	33–100	32–96	31–93	30–90	29–88	28–85	28–83
3.30	81–242	72–215	65–194	59–177	55–164	51–153	48–143	45–135	43–128	41–122	39–116	37–112	36–107	34–103	33–100	32–96	31–93	30–90	29–88	28–85
3.40	83–250	74–221	66–199	61–182	56–169	52–157	49–148	46–139	44–132	42–126	40–120	38–115	37–110	35–106	34–103	33–99	32–96	31–93	30–90	29–88
3.50	86–257	76–228	68–205	63–188	58–174	54–162	51–152	48–143	45–136	43–129	41–124	39–118	38–114	36–109	35–106	34–102	33–99	32–96	31–93	30–90
3.60	88–264	78–234	70–211	64–193	60–179	56–167	52–156	49–147	47–140	44–133	42–127	41–122	39–117	38–113	36–109	35–105	34–102	33–98	32–96	31–93
3.70	91–272	80–241	72–217	66–199	61–184	57–171	54–161	51–152	48–144	46–137	44–131	42–125	40–120	39–116	37–112	36–108	35–104	34–101	33–98	32–95
3.80	93–279	82–247	74–223	68–204	63–189	59–176	55–165	52–156	49–148	47–140	45–134	43–128	41–123	40–119	38–115	37–111	36–107	35–104	34–101	33–98
3.90	95–286	85–254	76–229	70–209	65–194	60–180	56–169	53–160	50–151	48–144	46–138	44–132	42–127	41–122	39–118	38–114	37–110	36–107	35–104	34–101
4.00	98–294	87–260	78–235	72–215	66–198	62–185	58–174	55–164	52–155	49–148	47–141	45–135	43–130	42–125	40–121	39–117	38–113	36–109	35–106	34–103
4.10	100–301	89–267	80–241	73–220	68–203	63–190	59–178	56–168	53–159	51–152	48–145	46–139	44–133	43–128	41–124	40–119	39–116	37–112	36–109	35–106
4.20	103–308	91–273	82–246	75–225	69–208	65–194	61–182	57–172	54–163	52–155	49–148	47–142	45–136	44–131	42–127	41–122	39–118	38–115	37–111	36–108
4.30	105–316	93–280	84–252	77–231	71–213	66–199	62–187	59–176	56–167	53–159	51–152	48–145	47–140	45–134	43–130	42–125	40–121	39–118	38–114	37–111
4.40	108–323	95–286	86–258	79–236	73–218	68–204	64–191	60–180	57–171	54–163	52–155	50–149	48–143	46–138	44–133	43–128	41–124	40–120	39–117	38–114

photosensitizers with the absorption of longer wavelengths in the red part of the spectrum, stage T $\geq$ 2 tumours can also be treated with PDT. However, in this situation, by the use of an intensified-PDT effect, also in normal submucosa, as well as the muscles of the bladder, an increased amount of contraction of the bladder (intolerable!) can be expected. This problem can be solved by the use of a photosensitizer with a high tumour selectivity, which does not induce photodynamic reaction within normal body tissue.

During clinical trials on the bladder, aspects of side-effects and quality of life are rapidly gaining importance as other efficient alternative forms of therapy for specific tumours, apart from PDT, are now available (e.g. BCG immunostimulation). The assessment of this method, on account of the assumed high therapeutical efficiency of PDT, at least in the urological sector, is concerned mainly with the comparison of side-effects, repetition-rate of therapy and the financial situation, rather than with the curative effect *per se*.

The specific problems of the frequently occurring (up to 80%) multifocal spread in bladder carcinoma necessitates the irradiation of all regions of the bladder, on account of the multiple occurrence of tumour sections (> 60%) which remain undetected during endoscopic examinations (severe pre-cancerous atypia, carcinoma *in situ* [CIS]). At least, within the scope of clinical trials, on account of insufficient tumour selectivity of the available photosensitizers and empirically chosen dosages of substances, the utilization of irradiation modalities with homogeneous irradiation of the bladder and a dosimeter suitable to perform on-line dosimetry of light distribution in the bladder, at the level of bladder mucosa, is necessary. The clinical routine application, based on the experience gained in clinical trials and, in particular, from the administration of photosensitizers with an improved tumour selectivity will make it possible to dispense with this complicated method [4,6,8,16,27,32,37].

The aforementioned remarks concerning PDT in tumours of the bladder are based on experience acquired by D. Jocham and his team in Munich, who, since 1977, have carried out experimental research work [29], and since 1984, clinical work on therapy with PDT in carcinoma of the bladder [16]. Following D. Jocham's departure to Lübeck, the work is being continued in Munich as well as in Lübeck [24,25]. The up-to-date data show that CIS is sensitive to PDT (Table 15.1).

In the meantime, in Canada Photofrin® has been licensed as a photosensitizer in PDT in the prophylaxis of recurrent superficial urothelial carcinoma of the bladder [11,33]. In the Netherlands, Photofrin® has been licensed for PDT in obstructive bronchial and oesophagus carcinoma.

In December 1995, Photofrin® was approved, for PDT of oesophagus carcinoma, in the USA.

Multi-centre randomized Phase III trial (Germany, Austria)

At the present time, a multi-centre Phase III trial on the prophylaxis of recurrent superficial urothelial carcinoma of the bladder and therapy of CIS with PDT versus a typical immunotherapy using bacillus Calmette–Guérin (BCG) is being undertaken, under the responsibility of D. Jocham, Lübeck, Germany.

In the following, the trial protocol is described as far as technical aspects are concerned.

PDT: basic technique

Concept of irradiation

Radiation treatment is undertaken by means of a bladder catheter fitted with two transparent concentric balloons. The outer balloon is laid against the bladder wall and is responsible for the positioning of the catheter. The inner balloon is filled with scattering medium and functions as a centrally positioned isotropic emitter. The light supply is provided from the centre of the inner balloon by means of a fibre with a cone-shaped tip. The scattering medium is supplied with light from the light supply fibre, radiating perpendicular to the catheter axis. The space between both balloons is filled with optically clear water. In order to remove blood and urine, during the treatment, the area between outer balloon and bladder wall is flushed with clear water. The water flows out of the catheter tip through a drainage canal and flows out of the bladder over the area between catheter-shaft and insertion tube.

Dosimeter concept

Light dosimetry is undertaken by means of a light detector, which measures the irradiation during therapy. The light detector is comprised of a detector fibre with a cone-shaped tip which is placed in the catheter tube, between the entrance to and centre of the bladder, and measures the light backscattered from a circular zone on the bladder wall. It can be assumed that the light registered from this zone is representative for the complete surface of the bladder. The light registered by the detector fibre is guided to the dosimeter, which calculates the light dosage.

Concept of the light dosimeter

The concept of light dosimetry for the application in question differs, to a large extent, from the majority of treatment with PDT. Usually, the light power per tissue area is specified as irradiance. Usually, only the primary amount of light is stated, i.e. light which is directly aimed at tissue from the applicator, but not the amount produced by backscattering from the tissue. In order to measure the irradiance, a light detector can be utilized. However, the radiation on surface tissue is at the highest with a vertical incidence, rather than in the case of light incidence on surface tissue at an angle, as a smaller cross-sectional area is presented. On the other hand, the therapeutic effect of light on a cell is independent of the direction of incidence. Therefore, the therapy-relevant slice is not the irradiance but the fluence rate. The fluence rate is defined as the power of radiation, which projects at a small detector with a spherical sensitive surface, divided by the cross-sectional surface of the detector. The same unit as for the irradiance is used for the fluence rate. These units, however, are not identical. The irradiation is the product of irradiance and duration of treatment, and the light dosage is the product of fluence rate and duration of treatment. As the fluence-rate flow in tissue can only be measured by means of complicated, invasive methods, the statement of primary irradiance and irradiation is established in PDT. In doing so, it is assumed that the irradiance and the fluence rate differ by a factor independent of the patient, but this factor varies drastically from patient to patient. In the case of superficial tumours of the bladder, the area of irradiation lies directly on the surface of tissue. The fluence rate in this area can be measured easily and for this reason is taken for dosimetry for the applicator under discussion.

The detector installed in the applicator measures only the scattered amount of fluence rate. The dosimeter displays the portion comprised of primary and scattered amounts, whereby a primary amount of light coming directly from the central supply of light can be estimated to be 16%. As the primary amount is influenced by patient-specific variations, deviations occur between the displayed and actual fluence rate. On account of the primary portion of light of only 16%, these deviations are less than ± 10%.

Realization: substance, application and patient care

Photofrin® (dihematoporphyrin ester/ether) 1.5 mg/kg bodyweight will be supplied by QLT. An opened vial, under sterile conditions, can be stored in a refrigerator at 4°C for 24 hours. During the preparation of the substance it should be protected from light in such a manner that the contents are dissolved in 30 ml of 5% dextrose and immediately following preparation slowly injected intravenously as a bolus within 3–5 minutes (PDT-day 1). Should, by mistake, an extravascular application be carried out, the injection area must be cooled with ice and protected from light.

On PDT-day 3 (40–50 hours following injection of Photofrin®) a cystoscopy, under anaesthesia, will be carried out; the capacity of the bladder must be determined after which treatment at 50–75% volume of the bladder capacity is undertaken. The argon-dye laser is turned to 630 ± 3 nm. Treatment of the entire bladder is carried out at a fluence rate of 150 J/cm^2.

Following treatment with PDT, the patient must be *observed* for a period of 24 hours, all side-effects are to be noted. Subsequent to injection with Photofrin®, patients must be protected from direct sunlight for 30 days, at least, and protected also from strong artificial light, or a light-protection cream should be applied to exposed areas of the body. In the case of patients with an over-sensitive skin, Cordes' lotion should be applied.

Preparation of the patient for radiation treatment

Preparation for the filling of the outer balloon (see Fig. 15.1)

In order to establish the filling volume of the outer balloon, it is necessary to determine the bladder volume of the patient during treatment. Additionally, the shape of the bladder must be checked by means of ultrasound. Should the shape of the bladder significantly differ from the normal spherical form, then it must be taken into consideration that the outer balloon does not form the shape of the bladder but must only have contact at various points with the wall of the bladder. Therefore, the filling volume of the balloon, in such cases, must be estimated smaller than the volume of the bladder.

The balloon is suitable for a filling volume of 100–500 ml. The remaining bladder volume will be taken up with the rinsing water. In order to fill the outer balloon, a suitable syringe should be available.

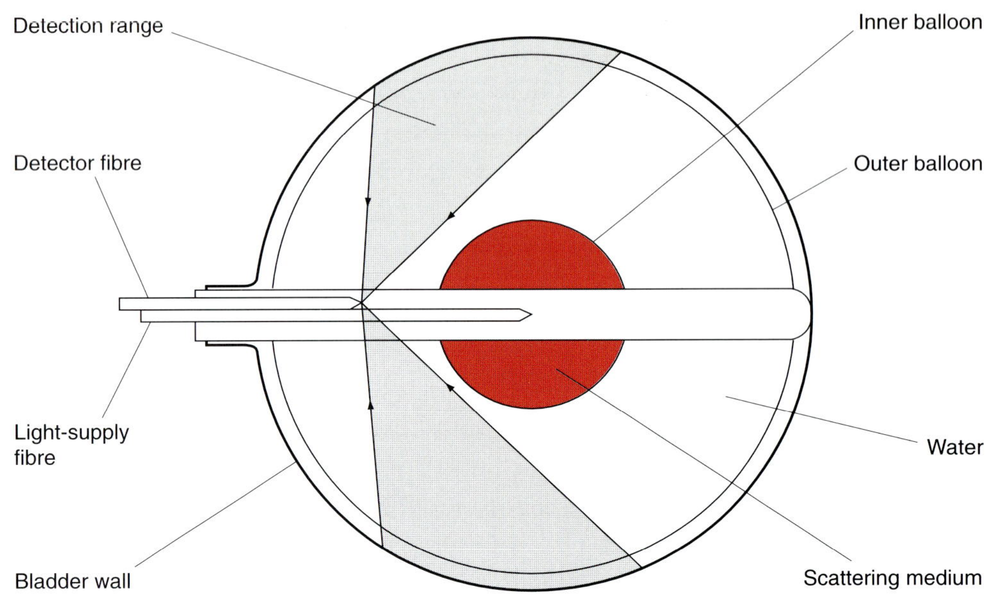

Figure 15.1. Double balloon catheter (Rüsch®, Germany) for PDT of the urinary bladder. The area marked as 'detection range' reflects the zone where light distribution and light intensity is monitored by the on-line dosimetry.

Preparation for the filling of the inner balloon

The inner balloon (connector is marked in red) is filled with 4 ml scattering medium. For this purpose, an emulsion with 0.5% fat content is utilized. Suitable emulsions are Lipovenous® (Fresenius AG, Oberursel) and Lipofundin® (Braun Melsungen, Melsungen). Only fat concentrations of 10% and 20% can be supplied. Therefore, the scattering medium must be prepared by mixing 1 part emulsion of 10% fat content with 19 parts of water or by mixing 1 part emulsion of 20% fat content with 39 parts of water.

If possible, the filling of the inner balloon must be undertaken without the occurrence of air bubbles. For this reason, the remaining air in the inner balloon should be removed by means of a syringe. Subsequently, the syringe must be filled with 4 ml scattering medium, from which the inner balloon is then repeatedly filled and emptied before insertion of the catheter; at the same time the syringe must be repeatedly ventilated. Finally, the balloon is again emptied. The filled syringe remains connected to the catheter up until commencement of radiation.

Fibre connection

In order to avoid confusion between light-supply fibre and detection fibre they are equipped with different plugs. The light-supply fibre plug is fixed onto the laser or laser-extension fibre (SMA-plug). The detection fibre is fitted to the dosimeter by means of a bajonet-plug (ST-plug). For this procedure, the fibre should be twisted so that the guide-pin in the plug fits into the socket, after which the bajonet-ring is locked. Extreme bending of the fibre (radius < 5 cm) is to be avoided. Extreme bending of the fibre, as well as pollution on the detection fibre can result in an overdosage of light during PDT. Therefore, the dust protection caps of the dosimeter fibre and dosimeter apparatus should only be removed immediately before assembly. Additionally, the cleanliness of the surface of the fibre tip must be visually checked. For the same reasons, the bajonet-plug on the dosimeter and the dust protection caps should be regularly checked on account of pollution. The cleansing of the inside of the bajonet-plug should only be undertaken by trained personnel.

Recording of the radiation conditions

In order to calculate the mean fluence rate during PDT, the duration of radiation should be measured. This is not necessarily identical with the remaining time displayed on the dosimeter at the commencement of PDT (see below). Therefore, a stopwatch should be available. In order to record eventually occurring variations in the fluence rate during PDT, it is possible to connect a recorder to the back of the dosimeter (BNC-plug). 1 V equals a fluence rate of 22 mW/cm^2.

Performance of irradiation

Installation of the catheter

Before insertion of the catheter, it must be established by means of cystoscopy that the bladder will be expanded at the planned filling volume, after which the catheter can be inserted. The outer balloon must be wrapped around the catheter shaft, and by insertion the catheter should be appropriately twisted (the use of a lubricant is recommended). Additionally, the insertion sluice must be withdrawn up to the end of the catheter, so that this area is watertight and the rinsing water can only drain off through the side-tube. Otherwise, the danger could arise that the inserted sluice may touch the outer balloon and in this way prevent the draining out of the rinsing water. Subsequently, the inner balloon should be filled with scattering medium, the outer balloon filled with the previously determined amount of water, and rinsing commenced. During this procedure, large air bubbles in the area between the outer balloon and bladder wall should be avoided and the pressure of the water should be kept low to prevent the forming of water-filled areas between the outer balloon and the bladder wall. The position of the balloon catheter must be controlled by means of ultrasound and should be photo-documented.

Starting the dosimeter (see below)

The dosimeter is switched on and the display mode switch is set at 'desired dosage (J/cm^2)' (Fig. 15.2) for which on the right display a value of 150 J/cm^2 should be set. It is recommended that this setting should be locked with the help of the locking lever. Immediately before commencement of treatment, the 'reset/start' button should be pressed.

Commencement of treatment and dosimetry check

Immediately prior to commencement of irradiation therapy, the light power, leaving the tip of the extension fibre, should be measured with an appropriate power meter. Immediately following commencement of therapy, the fluence rate should be read

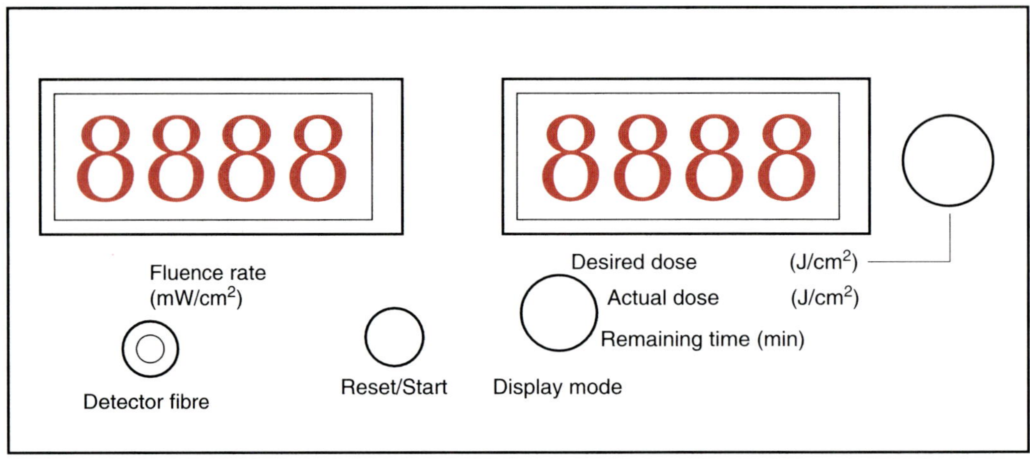

Figure 15.2. Starting the dosimeter.

from the display situated on the left of the dosimeter and on the right display, the prognosis for the irradiation time can be read. Finally, in accordance with the tables showing irradiation times, it should be checked whether the stated time lies within the estimated range. A value outside this range indicates a critical dosimetry situation. Possible reasons for this situation are, for example, damaged or polluted fibres, extreme deviations of the bladder from the usual spherical shape, or blood. The normal irradiation time is usually approximately half of the stated maximum value.

During the course of irradiation therapy

During irradiation therapy, the fluence rate on the bladder wall can be read in mW/cm^2 from the display on the left of the dosimeter (Fig. 15.2). The right display shows, according to the setting of the display mode switch, as well as the 'desired dosage (J/cm^2)', the 'actual dosage (J/cm^2)' (i.e. the light dosage already applied) and, additionally, the 'remaining time (min)'; a prognosis of the time duration until completion of the irradiation treatment, providing the light conditions remain unchanged. In order to achieve the shortest possible irradiation time, the treatment should be performed using the maximal available laser power. However, a fluence rate of 200 mW/cm^2 should not be exceeded.

Termination of irradiation treatment

When the set 'desired dosage (J/cm^2)' has been reached, an acoustic signal can be heard. The laser light can be switched off, the duration of irradiation documented and the bladder catheter removed. After disconnecting the detector fibre, the dust protection caps, on the dosimeter, should in all circumstances be replaced.

Time schedule of the Phase III trial

Patient recruitment was commenced in February 1995. The statistical evaluation of the trial ($n = 200$ patients), as well as the preparation of a report on the trial will be carried out, at least, 4 years subsequent to the commencement of the trial.

Experimental research: PDT (principles of action)

Independent of clinical work, research work on the principles of photodynamics is being pursued intensively.

Special scientific interest is being aimed at finding an explanation for the principles of action of PDT. The main point of discussion, at a cellular level, is that as opposed to ionic irradiation or to numerous cytostatic drugs, PDT acts not in the region of the cellular nucleus, but on the level of the cell membrane and cytoplasmic structures, e.g. mitochondria, lysosomes and endoplasmic reticulum. In the presence of oxygen, singlet oxygen is formed, which is a highly responsive and short-lived form of oxygen. In the double-binding chemical reaction organo-peroxide is formed, which can degrade organic membranes. At the same time, sensitized conglomerate can be observed in the region of the tumour neovascularization, resulting in a vasoconstriction from which hypoxia in tumour tissue is achieved.

On account of the short life and short depth of penetration of singlet oxygen, the apparent contradiction of the mechanism of effects can be explained by the interval of time. The exact process of photodynamic cytotoxicity is, however, still not clear [12,21,29,34].

Experimental research: photosensitizers

New substances to be used as photosensitizers in PDT are being tested more extensively. In order to obtain a maximum penetration of body tissue, with a minimum interference of absorption by naturally occurring biological chromophore, the photosensitizer should reach its absorption peak in the region of 600–800 nm. Porphyrin derivatives show a 35 times higher absorption at 363 nm than at 626 nm. However, in the red area, the peak of absorption is low, achieving a therapeutically effective depth of light transmission of 5–10 mm. Synthetic chromophore, such as mono-1-aspartyl derivative of chlorine E-6, disulfonated aluminium-phthalocyanine, zinc-phthalocyanine, tin- and zinc-derivatives of the octaethylporphyrin and pheophorbide are biochemically defined and achieve an ideal absorption maxima in the red area and are retinated, at varying amounts, in the tumour area [12].

However, as *in vitro* tests in the separate experimental set-ups show considerable differences, a comparison of the substances on account of the photodynamic potentials, especially in tumour of the bladder, is not possible at the present time.

Similar to the situation in other medical disciplines, a co-ordination of research work is urgently required. In Germany, such co-operation is taking place under the auspices of the BMBF (Federal Department of Science and Technology) (GSF/VDI) by the sponsoring of clinical trials (Co-ordination: D. Jocham, Lübeck) — see above.

Experimental research: modalities of irradiation

As a local treatment of the complete tumour-invaded region of the bladder, a homogeneous irradiation of the complete organ is absolutely necessary. As side-effects occur on account of the light dosage, an exact dosimetry can be achieved by means of the on-line method. As a therapeutic method of integral irradiation therapy inaugurated by Jocham *et al.* PDT has gained importance [3,5,6,8,11,14,16,19,25,27,28,32,37]. Trials have been performed, ranging from specialized rigid endoscopes, which allow the positioning of a spherical irradiator in accordance with the measurement values of three mobile isotropic detectors, up to a relatively simple double balloon catheter, whereby a homogeneous irradiation of the complete bladder is possible by using the inner balloon, filled with light-diffusion medium as an isotropic irradiator, whereas the outer balloon fixates the irradiator to the centre of the bladder.

In accordance with our own needs, special flexible bladder catheters with a large isotropic irradiation area have been developed for the relatively simple routine urological application of treatment; these catheters are better suited for PDT treatment as, for example, catheters with just a bulb-shaped fibre, acting as light distributor. The utilization of such catheters is emphasized by the uncomplicated method of insertion of the catheter, as neither anaesthesia nor a control of the position during irradiation is necessary, as in the case of a freely-movable bulb-shaped fibre (see above).

Regarding light dosage, related side-effects of PDT therapy, increased consideration must be given to light dosimetry.

Photodynamic fluorescence diagnosis

Photodynamic diagnosis (PDD) of tumour cells with fluorescent marker supports the endoscopic detection of tumour areas, which, up until now, have remained undetected. In the discipline of urology PDD is the method of choice in the detection of CIS of the bladder. Whereas the utilization of intravenously applied Photofrin® or Photosan 3® as a fluorescent tumour marker necessitated a highly complicated technical procedure in imaging [1,2,18], PDD has been relatively simplified on account of the introduction of delta-aminolevulinic acid, which can be instilled topically into the bladder [21–24]. Clinical results gained from pilot studies justify the further evaluation of PDD by means of urological clinical trials.

References

1   Baumgartner R, Fuchs N, Jocham D, Stepp H, Unsöld E. Pharmacokinetics of fluorescent polyporphyrin photofrin II in normal rat tissue and rat bladder tumor. *Photochem Photobiol* 1992; **55**: 569–74.
2   Baumgartner R, Kriegmair M, Jocham D *et al. Proc SPIE* 1992; **1641**: 107.
3   Baumgartner R, Beyer W, Friedsam G, Jocham D, Noack A, Sroka R, Stepp H, Unsöld E. Fiber optic probes for tissue illumination in photodynamic diagnosis (PDD) and therapy (PDT). *SPIE Optical Fibers in Medicine VII* 1992; **1649**: 91.
4   Benson RC Jr. Treatment of diffuse transitional cell carcinoma in situ by whole bladder hematoporphyrin derivative photodynamic therapy. *J Urol* 1985; **134**: 675.
5   Benson RC Jr. Integral photoradiation therapy of multifocal bladder tumours. *Eur Urol* 1986; **12** (Suppl 1): 47–53.
6   Beyer W, Pongratz T, Hofstetter AG, Jocham D, Unsöld E. Light dosimetry for photodynamic therapy of superficial tumors in the bladder. *Proc SPIE* 1993; **2078**: 52.

7   Boulnois J-L. Photophysical processes in recent medical laser developments: a review. *Laser Med Sci* 1986; **1**: 47.

8   D'Hallewin MA, Baert L, Marijnissen JPA, Star WM. *J Urol* 1992; **148**: 1152.

9   Dougherty TJ, Marcus SL. Photodynamic therapy. *Eur J Cancer* 1992; 28A: 1734–42.

10 Dugan M, Crawford E, Nseyo U. *Proc Ann Meet Am Soc Clin Oncol* 1991; **10**: 554.

11 Dugan M, Crawford E, Nseyo U et al. A randomized trial of observation (obs) vs photodynamic therapy (PDT) after transurethral resection (TUR) for superficial papillary bladder carcinoma. *Proc ASCO* 1991; **10**: 173.

12 Gomer CJ. Preclinical examination of first and second generation photosensitizers used in photodynamic therapy. *Photochem Photobiol* 1991; **54**: 1093–107.

13 Harty JI, Amin M, Wieman TJ, Tseng MT, Ackerman D, Broghamer W. Complications of whole bladder dihematoporphyrin ether photodynamic therapy. *J Urol* 1989; **141**: 1341–6.

14 Hisazumi H, Miyoshi N, Naito K, Misaki T. Whole bladder wall photoradiation therapy for carcinoma in situ of the bladder: a preliminary report. *J Urol* 1984; **131**: 884.

15 Jocham D, Staehler G, Chaussy Ch, Hammer C, Löhrs U. Laserbehandlung von blasentumoren nach photosensibilisierung mit hämatoporphyrin-derivat. *Urologe* 1981; **20**: 340–3.

16 Jocham D, Staehler G, Baumgartner R, Unsöld E. Die integrale photodynamische therapie beim multifokalen blasenkarzinom. Erste klinische erfahrungen. *Urologe* 1985; **24**: 316–19.

17 Jocham D, Schmiedt E, Baumgartner R, Unsöld E. Integral laser photodynamic treatment of multifocal bladder carcinoma photosensitized by hematoporphyrin derivative. *Eur Urol* 1986; **12** Suppl 1: 43–6.

18 Jocham D, Baumgartner R, Fuchs N, Lenz H, Stepp H, Unsöld E. Die fluoreszenzdiagnose porphyrin-markierter urothelialer tumoren. *Urologe* 1989; **28**: 59–64.

19 Jocham D, Baumgartner R, Stepp H, Unsöld E. Clinical experience with the integral photodynamic therapy of bladder carcinoma. *Photochem Photobiol* 1990; **6**: 183–7.

20 Kelly JF, Snell ME. Hematoporphyrin derivative: a possible aid in the diagnosis and therapy of carcinoma of the bladder. *J Urol* 1976; **115**: 150.

21 Kennedy JC, Pottier RH, Pross DC. Photodynamic therapy with endogenous protoporphyrin. IX. Basic principles and present clinical experience. *Photochem Photobiol* 1990; **6**: 143–8.

22 Kriegmair M, Baumgartner R, Hopstetter A. Intravesikale instillation von delta-aminolävulinsäure (ALA): eine neue methode zur photodynamischen diagnostik und therapie. *Lasermedizin* 1992; **8**: 83.

23 Kriegmair M, Baumgartner R, Lumper W, Riesenberg R, Stocker S, Hofstetter A. Fluorescence cystoscopy following intravesical instillation of aminolevulinic acid (ALA). *J Urol* 1993 ;**149**: 240A.

24 Kriegmair M. Baumgartner R, Knüchel, Ehsan A, Steinbach P, Lumper W, Hofstädter F, Hofstetter A. Photodynamische diagnose urothelialer neoplasien nach intravesikaler instillation von 5-aminolävulinsäure. *Urologe* 1994; **33**: 270–5.

25 Kriegmair M, Waidelich R, Baumgartner R, Lumper W, Ehsan A, Hofstetter A. Die photodynamische therapie (PDT) des oberflächlichen harnblasenkarzinoms. Eine alternative zur radikalen zystektomie? *Urologe* 1994; **33**: 276–80.

26 Manyok MJ. Photodynamic therapy: principles and urologic applications. *Semin Urol* 1991; **9**: 192.

27 Manyak MJ. Cole JW, McNellis RJ, Smith PD. Downstaging of BCG-resistant carcinoma in situ of the bladder by photodynamic therapy with intravesical diffusion medium. *J Urol* 1982; **147**: 374A.

28 Marynissen JPA, Jansen H, Star WM. Treatment system for whole bladder wall photodynamic therapy with in vivo monitoring and control of light dose rate and dose. *J Urol* 1989; **142**: 1351–5.

29. Moan J, Berg K. Photochemotherapy of cancer: experimental research. *Photochem Photobiol* 1992; **55**: 931.

30. Naito K, Hisazumi H, Uchibayashi T, Amano T, Hirata A, Komatsu K, Ishida T, Miyoshi N. Integral laser photodynamic treatment of refractory multifocal bladder tumors. *J Urol* 1991; **146**: 1541–5.

31 Nseyo UO, Dougherty TJ, Boyle DG, Potter WR, wolf R, Huben R, Pontes JE. Whole bladder photodynamic therapy for transitional cell carcinoma of bladder. *Urology* 1985; **26**: 274.

32 Nseyo UO, Lundahl SL, Merrill DC. Whole bladder photodynamic therapy: critical review of present-day technology and rationale for development of intravesical laser catheter and monitoring system. *Urology* 1990; **36**: 398.

33 Nseyo UO, Crawford ED, Shumaker BP, Hoodin AO, Marcus SL, Dugan MH. A Phase II multicenter trial of photodynamic therapy as treatment for refractory carcinoma *in situ*. *J Urol* 1993; **149**: 281A.

34 Pope AJ, Bown SG. Photodynamic therapy. *Br J Urol* 1991; **68**: 1–9.

35 Prout GR Jr, Lin C-W, Benson R, Nseyo UO, Daly JJ, Griffin PP, Kinsey J, Tian M-E, Lao Y-H, Mian Y-Z, Chen X, Ren F-M, Qiao S-J. Photodynamic therapy with hematoporphyrin derivative in the treatment of superficial transitional-cell carcinoma of the bladder. *N Engl J Med* 1987; **317**: 1251.

36 Shumaker BP, Hetzel FW. Clinical laser photodynamic therapy in the treatment of bladder carcinoma. *Photochem Photobiol* 1987; **46**: 899–901.

37 Hirazumi H, Miyoshi N, Misaki T. A trial manufacture of a motor-driven laser light scattering optic for whole bladder wall irradiation. In: *Porphyrin localization and treatment of tumors*. Alan R. Liss, Inc., 1984: 239–47.

CHAPTER 16

Unresponsive superficial bladder cancer

P. Bassi, N. Piazza, G. Abatangelo,
G. Pappagallo and F. Pagano

The problem: 'art rather than science'

For more than four decades intravesical therapy has been applied by urologists to prevent and/or reduce tumour recurrences of superficial bladder cancer as well as tumour progression. Although different drugs and regimens have been used, the best therapeutical approach has yet to be defined [1].

A proportion of patients fail to respond to the conservative approach and although their disease does not progress it recurs several times. In the long run the clinical management of this population, considered unresponsive to intravesical therapy, differs widely due to the lack of scientific data and, consequently, the lack of clear clinical guidelines. As a matter of fact, the clinical approach to the treatment of these patients relies more on personal feeling than on objective evidence ('art rather than science'). Several questions arise when facing this problem: (1) *what* precisely is unresponsive superficial bladder cancer? (2) *when* is superficial bladder cancer considered unresponsive? (3) Is there or should there be a *rational approach* to unresponsive superficial bladder cancer? Unfortunately no scientific answers to these questions are available to date [2–4].

By convention, in this chapter, a persistent or a recurrent, multifocal superficial bladder tumour after unsuccessful intravesical therapy is considered unresponsive. This is a practical definition that reflects the clinical routine and the clinical problem. Patients with monofocal and/or infrequent recurrent disease have been excluded.

There are two therapeutical approaches to unresponsive superficial bladder cancer: the conservative and the aggressive. There are no scientific data to support a clear advantage of one approach over the other. As a result, the clinical choice exclusively continues to be based on the urologist's personal experience.

The aggressive approach

Radical cystectomy has been proposed by several authors as the therapeutical alternative for patients with unresponsive bladder cancer [5–7]. Surprisingly only a few reports have paid specific attention to the indications for surgery or the impact that radical cystectomy has on superficial bladder cancer and survival. Furthermore, the indications for surgery reported in the literature are equivocal and differ widely, particularly with regard to the pivotal definition of unresponsive bladder cancer. Only in the more recent Paulson series, did the authors clearly define unresponsive superficial bladder cancer [7].

Predictably, radical surgery for superficial bladder cancer, regardless of the indications, has shown favourable responses in terms of survival (Table 16.1). Furthermore, the increasing possibility of performing continent urinary diversions has led a number of urologists adopting a radical approach. However, in spite of continent urinary diversions and nerve-sparing techniques, a normal functioning, tumour-free bladder obtained by using conservative measures is still preferable to the most expertly performed bladder substitution procedure. The operative morbidity and mortality of radical cystectomy must also be taken into account.

The question, however, is not whether radical cystectomy is successful in the treatment of superficial bladder cancer, but when is it indicated, particularly in patients with unresponsive tumours? Unfortunately, no study has answered this question.

Table 16.1 Survival after radical surgery for superficial bladder cancer.

Study	Patient (N)	% 5-year survival			Follow-up ($\bar{x}$) months	% Mortality
		pTa	pTis	pT1		
Bracken *et al.* [5]	109	←	75	→	?	2.7
Malkowicz *et al.* [6]	107	100	85	80	?	3
Amling *et al.* [7]	220	88	100	76	60	2.3
Personal data, 1995	108	–	70	74	56	1.4

The conservative approach

The optimal therapeutical approach to superficial bladder cancer relies on prognostic factors; unfortunately the conventional prognostic factors such as tumour stage, grade, focality, etc. cannot reliably identify *'ab initio'* responders from non-responders to the initial therapy. The most common therapeutical approach to patients with recurrent superficial bladder cancer is transurethral resection (TUR) and/or intravesical therapy. Unfortunately, the long-term impact in terms of risks/benefits of the repeated conservative treatment of patients with recurrent superficial bladder cancer is unknown.

None of the most common factors suggested (Table 16.2) are able to predict the response to treatment in the individual patient and particularly in patients with a 'chronic' disease such as *multi-recurrent* unresponsive superficial bladder cancer.

The response to intravesical therapy is undoubtedly a well-known prognostic factor. The most exhaustive data come from bacillus Calmette–Guérin (BCG) therapy trials. In a multivariate analysis of factors affecting tumour progression, Herr *et al.* [8] found that the prognostic risk groups were best defined 6 months after BCG therapy; positive cytology and positive cystoscopy as well as multifocality are independent

Table 16.2 Unfavourable prognostic factors of superficial bladder cancer.

- Stage 1
- Grade 3
- Multifocality
- Adjacent dysplasia/CIS
- No response to intravesical therapy
- Recurrent
- Tumour size

prognostic variables. Soloway [9] suggested that the 3-month evaluation after MMC therapy is a marker point for a change of therapy. The persistence of TCC prostate involvement after BCG therapy is associated with a high frequency of invasive or metastatic bladder cancer [10]. It must be underlined that these data and others relate to a single intravesical treatment.

The following step in clarifying the problem is to look at the patients who underwent second- (or more) line intravesical therapy. Once again, data available in the literature are sparse and anecdotal and come from small patient series (Tables 16.3 and 16.4). Catalona *et al.* [11] found that failure to respond to three or more courses of BCG therapy was associated with 30% and 50% of tumour progression and metastases, respectively. Furthermore, 42–60% of patients responded favourably to second-line intravesical chemotherapy after failure to respond to previous chemotherapy [12–15]. Moreover, two small series showed that intravesical chemotherapy is worthwhile after unsuccessful BCG therapy [16,17]. BCG therapy is also active as a second-line therapy in patients who have been unsuccessfully treated with intravesical chemotherapy with response rates ranging from 38–68% [18–20] and 84% of long-term relapses after previous successful BCG therapy can be effectively treated with further BCG therapy [21].

Table 16.3 Second-line intravesical therapy: percent responses.

Study	CHEMO. after CHEMOTHERAPY			
	Agent	Patients (*N*)	Treatment	% Response
Prout *et al.* [12]	MMC after TTPA	23	Prophyl/therapy	43
Issel *et al.* [13]	MMC after TTPA	57	Prophyl/therapy	42
Zincke *et al.* [15]	TTPA after MMC	5	Prophylaxis	60
Milani *et al.* [14]	MMC after ADM	31	Prophylaxis	62
	CHEMO. after BCG			
Pinon *et al.* [16]	MMC	4	Prophylaxis	100
Rintala *et al.* [17]	MMC	11	Prophyl/therapy	82

Abbreviations: ADM, Adriamycin; MMC, Mitomycin C; TTPA, Thiotepa.

Table 16.4 Second-line intravesical therapy: percent response.

	BCG after CHEMOTHERAPY			
Study	Previous agent	Patients (*N*)	Treatment	% Response
Soloway and Perry [18]	TTPA/MMC	30	Prophyl/Therapy	50
Lamm *et al.* [20]	MMC/TTPA	37	Prophylaxis	38
Pagano *et al.* [19]	MMC/ADM	28	Prophylaxis	68
	BCG after BCG			
Bassi *et al.* [21]	BCG	19	Prophyl/Therapy	84

Abbreviations: ADM, Adriamycin; MMC, Mitomycin C; TTPA, Thiotepa.

The above-mentioned data support the general statement that second-line intravesical therapy works even though no data are available about more than two intravesical treatments or, specifically, about the optimal time to change therapy.

When to change therapy? The scientific answer

'Perseverare autem diabolicum?' [22]. In other words, is repeated intravesical therapy justified in patients with multifocal and multi-recurrent superficial bladder cancer? If so in which patients and when should therapy be changed?

In order to answer these questions we reviewed our experience of 148 patients with multifocal and multi-recurrent or persistent superficial bladder tumours who underwent multiple TUR and/or two or more intravesical treatments because of multifocal disease (stages Ta, T1, Tis, G1–3) without prostate or upper urinary tract transitional-cell carcinoma involvement. Patient characteristics are listed in Table 16.5.

The patients were given the most commonly used intravesical agents (Mitomycin C, doxorubicin, epirubicin, BCG, mitoxantrone) with recognized therapeutical regimens. All visible papillary tumours were resected and cold biopsies of normal and abnormal appearing bladder mucosa were routinely taken during every cystoscopy. Response criteria for the prophylaxis group were: no recurrence (negative histology and bladder washing cytology), recurrence (positive histology and/or bladder washing cytology) and progression (muscle invasion and/or metastases). In the therapy group, complete response (negative histology and bladder washing cytology), no response (positive histology and/or bladder washing cytology) and progression (muscle invasion and/or metastases) were considered as well.

The patient series was statistically evaluated by univariate (Log-rank test) and multivariate analyses (MPLR stepwise selection procedure and L-ratio Cox's test). The primary endpoint was progression-free survival (PFS) which was evaluated according to the following variables: initial stage, initial grade, 'dynamic' stage (considered as: to have initially been diagnosed as stage T1, to have developed a stage T1 in the long run or to have never been diagnosed as stage T1), 'dynamic' grade (considered as: to have initially been diagnosed as grade-3 tumour, to have developed a grade-3 tumour in the long run or to have never been diagnosed as grade-3 tumour) and number of positive cystoscopies at the 3-year follow-up.

Table 16.5 Patient characteristics (148 pts).

Initial stage		Initial grade	
Patients (*N*)	%	Patients (*N*)	%
Ta, 90	61	G1, 19	13
Tis, 34	23	G2, 84	57
T1, 24	16	G3, 45	30
Median follow-up		52 months (10–134)	
i.v. chemotherapy		134/138 pts (90.5%)	
i.v. immunotherapy		133/148 pts (90%)	
No. i.v. treatments		× 2 = 78 pts (53%)	
		× 3 = 40 pts (27%)	
		× 4–5 = 50 pts (20%)	
Median TUR number		9 (3–20)	
Median i.v. treatments		2 (2–5)	

Initial stage and dynamic stage

The univariate analysis showed that Ta and Tis stages had a similar prognosis when compared to stage T1 (Fig. 16.1). The patients who never had a T1 tumour had a higher progression-free survival rate than those who eventually developed a T1 tumour and more, even more so, than those in whom a T1 tumour was initially diagnosed, as shown by the multivariate analysis (Fig. 16.2).

Initial grade and dynamic grade

No statistically significant differences were shown between G1, G2 and G3 tumours at the univariate analysis ($p = 0.0700$). However, coupling G1 and G2 tumours, a statistically significant difference was observed (Fig. 16.3) in comparison with grade-3 tumours. The multivariate analysis, indeed, showed the progression-free survival to be superior in patients who never had a G3 tumour in comparison with that observed in patients who developed a G3 tumour in the long run or in those in whom a G3 tumour had been initially diagnosed (Fig. 16.4).

3-year positive cystoscopies number

Both univariate and multivariate (Fig. 16.5) analysis showed that the patients with less than three positive cystoscopies at the 3-year follow-up had a better prognosis when compared with that recorded in patients with three or more positive cystoscopies at the same follow-up.

Risk factors and risk categories

The above-mentioned statistical evaluations led to the selection of three independent predictive factors as listed in Table 16.6 and subsequently to the identification of three

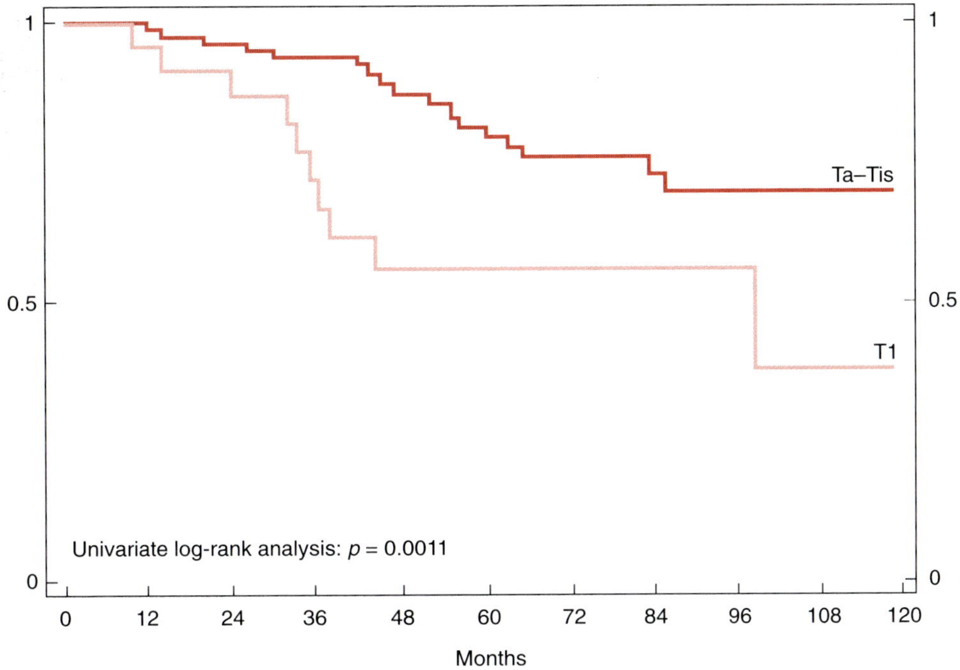

Figure 16.1. Progression-free survival (PFS) according to initial tumour stage.

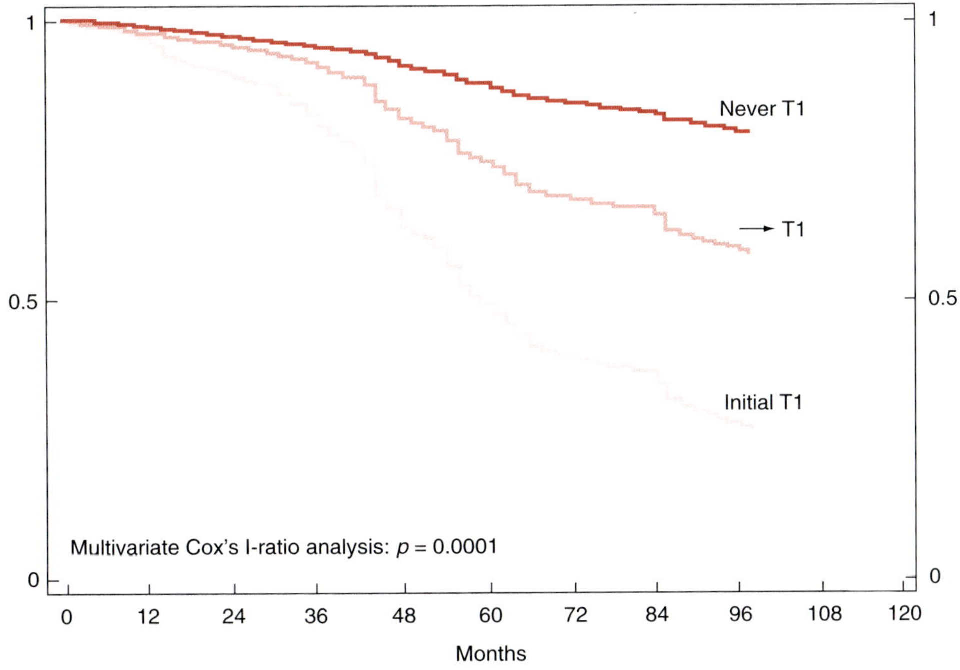

Figure 16.2. Progression-free survival (PFS) according to 'dynamic' tumour stage.

risk categories (Table 16.7) for tumour progression: low, moderate and high risk. The definition of three risk factors for tumour progression subsequently led to the identification of 18 more combinations of risk factors, which were then reduced to six combinations by applying the mentioned risk categories. A further attempt to reduce the number of prognostic levels was made as shown in Fig. 16.6. The comparison of

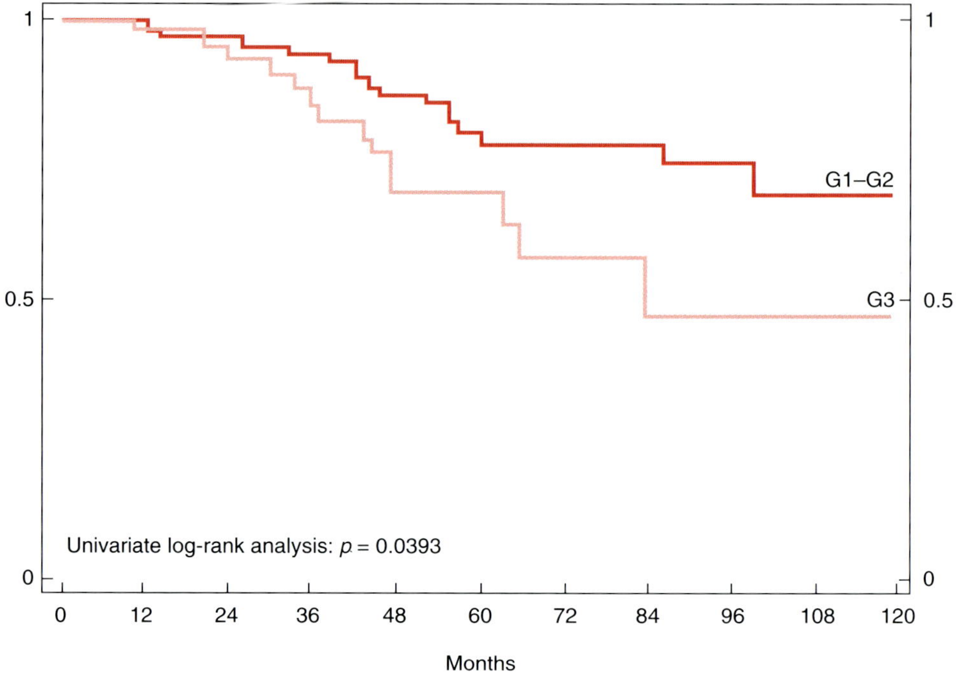

Figure 16.3. Progression-free survival (PFS) according to initial tumour grade.

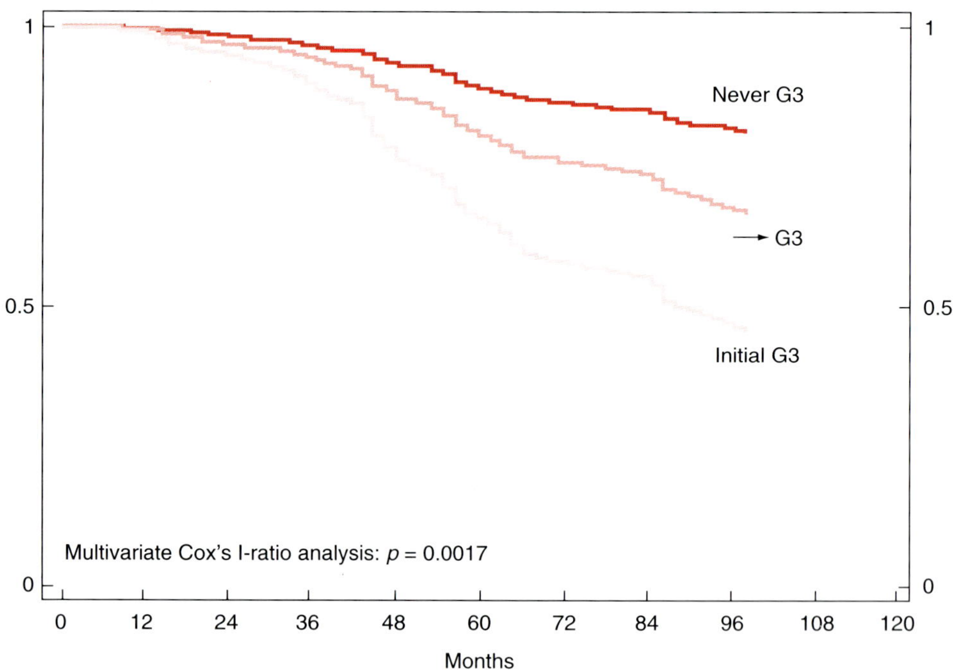

Figure 16.4. Progression-free survival (PFS) according to 'dynamic' tumour grade.

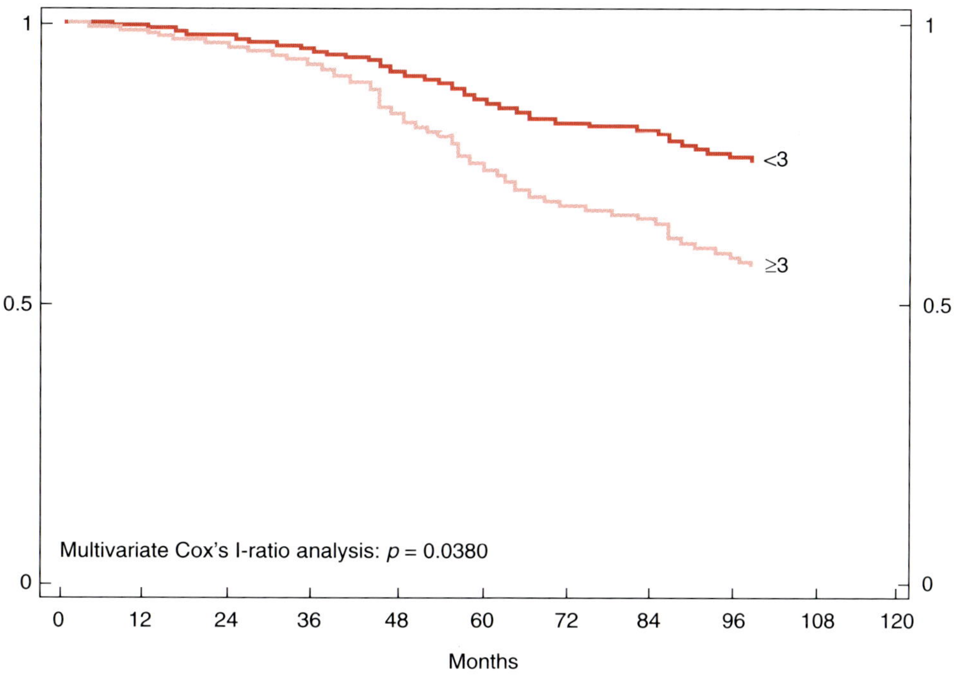

Figure 16.5. Progression-free survival (PFS) according to the number of positive cystoscopies at 36-month follow-up recurrences.

Table 16.6 Risk factors: *p* values.

Covariates	Univariate	Multivariate
'Dynamic stage'	< 0.0001	0.0001
'Dynamic grade'	0.0026	0.0017
No. positive cystoscopies at 3-year follow-up	0.0043	0.0380

Table 16.7 Risk categories as from multivariate and stepwise selection analyses.

	Risk groups		
Risk factor	Low risk	Moderate risk	High risk
'Dynamic' T	Never T1	→ T1	Initial T1
'Dynamic' G	Never G3	→ G3	Initial G3
No. positive cystoscopies at 3-year follow-up	< 3	≥ 3	–

these curves to those of the survival estimates resulting from the Kaplan–Meier test confirmed the prognostic value of this selection (Fig. 16.7).

Patients with no risk factors or one moderate risk factor had a better prognosis (low-risk category, 90% 5-year progression-free survival) in comparison with that observed in a high-risk population who had two high-risk factors or one high-risk + two moderate-

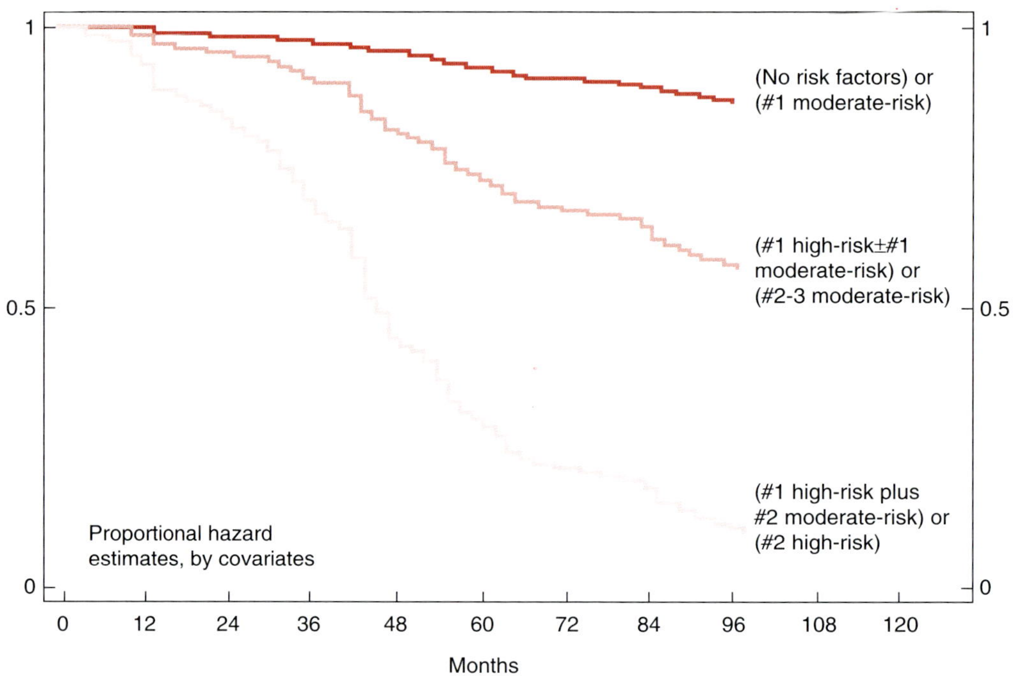

Figure 16.6. Progression-free survival (PFS) according to risk factors (three prognostic levels).

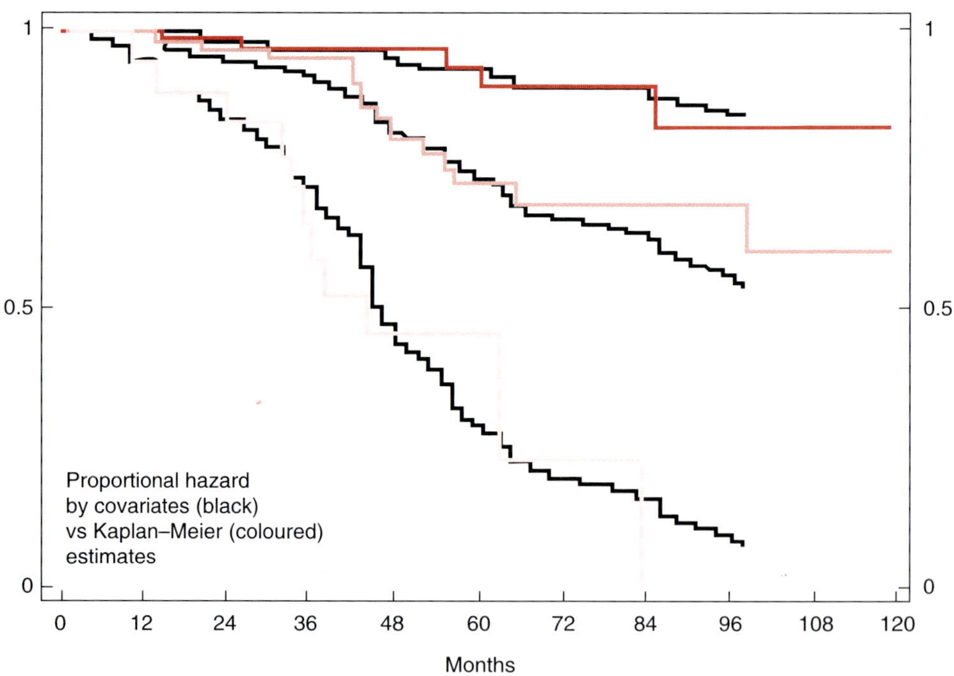

Figure 16.7. Progression-free survival (PFS) according to risk factors (three prognostic levels).

risk factors (high-risk category, 30% 5-year progression-free survival). An intermediate-risk category with a 75% 5-year progression-free survival is characterized by one high-risk + 1 moderate-risk factor or by two to three moderate-risk factors.

Conclusions

Three independent prognostic factors for tumour progression have been identified through the statistical evaluation of a series of patients who underwent repeated conservative treatments (TUR, chemo-immunotherapy) for multifocal and multi-recurrent superficial bladder cancer: 'dynamic' stage, 'dynamic' grade and number of positive cystoscopies at the 3-year follow-up. A practical and scientifically based-risk category system has been found to guide decisions regarding therapy.

References

1   Lamm DL. Long-term results of intravesical therapy for superficial bladder cancer. *Urol Clin N Am* 1992; **19**(3): 573–80.

2   Badalament RA, Ortolano V, Burgres JK. Recurrent or aggressive bladder cancer. *Urol Clin N Am* 1992; **19**(3): 485–98.

3   Hudson MLA. When intravesical measures fail. *Urol Clin N Am* 1992; **19**(3): 601–9.

4   Vogeli T, Ackermann R. When does superficial bladder cancer resist intravesical therapy? *Sem Urol* 1990; **8**: 248–53.

5   Bracken RB, McDonald MW, Johnson DE. Cystectomy for superficial bladder cancer. *Urology* 1981; **18**: 459–65.

6   Malkowicz SB, Nichols P, Lieskovsky G *et al.* The role of radical cystectomy in the management of high grade superficial bladder cancer (PA, P1, P1s and P2). *J Urol* 1990; **144**: 641–6.

7   Amling CL, Thrasher JB, Frazier HA *et al.* Radical cystectomy for stages Ta, Tis, T1 transitional cell carcinoma of the bladder. *J Urol* 1994; **151**: 31–6.

8   Herr HW, Badalament RA, Amato VP. Superficial bladder cancer treated with bacillus Calmette–Guérin: a multivariate analysis of factors affecting tumor progression. *J Urol* 1989; **141**: 22–8.

9   Soloway MS. Treatment of superficial bladder cancer with intravesical Mitomycin C: analysis of immediate and long-term response on 70 patients. *J Urol* 1985; **134**: 1007–12.

10 Montie JE, Wood DP Jr. The significance and the management of transitional cell carcinoma of the prostate. *Semin Urol* 1990; **8**: 262–9.

11 Catalona WJ, Hudson MA, Gillen DP, Andriole GL, Ratliff TL. Risks and benefits of repeated courses of intravesical bacillus Calmette–Guérin therapy for superficial bladder cancer. *J Urol* 1987; **137**: 220–4.

12 Prout GR Jr, Griffin PP, Nocks BN. Intravesical therapy of low stage bladder carcinoma with Mitomycin C: comparison of results in untreated and previously treated patients. *J Urol* 1982; **127**: 1096–102.

13 Issel BF, Prout GR, Soloway MS. Mitomycin C intravesical therapy in noninvasive bladder cancer after failure on thiotepa. *Cancer* 1984; **53**: 1025–30.

14 Milani C, Bassi P, Meneghini A *et al.* Mitomycin C in multiple superficial bladder cancer: short-term therapy, long-term results. *Urol Int* 1992; **48**: 154–6.

15 Zincke H, Benson RC Jr, Hilton JF. Intravesical thiotepa and Mitomycin C treatment immediately after transurethral resection and later for superficial bladder cancer: a prospective, randomized, stratified study with crossover design. *J Urol* 1985; **134**: 1110–16.

16 Pinon AA, Suarez GM, Politano VA. Experience with second and third line intravesical chemotherapy agents after initial agent failures. *J Urol* 1988; **139**: 320A.

17 Rintala E, Jauhiainen K, Alfthan O *et al.* Intravesical chemotherapy (Mitomycin C) versus immunotherapy (bacillus Calmette–Guérin) in superficial bladder cancer. *Eur Urol* 1991; **20**: 19–25.

18 Soloway MS, Perry A. Bacillus Calmette–Guérin for treatment of superficial transitional cell carcinoma of the bladder in patients who have failed thiotepa and/or Mitomycin C. *J Urol* 1987; **137**: 871–3.

19 Pagano F, Bassi P, Milani C. A low dose bacillus Calmette–Guérin regimen in superficial bladder cancer therapy: is it effective? *J Urol* 1991; **146**: 32–6.

20 Lamm DL, Grissmann J, Blumenstein B *et al.* Adriamycin versus BCG in superficial bladder cancer: a Southwest Oncology Group Study. *Prog Clin Biol Res* 1989; **310**: 263–70.

21 Bassi P, Milani C, Piazza N *et al.* Effectiveness of a rescue bacillus Calmette–Guérin (BCG) therapy in patients who relapsed after successful response to BCG therapy of superficial bladder cancer. *J Urol* 1992; **147**: 372A.
22 Saint Agostino. De Civitate Dei (Sermon 164,14). Milan: Garzanti Editore 1982.

CHAPTER 17

Automated nuclear morphological grading

H.G. van der Poel, J.A. Witjes, J.A. Schalken
and F.M.J. Debruyne

Introduction

The biology of tumour development is characterized by many cellular and nuclear changes. Many of these changes, which can be observed using light microscopy, have been widely applied for the grading of malignancies. The causes of the morphological changes are ill-understood. The nuclear matrix is putatively the framework of the nucleus determining nuclear appearance. The changes occurring in nuclear and cellular morphology may be applicable for automated grading. The application of quantitative analysis of cellular and nuclear morphology for clinical decision-making will be reviewed.

Nuclear matrix and nuclear morphology

In 1974, Berezny and Coffey [1] observed disruption of the nuclear structure of isolated rat-liver nuclei by mild digestion with proteases; however, other chemical treatments were of no influence on nuclear morphology. Upon removing chromatin, DNA, RNA, and phospholipids from the nucleus, they found a spherical residual particle for more than 98% consisting of polypeptides and accounting for less than 15% of the mass of an entire cell nucleus. The major function of this nuclear matrix is organization of the DNA into loop domains. Matrix-associated topoisomerase-II activity for instance modulates DNA topology. The nuclear matrix plays a role in RNA synthesis by association of the transcribed genes to the matrix and binding RNA processing intermediates [2,3,4,5]. The mechanism by which the nuclear matrix structures nuclear shape is called tensegrity. This is defined as a dynamic structure based on a framework composed of compression elements and tension cables [5].

The nuclear matrix is cell-type specific [2,3]. Moreover, extracellular factors determine the composition and morphology of the nuclear matrix [4,5,6]. Recent studies have shown differences in nuclear-matrix protein composition in transitional-cell cancer compared to composition in normal bladder mucosa, illustrating the role of the nuclear matrix in tumour development [7].

The nuclear matrix determines nuclear morphology and regulates gene expression. Mulder *et al.* [8] described the genetic changes in colorectal cancer and correlated these changes with nuclear morphology. The nuclear shape and chromatin-pattern features established in light microscopic images were predominantly associated with tumour progression in colon carcinoma and were not influenced by the individual molecular genetic alterations like allelic deletions in chromosomes *5q, 18p, 17p* and mutations in the *ras* gene. Nuclear-chromatin texture, however, was inversely related to fractional allelic loss, a measure of overall genetic change in the cell. Moreover, for urothelium it was shown that extracellular components influence nuclear-matrix organization and in this way may regulate the epithelium [6]. These findings suggest that, in normal as well as cancerous tissue, genetic and epigenetic changes determine nuclear morphology. Hence, nuclear morphology could be applied to monitor the summation of genetic and epigenetic changes in tumour development.

Image analysis techniques

Computer development has led to the availability of image-analysis equipment at relatively low costs. Image-analysis systems are normally composed of a light or fluorescence microscope and a charge-coupled device (CCD) camera for image acquisition. Image processing and analysis are often performed with a (personal) computer using a frame-grabber board. The microscope can be equipped with an automated cross-table for computer-directed selection of areas of interest. Moreover, autofocus methods can be applied.

Using different staining techniques, objects of interest can be differentiated. The Feulgen–Schiff staining method is used for analysis of nuclear morphology and chromatin analysis [9]. Since DNA is stained using this method it is also well suited for analysis of nuclear DNA content. Furthermore, *in situ* hybridization methods and immunostainings can be quantified by image-analysis techniques [10]. In this review nuclear morphological analysis by image analysis in transitional-cell carcinoma of the bladder will be discussed on the basis of recent literature. Earlier studies have been reviewed elsewhere [11].

The basic principle of image-analysis techniques is to digitize and quantify image information after image enhancement. By segmentation of the image the present object(s) can be identified using criteria for background and objects such as grey value or size. After segmentation morphological operations can be performed to obtain information on shape and size of the object.

Shape descriptors

A commonly applied shape descriptor, the nuclear roundness factor, basically presents the ratio of nuclear surface area divided by nuclear contour length (i.e. perimeter). A drawback of the (nuclear) roundness factor is that it confuses roundness and circularity [12]. Hence, it is less suited for discrimination between ellipsoid and irregular round objects. The so-called Freeman-chain code of the perimeter pixels enables a wide variety of morphometric analyses [13,14]. The spectrum of shape descriptors is extensive. Dependent on smoothing procedures, large- or small-form deviations can be quantified. Moreover, discrimination between concavities and convexities can be made. Detailed information of shape can be obtained [13]. From histological interpretation, it is known that for each tissue type specific nuclear-shape changes occur in malignant development. Hence, selection of the shape descriptors to apply will always be necessary dependent on shape changes to be discriminated.

For bladder cancer we assumed elongation of the nucleus to be the initial step in malignant development, since it is found in most low-grade tumours. Histological sections contain entire as well as cut nuclei. Hence, section thickness and the direction of tissue resection determine the way the nuclei present in a histological slide. To avoid this problem digestion of cells to cytological material can be performed [15].

To recalculate the nuclear volume, assuming that not every nucleus is entirely included in the section but rather presented as a slice of it, several mathematical approaches have been applied [16,17]. The use of these corrections did not prove to be of additional prognostic value for bladder cancer.

DNA ploidy analysis

During the cell cycle nuclear DNA content varies. These changes and the distribution of cells over the different stages of the cycle can be analysed using the DNA histogram of the population. The DNA content of each nucleus is analysed using the integrated optical density of a DNA stoichiometric staining (e.g. Feulgen). It should be noted here that (fluorescence) *in situ* hybridization techniques can be analysed by image-analysis techniques enabling more accurate determination of chromosomal aberrations in cancer [10,18].

Nuclear chromatin analysis

Chromatin texture analysis comprises the description of distribution of intranuclear material. Material processing highly influences chromatin appearance in cytology and histology [19]. Therefore, absolute values only apply to well-standardized populations. Examples of texture descriptors are Markovian-matrix analysis, run-length analysis, and variance in optical density [17,20,21].

Histology

Quantitative studies in bladder cancer can basically be divided into cytological and histological methods.

For histologically automated tumour grading several multivariate studies have been published. Blomjous *et al.* [22] proposed an interactive nuclear-selection system for the histological grading of bladder cancer; a mean value over 95 μm^2 of the largest selected nuclei was correlated with an increased progression rate. In T1–T2 low-grade cancers, however, Lipponen *et al.* [23] found the mean nuclear size of the 10 largest selected nuclei only of predictive value in combination with the mitotic/volume index, indicating that proliferation rather than nuclear size was of predictive value [24,25,26]. Sowter *et al.* [27,28] proposed a grading system based on both subjective histological grading and nuclear-size analysis, whereas Borland *et al.* (1993) [29] found nuclear shape useful for predicting progression after cystectomy.

Including tissue architecture de Meester *et al.* [30] developed a system for the automated grading of histological bladder tumour material. The system, however, was sensitive to the area selected and was not tested against clinical outcome. Lipponen *et al.* [26] suggest D_{max}, the longest nuclear axis, as a prognostic clinical marker in pTa–pT1 papillary bladder cancer. A comparable multivariate analysis on histological material was performed by Colombel *et al.* [31,32]. Again, a combination of several nuclear features resulted in prognostic information regarding tumour recurrence and progression for superficial as well as invasive tumours [31]. They advocated the use of their system mainly in superficial cancers.

A different approach to histological grading was applied by van Velthoven *et al.* [15]. Instead of using histological sections, pronase digested, re-suspended material was used. The chromatin pattern of each Feulgen-stained nucleus was quantified. In combination with ploidy analysis this yielded a 91% correct prediction of tumour recurrence. Similar evidence of the value of chromatin-pattern characterization for the grading of tumours was provided by Choi *et al.* [33]. Before widespread clinical application is feasible, however, study is needed to determine the influence of digestion techniques on chromatin patterns.

In summary, early studies focused on nuclear size as a prognostic marker. When more sophisticated systems became available the complexity of morphological features increased. Multivariate analysis showed that a combination of nuclear shape and chromatin features probably add to clinical findings. Although all of these studies support the value of quantitative analysis methods for interpretation of microscopic images, none compared the method to a range of other markers. Hence, before imaging methods become of clinical value, studies comparing different prognosticators are required; however, the currently available methods can support pathological diagnosis. In particular, reproducibility increases using quantitative methods. Moreover, cell-to-cell analysis of, for example, DNA ploidy may aid in more accurate sub(grading), e.g. grade-2 tumours.

Cytology

From 1975 to 1989 several publications appeared from the Montefiore Medical Center in New York on computer-image analysis of voided urine cytology [34,35]. A system was constructed for the automatic grading of urinary cytology based on the cell-to-cell reference of a panel of observers. Sensitivity of the system was 84% for the detection of urothelial-cell carcinoma, as compared to 63% for visual cytology of the same cases [32]. A special algorithm reduced the number of cells necessary for analysis. Although promising results were obtained, as yet, widespread clinical application is not obtained.

In an analysis of 32 nuclear features analysed in bladder-wash material from patients with superficial bladder cancer, nuclear shape and the 2c-deviation index [36] were found to correlate to tumour grading [37,39]. This quantitative cytology system (QUANTICYT®) was tested in a study population of 1412 patients. With the help of the system, bladder-wash samples were divided into low, intermediate, and high risk (Fig. 17.1) referring to the subsequent risk for tumour recurrence or progression (Fig. 17.2). A report form was designed to present results from consecutive samples graphically in order to detect changes in the morphometric characteristics in the bladder-wash sample (Fig. 17.3).

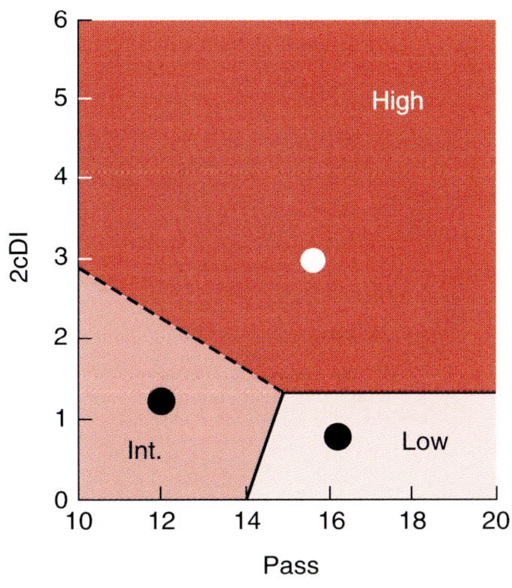

Figure 17.1. Risk groups as defined by the QUANTICYT® system on basis of the nuclear shape (MPASS) and 2cDI (Low risk, Intermediate risk, High risk).

(a)

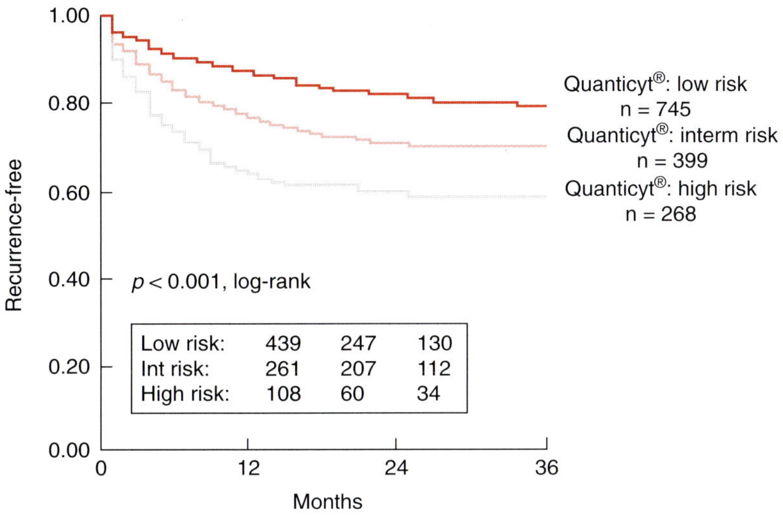

(b)

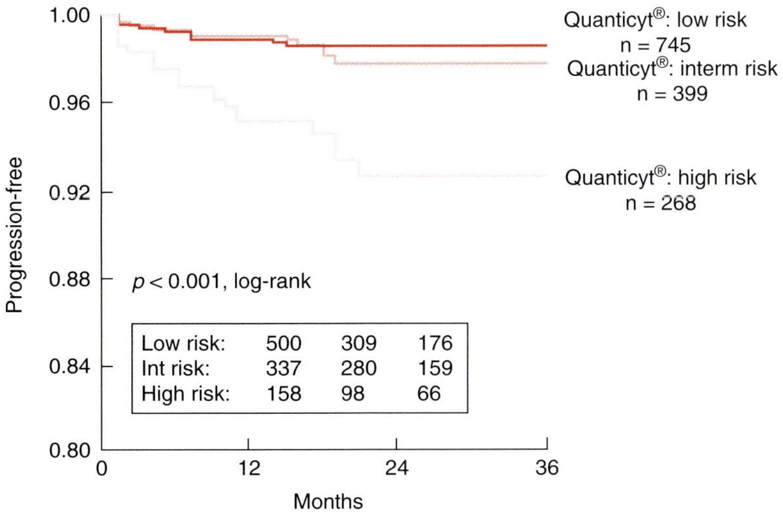

Figure 17.2. (a) Recurrence and (b) progression by QUANTICYT® risk groups (n = 1412).

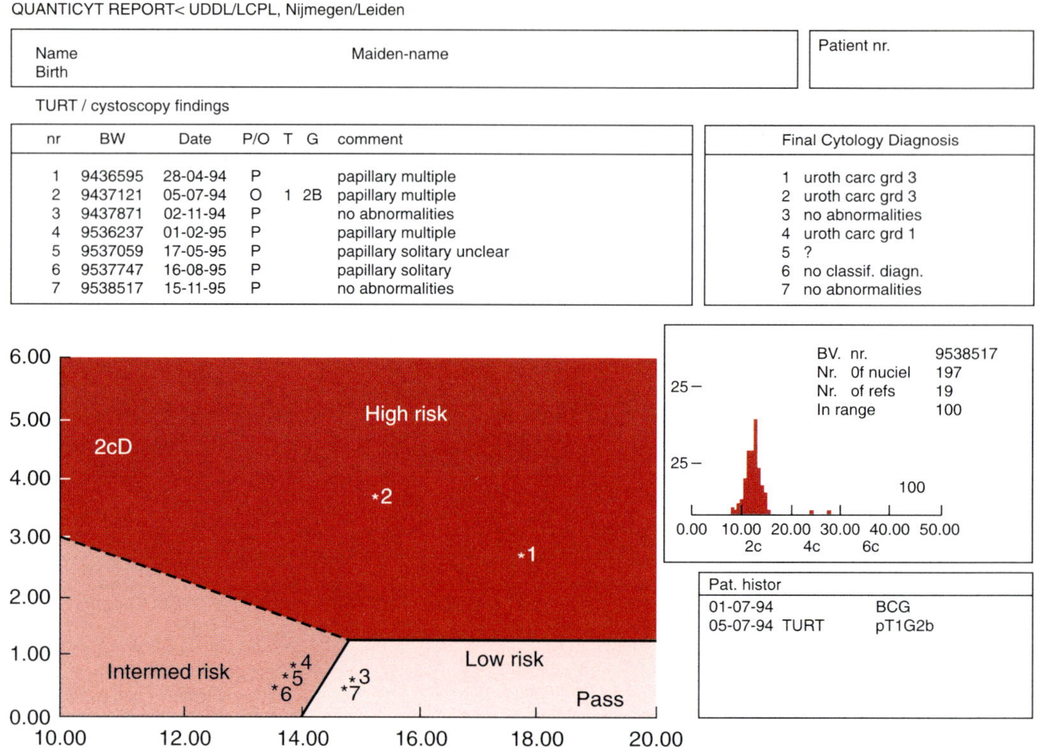

Figure 17.3. Example of a report form from the QUANTICYT® system.

Analogous to the system described by Koss *et al.* [34,35] the QUANTICYT® system automatically analyses nuclei in light-microscopic images. In contrast to the system of Koss *et al.*, the QUANTICYT® system used the histological findings and follow-up data (tumour recurrence and progression) as references, instead of cytology grading. Moreover, bladder-wash samples were applied instead of voided urine.

Cytological material enables the analysis of entire cells and nuclei with little distortion of the image by background objects like intercellular material or sectioning artifacts. Assuming random distribution of cells in the cytology medium renders the sample even more accessible to automated analysis compared to histological material.

DNA ploidy and bladder cancer

For both cytology and histology, nuclear size proved to be an important prognostic factor. Is the increase in nuclear size caused by an increase in nuclear DNA content? This is only partly true. Fosså and Kaalhus [39] demonstrated an increase of nuclear size with aneuploidy, but found large nuclei in more differentiated cells in comparable ploidy classes; this was explained by a decrease in chromatin concentration.

By flow cytometry, aneuploidy in general was found to be associated with more malignant behaviour [40,41]. Quantitative light microscopy in histology proved to be more sensitive for small populations of aneuploid cells compared to flow cytometry [42]. For cytological material, where enzymatic digestion of the material prior to flow cytometry is not required, image techniques were not inferior to flow cytometry [43].

Moreover, image-analysis methods provide the possibility of simultaneous DNA analysis, morphometry, and visual interpretation of each cell or cluster of cells.

Bass *et al.* [44–47], developed a fluorescence method for the ploidy analysis in bladder cytology. Sensitivity of ploidy analysis of (urine) cytology for low-grade diploid cancers is low and this renders ploidy analysis alone less applicable for the follow-up of patients with superficial bladder cancer. In combination with nuclear shape [38] or nuclear size [23], ploidy analysis can be a more valuable prognostic tool.

Follow-up of bladder cancer patients

To assess the possible role of new markers in the clinical diagnosis and follow-up of patients with superficial bladder cancer, the tools used need to be addressed. Cystoscopy and urine cytology comprise the basic elements in the follow-up of patients diagnosed with superficial bladder cancer. Cystoscopy is unpleasant to the patient and may underestimate small lesions of carcinoma *in situ*, whereas (urinary) cytology shows low sensitivity in low-grade lesions and low inter- and intra-observer reproducibility [48].

Several clinical factors predict the chance of tumour recurrence. Multiplicity, tumour grade and stage, and earlier tumour-recurrence rate are correlated with tumour recurrences, despite intravesical instillation treatment [49,50]. Hall *et al.* [51] proposed a follow-up plan, based on multiplicity and recurrence at 3 months after resection, two indicators of increased recurrence rate. Hence, available clinical data can aid in the planning of follow-up schemes. Cystoscopy remains the 'gold standard' in the detection of tumour recurrences. A reliable marker on cytological material could replace cystoscopy in patients with low risk for tumour recurrence and thus reduce costs and patient inconvenience. Moreover, predicting tumour recurrences more reliably can aid in the stratification for (intravesical) treatment modalities.

In the low-risk group of patients, as defined by Kurth *et al.* [50] on clinical parameters, 7% of tumours still progress to invasive disease within 3 years of diagnosis; this group comprised 52% of their patient population, whereas the high-risk group comprised only 6.7% of the patients of whom 42% progressed. Hence, the absolute number of progressive tumours in the low-risk group is still higher than the absolute number in the high-risk group. These data indicate that changing treatment and follow-up schemes, based on relative risk alone, underestimates the potential risk of the less aggressive, but more frequent, cancers and may put an equal number of patients at risk of late detection of progression, as are found in time by meticulous follow-up of the high-risk patient group. Two factors are important to overcome this dilemma: (1) more accurate prognostic markers, and (2) a reliable tool for the monitoring of bladder mucosal changes during patient follow up, in particular in the less progressive cancers.

Follow-up schemes and automated-image analysis

Since the majority of patients who experience tumour recurrences do so within 2 years of transurethral resection (TUR) of a tumour, cystoscopy frequency is traditionally recommended to be every 3 or 4 months for the first 1–2 years. The chance of developing tumour progression due to later detection and thus resection of

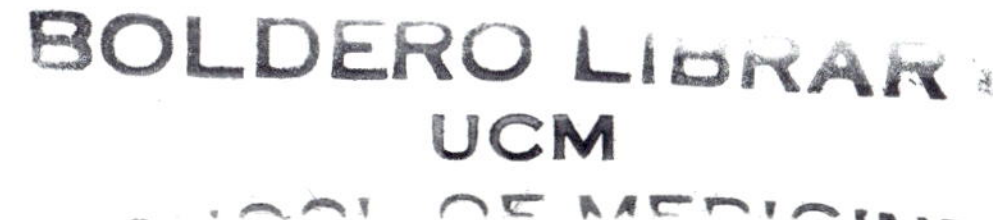

tumour recurrences is not known. Moreover, tumour characteristics seem to change over time, making prediction of tumour behaviour in an early phase of disease more difficult [52].

A clear report is mandatory for clinical integration of an automated-imaging system. A high frequency of follow-up cystoscopies may not be necessary in large groups of 'low-risk' patients. The presence of small lesions of low-malignancy grade may be efficiently treated expectively or with laser coagulation. In these cases information on malignancy grade of the bladder mucosa and the present lesions can be provided by automated image analysis-supported cytology.

Future studies will have to answer the question regarding whether cystoscopy frequency can be reduced by applying automated image analysis methods. In particular, in low-grade superficial lesions, automated image analysis of cytologic material can play a role since few reliable markers exist for these tumours. Quantitative analysis enables comparison of subsequent samples which can give an early measure of malignant mucosal changes indicating the need for earlier resection or (random) biopsies.

Automated image analysis is an easily accessible technique for use in daily practice. Urologists acquainted with markers of DNA ploidy and morphology can apply the method to support decision making. Only with effective collaboration between urologists and pathologists will new methods find their way into daily practice and optimize clinical decision making.

References

1   Berezny R, Coffey DS. Identification of a nuclear protein matrix. *Biochem Biophys Res Commun* 1974; **60**: 1410.

2   Fey EG, Penman S. Nuclear matrix proteins reflect cell type of origin in cultured human cells. *Proc Natl Acad Sci* 1988; **85**: 121.

3   Getzenberg RH. Nuclear matrix and the regulation of gene expression: tissue specificity. *J Cell Biochem* 1994; **55**: 22.

4   Pienta KJ, Murphy BC, Getzenberg R, Coffey DS. The effect of extracellular matrix interactions on morphologic transformation *in vitro. Biochem Biophys Res Commun* 1991; **179**: 333.

5   Pienta KJ, Partin AW, Coffey DS. Cancer as a disease of DNA organization and dynamic cell structure. *Cancer Res* 1989; **49**: 2525.

6   Gordon JN, Shu WP, Schlussel RN, Droller MJ, Liu BC. Altered extracellular matrices influence cellular processes and nuclear matrix organization of overlying human bladder urothelial cells. *Cancer Res* 1993; **53**: 4971.

7   Miyanaga N, Akaza H, Ohtani M *et al.* Nuclear matrix proteins as a urine marker for transitional cell carcinoma of the bladder. A preliminary report. *J Urol* 1995; **153**: 457A.

8   Mulder JW, Offerhaus GJ, de Feyter EP *et al.* The relationship of quantitative nuclear morphology to molecular genetic alterations in the adenoma–carcinoma sequence of the large bowel. *Am J Pathol* 1992; **141**: 797.

9   Feulgen R, Rossenbeck M. Mikroskopisch-chemischer Nachweiss einer Nucleinsäure vom Typhus der Thymonucleinsäure und die darauf beruhrende elektive Färbung von Zellkernen in mikroskopische Präparaten. *Hoppe Seyler's Z Physiol Chem* 1924; **135**: 203.

10 Cajulis RS, Haines GK, Frias-Hidvegi D, McVary K, Bacus JW. Cytology, flow cytometry, image analysis, and interphase cytogenetics by fluorescence *in situ* hybridization in the diagnosis of transitional cell carcinoma in bladder washings: a comparative study. *Diagn Cytopathol* 1995; **13**: 214.

11 van der Poel HG, Schaafsma HE, Vooijs G, Debruyne FMJ, Schalken JA. Quantitative light microscopy in urologic oncology. *J Urol* 1992; **148**: 1.

12 Serra J. *Image analysis and mathematical morphology.* London: Academic Press, 1982; 366.

13 Bengtsson E, Eriksson O, Holmquist J *et al.* Segmentation of cervical cells: detection of overlapping cell nuclei. *Comp Graph Image Proc* 1981; **16**: 382.

14　Bowie JE, Young IT. An analysis technique for biological shape. II. *Acta Cytol* 1977; **21**: 455.

15　van Velthoven R, Petein M, Oosterlinck WJ *et al.* The use of digital image analysis of chromatin texture in Feulgen-stained nuclei to predict recurrence of low grade superficial transitional cell carcinoma of the bladder. *Cancer* 1995; **75**: 560.

16　Bins M, Takens F. A method to estimate the DNA content of whole nuclei from measurements made on thin tissue sections. *Cytometry* 1985; **6**: 234.

17　van der Poel HG, Boon ME, Kok LP *et al.* Morphometry, densitometry, and pattern analysis of plastic-embedded histologic material from urothelial cell carcinoma of the bladder. *Anal Quant Cytol Histol* 1991; **13**: 307.

18　Persons DL, Takai K, Gibney DJ *et al.* Comparison of fluorescence *in situ* hybridization with flow cytometry and static image analysis in ploidy analysis of paraffin-embedded prostate adenocarcinoma. *Hum Pathol* 1994; **25**: 678.

19　Boon ME, van der Poel HG, Tan CJ, Kok LP. Effect of embedding methods versus fixative type on karyometric measures. *Anal Quant Cytol Histol* 1994; **16**: 131.

20　Nafe R, Roth S, Rathert P. Fourier analysis as a planimetric procedure — application to malignant and normal urothelial cells with reactive changes. *Exp Pathol* 1991; **43**: 155.

21　Pressman NJ, Haralick RM, Tyrer HW, Frost JK. Texture analysis for biomedical imagery. In: Fu KS, Pavlides T (eds) *Biomedical Pattern Recognition and Image Processing*. Berlin: Dahlem workshop, 1979.

22　Blomjous CEM, Vos W, Schipper NW *et al.* The prognostic significance of selective nuclear morphometry in urinary bladder carcinoma. *Hum Pathol* 190; **21**: 409.

23　Lipponen PK, Eskelinen MJ, Sotarauto M. Prediction of T1-2 G1-2 transitional cell bladder cancer; evaluation by histoquantitative methods. *Scand J Urol Nephrol* 1991; **25**: 129.

24　Lipponen PK. The prognostic value of basement membrane morphology, tumour histology and morphometry in superficial bladder cancer. *J Cancer Res Clin Oncol* 1993; **119**: 295.

25　Lipponen PK. Stereologically measured nuclear volume in comparison to two-dimensional nuclear morphometry, mitotic index and flow cytometry in predicting disease outcome in bladder cancer. *Anticancer Res* 1993; **13**: 529.

26　Lipponen PK, Eskelinen MJ, Jauhiainen K *et al.* Prediction of superficial bladder cancer by nuclear image analysis. *Eur J Cancer* 1992; **29a**: 61.

27　Sowter C, Slavin G, Sowter G, Rosen D, Hendry W. Morphometry of bladder carcinoma: morphometry and grading complement each other. *Anal Cell Pathol* 1991; **3**: 1.

28　Sowter C, Sowter G, Slavon G, Rosen D. Morphometry of bladder-carcinoma: definition of a new variable. *Anal Cell Pathol* 1990; **2**: 205.

29　Borland RN, Partin AW, Epstein JI, Brendler CB. The use of nuclear morphometry in predicting recurrence of transitional cell carcinoma. *J Urol* 1993; **149**: 272.

30　de Meester U, Young IT, Lindeman J, van der Linden HC. Towards a quantitative grading of bladder tumors. *Cytometry* 1991; **12**: 602.

31　Colombel M, de Launoit Y, Bellot J *et al.* Prognostic evaluation of morphonuclear parameters in superficial and invasive bladder cancer. *Br J Urol* 1995; **75**: 364.

32　Colombel MC, Pous MF, Abbou CC *et al.* Computer assisted image analysis of bladder tumour nuclei for morphonuclear and ploidy assessment. *Anal Cell Pathol* 1994; **6**: 137.

33　Choi HK, Vasko J, Bengtsson E *et al.* Grading of transitional cell bladder carcinoma by texture analysis of histological sections. *Ann Cell Pathol* 1994; **6**: 327.

34　Koss LG, Bartels PH, Wied GL. Computer-based diagnostic analysis of cells in the urinary sediment. *J Urol* 1980; **123**: 846.

35　Sherman AB, Koss LG, Wyschogrod D *et al.* Bladder cancer diagnosis by computer image analysis of cells in the sediment of voided urine using a video scanning system. *Anal Quant Cytol Histol* 1986; **8**: 177.

36　Böcking A, Adler CP, Common HD *et al.* Algorithm for a DNA cytophotometric diagnosis and grading of malignancy. *Anal Quant Cytol* 1984; **6**: 1.

37　van der Poel HG, Oosterhof GON, Debruyne FMJ, Schalken JA. Image analysis in superficial transitional cell carcinoma of the bladder. *Sem Urol* 1993; **11**: 164.

38　van der Poel HG, Oosterhof GON, Schaafsma HE *et al.* Karyometry of bladder washings for the follow up of patients with transitional cell carcinoma of the bladder. In: Schröder FH (ed) *EORTC Genitourinary Group Monograph 11: Recent Progress in Bladder and Kidney Cancer.* 1992; 9.

39　Fosså SD, Kaalhus O. Nuclear size and chromatin concentration in transitional cell carcinoma of the human urinary bladder. *Beitr Path Bd* 1976; **157**: 109.

40　Borchers H, Planz B, Jakse G, Böcking A. DNA aneuploidy in G1-urothelial carcinomas of the urinary bladder. *Urol Int* 1994; **52**: 145.

41　Tribukait B, Gustafson H, Esposti PL. The significance of ploidy and proliferation in the clinical and biological evaluation of bladder tumors: a study of 100 untreated cases. *J Urol* 1982; **54**: 130.

42 Clemo FA, Crabtree WN, Walker E, DeNicola DB. Comparison of image analysis and flow cytometric measurements of DNA content of canine transitional cell carcinomas. *Anal Quant Cytol Histol* 1993; **15**: 418.

43 Chabanas A, Rambeaud JJ, Seigneurin D *et al.* Flow and image cytometry for DNA analysis in bladder washings: improved concordance by using internal reference for flow. *Cytometry* 1993; **14**: 943.

44 Bass RA, Hemstreet GP, Honker NA, Hurst RE, Doggett RS. DNA cytometry and cytology by quantitative fluorescent image analysis in symptomatic bladder cancer patients. *Int J Cancer* 1987; **40**: 698.

45 Bi W, Rao JY, Hemstreet GP *et al.* Field molecular epidemiology. Feasibility of monitoring for the malignant bladder cell phenotype in a benzidine-exposed occupational cohort. *J Occup Med* 1993; **35**: 20.

46 Bonner RB, Hemstreet GP, Fradet Y *et al.* Bladder cancer risk assessment with quantitative fluorescence image analysis of tumor markers in exfoliated bladder cells. *Cancer* 1993; **72**: 2461.

47 Hemstreet GP, Rollins S, Jones P *et al.* Identification of a high risk subgroup of grade 1 transitional cell carcinoma using image analysis based deoxyribonucleic acid ploidy analysis for tumor tissue. *J Urol* 1994; **146**: 1525.

48 Sherman AB, Koss LG, Adams SE. Interobserver and intraobserver differences in the diagnosis of urothelial cells. Comparison with classification by computer. *Anal Quant Cytol Histol* 1984; **6**: 112.

49 Kiemeney LA, Witjes JA, Heijbroek RP *et al.* Predictability of recurrent and progressive disease in individual patients with primary superficial bladder cancer. *J Urol* 1993; **150**: 60.

50 Kurth KH, Denis L, Bouffioux Ch *et al.* Factors affecting recurrence and progression in superficial bladder tumours. *Eur J Cancer* 1995; **31A**: 1840.

51 Hall RR, Parmar MKB, Richards AB, Smith PH. The cystoscopic follow up of patients with Ta,T1 bladder carcinoma and the role of adjuvant intravesical therapy: a proposal. *Br Med J* 1994; **308**: 257.

52 van der Poel HG, van Caubergh RD, Boon ME, Debruyne FJM, Schalken JA. Karyometry in recurrent superficial transitional cell tumors of the bladder. *Urol Res* 1992; **20**: 375.

CHAPTER 18

T1 bladder tumour: conservative treatment

W.R. Fair and G. Dalbagni

The problem facing the clinician dealing with patients who have T1 transitional carcinoma of the bladder is essentially that of a management 'tightrope' in that the clinician must balance the respective benefits of early bladder removal or conservative therapy versus the risk of disease progression.

The arguments for conservative therapy of T1 bladder cancer are as follows:

1. The inaccuracy of surgical staging — including errors in detecting vascular-space invasion.
2. The effectiveness of alternative therapy.
3. The availability of potential molecular biological markers to predict those at risk of disease progression.
4. The results of aggressive therapy of T1 disease may reflect more the biology of the disease rather than the treatment.

Inaccurate surgical staging and errors in detecting vascular space invasion

Table 18.1 illustrates data comparing the accuracy of surgical staging with pathological staging [1]. In 166 patients surgically staged as T1 disease, 53% were staged inaccurately by transurethral resection (TUR) and imaging modalities. Most notable, 38 of the 166 (23%) thought to have T1 disease on histological examination of the tissue obtained by TUR were actually overstaged; thus those who would advocate early cystectomy, because of a diagnosis of T1 disease based on TUR results, may in fact be removing more than one in five bladders unnecessarily due to this overstaging.

Additionally, the finding of vascular invasion has been reported to be an adverse prognostic factor in patients with T1 disease [2]. However, in an elegant study by Larsen *et al.* [3], 36 specimens from 33 patients with T1 tumours were originally felt to have vascular invasion on conventional histology alone. The major criteria for patients in this study were strict in that no patient could have a history of prior muscle-invading tumour (T2 or greater); the presence of adequate muscularis propria negative for tumour in the TUR specimen was required and clear lamina propria invasion had to be demonstrated. Despite these strict entry criteria, and the

Table 18.1 Data presented by Thrasher and colleagues at Duke University. Staging accuracy.

	No.	T>P	(%)	P>T	(%)	≥ P2	(%)
Tis/Ta	54	11	(20%)	19	(35%)	6/54	(11%)
T1	166	38	(23%)	50	(30%)	50/166	(30%)
T2	213	28	(13%)	114	(54%)	185/213	(87%)

T>P 77/433 = 18%

P>T 183/433 = 43%

From Thrasher *et al.* [1]

observation on standard haematoxylin and eosin staining that all specimens showed vascular invasion, when immunohistochemistry for factor 8 expression was performed, only 5 of the 36 specimens (14%) were found to have vascular invasion. The negative control for this study involved 35 specimens from 28 patients with clinical T1 disease, but no evidence of vascular invasion. The authors found extensive resection artifacts around the tumour nest, which often could be confused with tumour involving the blood vessels.

Thus, the surgical staging and histochemical evaluation of the extent of lamina propria and blood-vessel invasion is subject to considerable error, and in my opinion the 23% risk of removing a bladder thought to have T1 disease, but pathologically actually free of lamina propria invasion, makes a strong argument for a trial of intravesical therapy followed by a re-staging TUR before cystectomy is considered.

The effectiveness of alternative therapy

Table 18.2 lists a compilation of 5-year survival rates following surgical therapy [4]. These data show that with the exception of TUR for T3 disease, the overall results of radical cystectomy are in general, no better than the judicious use of TUR or segmental cystectomy, especially in the management of T1 disease. The availability of

Table 18.2 Compilation of 5-year survival rates following surgical therapy.

Treatment	T-category			
	Tis, T1	T2	T3a	T3b
Transurethral resection	47–81%	57–59%	14–23%	2–7%
Segmental cystectomy	43–100%	43–80%	43–80%	0–38%
Simple cystectomy	27–88%	45–52%	16–40%	2–31%
Radical cystectomy	63–83%	50–88%	26–60%	6–40%

From Whitmore WF [4]

effective alternative therapy and the adequacy of TUR biopsy, plus urinary cytology enabling the clinician to evaluate the presence of disease following conservative therapy, make a strong argument for a conservative approach in dealing with patients with T2 disease.

The results of intravesical bacillus Calmette–Guérin (BCG) therapy appear to be clearly superior to intravesical chemotherapy in the treatment of T1 disease [5,6]. Table 18.3 lists a variety of reports showing the progression following BCG therapy [7–14]. In these 355 patients followed from 16 to 72 months, the overall progression rate was 12% (43/355). In a particularly elegant study, Baccon-Gibod and colleagues [15] compared the recurrence and progression rates in 50 patients with T1 disease treated by TUR alone, with 47 treated with TUR plus intravesical BCG. The recurrence rate in the patients treated with surgical resection alone was 90%; 23 of the 50 (46%) went on to progression, including 10 patients (20%) who developed distant metastases. In contrast, of the patients treated with TUR with BCG, progression was noted in only 10 (18%), and only four (8.5%) developed evidence of metastases. In a study of 29 patients treated at Memorial Sloan-Kettering Cancer Center (MSKCC), Herr *et al.* [16] reported on 29 patients treated with BCG followed between 5 and 9 years. Twenty-three of the 29 (79%) were free of disease at 6 months, and overall, 15 of the 29 (52%) progressed with a median time to progression of 29 months. Six of these patients developed muscle-infiltrating disease; one had metastases; and eight had local progression requiring further treatment. Overall, 10 of the 29 patients (35%) underwent cystectomy at a median time of 28 months. Although three patients died of disease at 15, 28 and 58 months, 26 of the 29 (90%) have survived for more than 5 years following treatment; 16 of the 26 survivors (62%) still retain their bladder. These data strongly argue for the use of BCG as initial therapy in the treatment of T1 disease.

Table 18.3 Reports showing the progression following BCG therapy.

Series	No. with T1	No. with progression (%)	Follow-up (months)
Herr *et al.* [7] 1988	13	5 (38%)	72
Sarosdy and Lamm [8] (1989)	40	4 (10%)	67
Steg *et al.* [9] (1990)	45	8 (18%)	16
Boccon-Gibod *et al.* [10] (1989)	47	10 (21%)	27
Pagano *et al.* [11] (1989)	98	7 (7%)	24
Martinez-Pineiro *et al.* [12] (1990)	49	1 (2%)	36
Schellhammer [13] (1990)	30	5 (17%)	33
Khanna *et al.* [14] (1990)	33	3 (9%)	24
Totals	355	43 (12%)	

The availability of potential molecular biological markers to predict those at risk of disease progression

The usefulness of various molecular biological markers as indicators of the natural history of bladder-tumour behaviour and as prognostic indicators is well appreciated. With respect to stage T1 bladder cancer, mutation or over expression of the tumour suppressor gene — *p53* — appears to be the single most valuable predictor of both progression and survival. Figure 18.1 depicts the progression in 77 patients treated with a variety of modalities at MSKCC. In this retrospective analysis the median follow-up period was 121 months. When stained with the monoclonal antibody 1801, tumours in which more than 20% of the cells stained positive for the mutated *p53* product had a 30% progression-free rate at 10 years, contrasted with 80% in those in which fewer than 20% of the cells were positive for mutated *p53*. In Fig. 18.2 survival is shown for the same group of patients, and again a significant survival advantage is demonstrated in patients whose tumours were negative for immunohistochemical evidence of *p53* overexpression. Figures 18.3 and 18.4 show the progression and survival curve in 32 patients who were considered non-responders to a 6-week course of BCG treatment. While *p53* expression pre-BCG treatment was not able to distinguish between those who would respond to therapy from those who would not, in 32 nonresponders (42%) the *p53* expression of the tumour present after BCG treatment showed a much poorer rate of progression and survival in patients whose tumours were positive for *p53* overexpression, as compared to those in whom fewer than 20% of the cells stain for mutated *p53* [17].

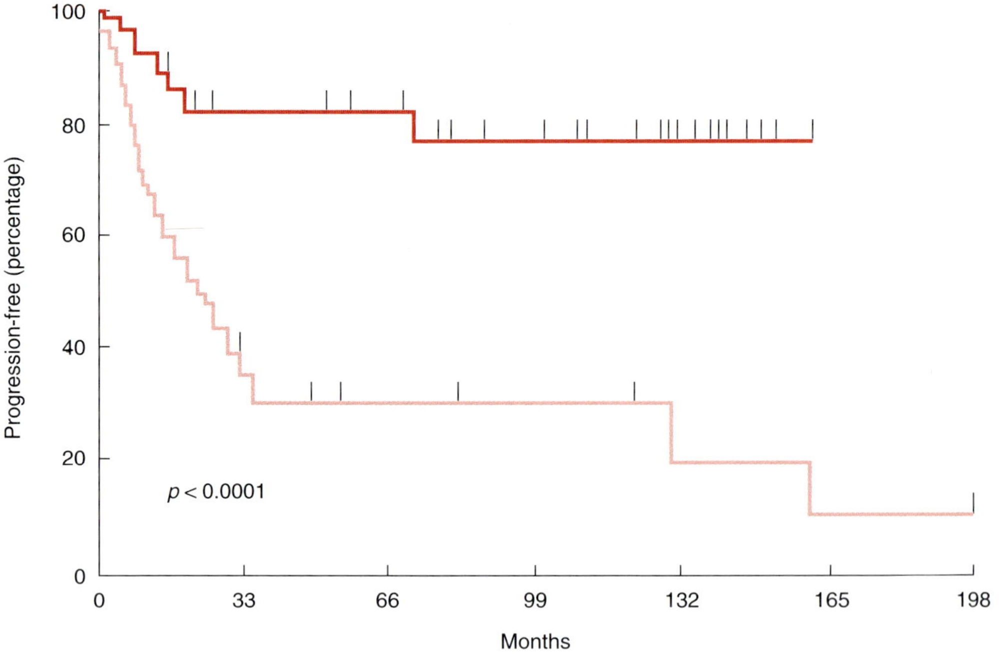

Figure 18.1. Progression in 77 patients treated with a variety of modalities at MSKCC. (Median follow-up = 121 months.) —— *< 20% p53 (+) N=33;* —— *> 20% p53 (+) N=44.*

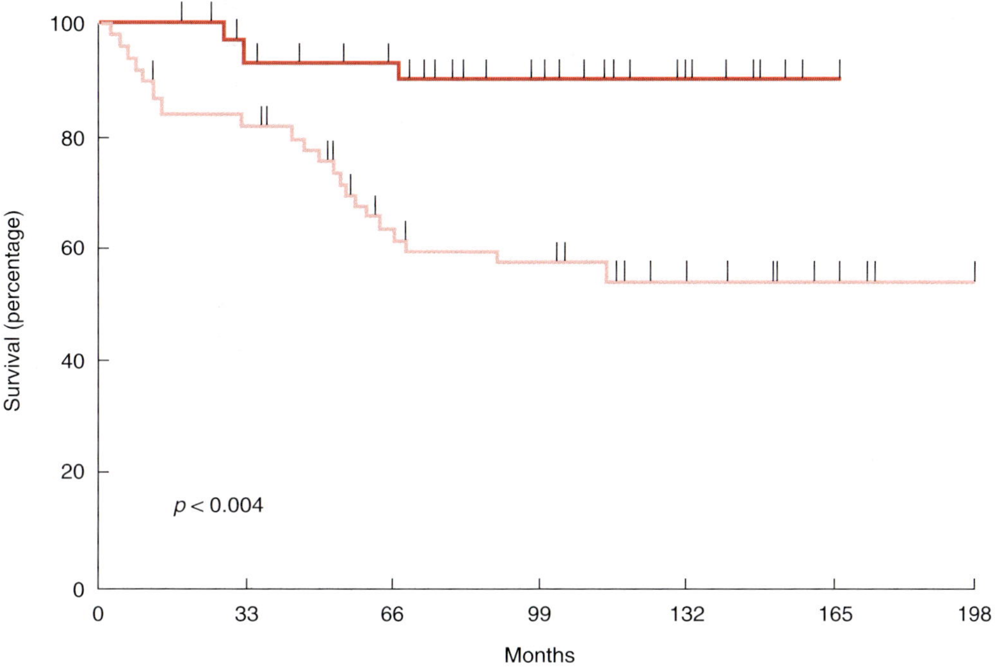

Figure 18.2. Survival is shown for the same group of patients, and again a significant survival advantage is demonstrated in patients whose tumours were negative for immunohistochemical evidence of p53 overexpression. —— *<20% p53 (+) N = 33;* —— *>20% p53 (+) N = 44.*

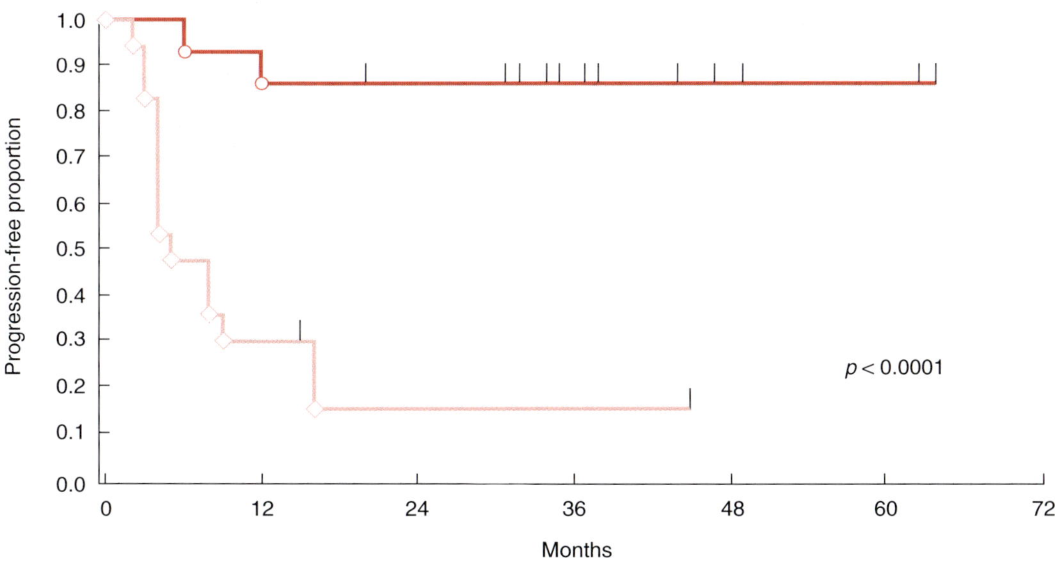

Figure 18.3. Progression in 32 patients who were considered non-responders to a 6-week course of BCG treatment. —— *p53 < 20% N=15;* —— *p53 > 20% N=17.*

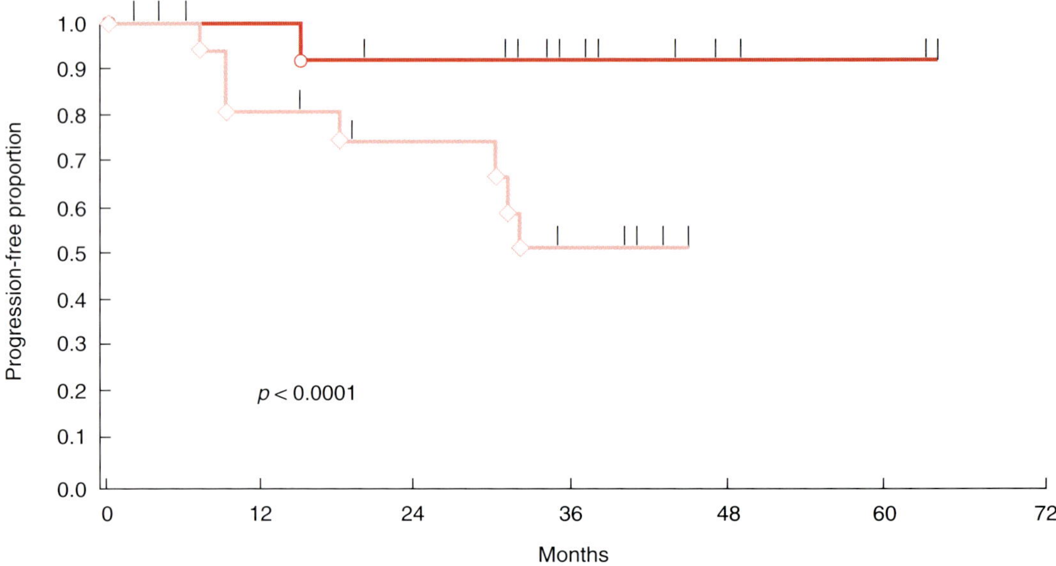

Figure 18.4. Survival curve in 32 patients who were considered non-responders to a 6-week course of BCG treatment. —— *p53 < 20% N=15;* —— *p53 > 20% N = 17.*

The results of aggressive therapy of T1 disease: the effect of early cystectomy or the biology of the disease?

With regard to bladder neoplasia 'the behaviour of the tumour is set before detection' (see Chapter 3). In comparing the recurrence rate of transitional-cell carcinoma in pathologically-staged pT1 following radical cystectomy, Skinner *et al.* [18], a group that has been a proponent of aggressive early therapy, reported that patients whose tumours showed no evidence of mutated *p53* on immunohistochemical staining had only a 9% recurrence rate following cystectomy. However, in those with evidence of *p53* overexpression, 64% of patients had recurrence following cystectomy (Table 18.4). Thus, this is a clear indication that the biology of the tumour, rather than the therapy, was the major factor in the subsequent recurrence, since all patients were treated by cystectomy.

The challenge for the basic scientist and clinician then is to identify further markers which may be utilized in a prospective fashion to identify those patients who

Table 18.4 Mutated p53 and TCC recurrence.

Initial stage	No. patients	p53 (−)	p53(+)
p1	45	9%	64%
p2	30	16%	56%
p3a	26	17%	71%

Esrig *et al* [18].

need aggressive treatment at the first appearance of a T1 tumour, while at the same time permitting a conservative bladder-sparing approach for those in whom the molecular biological markers indicate that a conservative approach, at least as initial therapy, may be warranted.

In conclusion, the present policy at MSKCC is one that has permitted maximum bladder preservation without carrying conservative therapy beyond the time at which cystectomy would no longer be considered curative. Our approach is for initial TUR followed by intravesical BCG therapy for most, if not all T1 tumours. The only exception is the uncommon presentation of a single small T1 lesion that is totally resected and in which follow-up cystoscopy and urinary cytology is negative. It is axiomatic that the primary lesions must be controlled for adjunctive therapy to be effective. A reappearance of a T1 lesion following TUR and intravesical BCG therapy is an indication for more aggressive therapy, and in these patients a radical cystectomy is indicated.

References

1   Thrasher JB, Frazier HA, Robertson JE, George SL, Paulson DF. Does a pT0 cystometry specimen confer any survival advantage? *J Urol* 1992; **147**(2): 403A.

2   Fossa SD, Reitan JB, Ous S, Odegaard A, Loeb M. Prediction of tumor projection in superficial bladder carcinoma. *Eur Urol* 1985; **11**: 1–5.

3   Larsen MP, Steinberg GD, Brendler CB, Epstein JI. Use of *Ulex europaeus* agglutinin I (UEAI), to distinguish vascular and "pseudo-vascular" invasion in transitional cell carcinoma of a bladder with lamina propria invasion. *J Mod Pathol* 1990; **3**: 83–8.

4   Whitmore WF Jr. Towards the rational management of bladder cancer: an overview. *Urology* 1988; **31**(Suppl.): 5–11.

5   Bassi P. Rationale and principles of intravesical therapy. *Second International Symposium on Bladder Cancer*, May 1995.

6   Brosman SA, Lamm DL. The preparation, handling and use of intravesical bacillus Calmette–Guérin for the management of Stage Ta, T1, carcinoma *in situ* and transitional cell cancer. *J Urol* 1990; **144**: 313–15.

7   Herr HW, Laudone VP, Badalament RA *et al*. BCG therapy alters the progression of superficial bladder cancer. *J Clin Oncol* 1988; **6**: 1450–5.

8   Sarosdy MF, Lamm DL. Long-term results of intravesical BCG therapy for superficial bladder cancer. *J Urol* 1989; **142**: 715.

9   Steg A, Belas M, Leleu C. Intravesical BCG therapy in patients with superficial bladder cancer. In: deKernion JB (ed) *Immunotherapy of Urological Tumors*. New York: Churchill–Livingstone, 1990; 107–12.

10 Boccon-Gibod L, Leleu C, Herve JM *et al*. Bladder tumors invading the lamina propria (Stage T1): Influence of endovesical BCG therapy on recurrence and progression. *Prog Clin Biol Res* 1989; **310**: 161.

11 Pagano F, Bassi P, Milam C *et al*. Low-dose BCG-Pasteur strain in the treatment of superficial bladder cancer: preliminary results. *Prog Clin Biol Res* 1989; **310**: 253.

12 Martinez-Pineiro JA, Leon JJ, Martinez-Pineiro L *et al*. BCG v doxorubicin v thiotepa: a randomized prospective study in 202 patients with superficial bladder cancer. *J Urol* 1990; **143**: 502.

13 Schellhammer P. BCG therapy for stage T1 superficial bladder cancer. *J Urol* 1990; **143**: 341A.

14 Khanna OP, Son DL, Mazer H. Multicenter study of superficial bladder cancer treated with intravesical BCG or Adriamycin. *Urology* 1990; **35**: 101.

15 Boccon-Gibod L, Leleu C, Herve JM, Belas M, Steg A. Bladder tumors invading the lamina propria (Stage A/T1): influence of endovesical bacillus Calmette–Guérin therapy on recurrence and progression. *Eur Urol* 1989; **16**: 401–4.

16 Herr HW, Badalament RA, Amato DA *et al*. Superficial bladder cancer treated with bacillus Calmette–Guérin: a multivariate analysis of factors affecting tumor progression. *J Urol* 1989; **141**(1): 22–9.

17 Lacombe L, Dalbagni G, Zhang ZF *et al.* Overexpression of the p53 protein in a high risk population of patients with superficial bladder cancer before and after BCG therapy: correlation to clinical outcome. *J Clin Oncol* 1996; **14**: 2646–52.

18 Esrig D, Spruck CH 3rd, Nichols PW *et al.* p53 nuclear protein accumulation correlates with mutations in the *p53* gene, tumor grade, and stage in bladder cancer. *Am J Pathol* 1993; **143**(5): 1389–97.

CHAPTER 19

T1 bladder tumour: the case for aggressive treatment

M.A.S. Jewett, P.A. Cybulski and G.R. Khakpour

Introduction

Patients with stage T1 transitional-cell carcinoma of the bladder are common and comprise approximately 20% of all patients presenting with transitional-cell carcinoma [1]. The proportion of patients with T1 in each institution's experience varies according to referral patterns and local pathological interpretation. Patient management is controversial and requires an understanding of prognostic factors [2–4]. Unfortunately, their individual prognostic ability tends to be poor [5]. The most important clinical prognostic factors in superficial bladder cancer remain histopathological [6]. Over-staging can occur in up to 31% of patients so that reports of natural history and treatment results may be favourably biased due to the inclusion of many pathological Ta tumours. Patients with T1 tumours are at significant risk and need to be managed with care.

Tumour progression is defined as the development of muscle-invasion metastases or progression of local disease which requires radical treatment; such treatment is often delayed. The high rate of progression in T1s is well established. With transurethral resection (TUR), with or without intravesical chemotherapy, progression occurs in approximately 30% [1,3–5,7–11] (Table 19.1). The current practice of using prophylactic bacillus Calmette–Guérin (BCG) has lowered these rates, but 10–15% still progress (Table 19.2). However, tumour progression has been reported in up to 82% of patients with recurrent stage-T1 disease, initially managed by TUR and an initial 6-week course of intravesical BCG, when evaluated after 3 months [12,13]. The median interval to progression was 8.4 months. This cohort may be highly selected, but demonstrates that some T1-tumour patients may do extremely poorly.

Table 19.1 Progression rates for T1 tumours treated by TUR with or without topical chemotherapy.

Reference	No. of patients	No. with progression (%)	Treatment	Min. F/U (yrs)
Heney *et al.* [1]	63	19 (30)	TURBT	3
Torti *et al.* [3]	51	14 (27)	TURBT	1
England *et al.* [4]	192	53 (28)	TURBT plus IVe chemotherapy	5
Jakse *et al.* [5]	77	14 (18)	TURBT	5
Williams *et al.* [7]	45	8 (18)	TURBT plus IVe chemotherapy	5
Hellsten *et al.* [8]	81	32 (39)	TURBT	5
Smith *et al.* [9]	103	29 (28)	TURBT plus IVe chemotherapy	5

IVe, intravesical.

Table 19.2 Overall recurrence and progression for T1 tumours with IVe BCG immunotherapy.

Result	No.	%
Complete response	27	62.8
Recurrence	8	18.6
Progression	8	18.6

Review of risk factors for progression

The relative importance of individual risk factors for progression and therefore the requirement for radical therapy for stage T1, continues to be a somewhat controversial issue. Data has been generated from patients treated by initial TUR with or without intravesical chemotherapy. They include tumour grade, recurrence rate at 3 months, BCG response, associated carcinoma *in situ* (CIS), tumour morphology, tumour size and biological markers.

Tumour grade

Urologists feel most comfortable with tumour grade as the primary prognostic factor in patients managed by resection with or without adjuvant intravesical chemotherapy. It is estimated that 25–40% of T1 patients have high grade (grade 3 or G3) tumour while G1 is extremely rare. Natural history data indicate that up to 50% of G3 patients progress [5]. There is a clear cut point in survival rates between the G1/G2 five-year survival data of approximately 90% and G3 survival of 43–64%. Therefore, approximately 10% of all new superficial bladder cancer patients will progress (from the 30% of the T1s who are in the T1 G3 subset destined to progress) and up to 57% will die by 5 years.

Recurrence at 3 months

Persistent or recurrent tumour at the 3-month follow-up cystoscopy after initial transurethral resection, is unfavourable and up to 56% of these patients will progress [2]. This finding is not supported by all studies and may in part reflect the practice patterns in the UK at the time, with the initial resections frequently conducted by general surgeons.

BCG response

The response to BCG treatment is predictive of ultimate progression, and appears to be an important prognostic factor to determine the next step in management. A second course of BCG is recommended by some, but the risk of progression increases [12]. In the most unfavourable experience to date, but in selected patients, Herr *et al.* reported that 82% of patients progressed to muscle invasion if there was persistent tumour after BCG-induction therapy [13]. This is particularly true for those that relapse within the prostate [13].

Associated CIS (Tis)

The presence of Tis in association with T1 increases the risk of progression to as high as 83% [14]. Occult urethral or prostatic disease at the time of diagnosis are also adverse prognostic signs.

Tumour morphology

The endoscopic morphology of the tumours appear to be another significant prognostic factor for recurrence. Solid-tumour masses have been reported to have higher recurrence rates but solid morphology is usually considered more predictive of invasion than of recurrence. The recurrence and progression rates for papillary tumours are less than for solid tumours [11].

Tumour size

The size of the tumour at first observation is important but not as critical as other factors, particularly in multivariant analysis. Tumours with a diameter larger than 1 cm have higher recurrence and progression rates [11].

Biological markers

Biological markers are clearly promising as prognostic factors [15,16]. DNA and chromosomal abnormalities, as studied by flow cytometry which measures the DNA content of cells, can quantitate the aneuploid-cell population and proliferative activity. Tumours with a triploid or tetraploid chromosome number and with more than one aneuploid-cell population have unfavourable pathological characteristics and patients have a poor prognosis. In general, however, flow cytometry has not been found clinically to be more valuable than conventional cytology, although some studies have reported that it is more accurate [1,11,16]. The detection of oncogenes and tumour-suppressor genes, particularly *p53* overexpression, has demonstrated a strong association between *p53* mutations, with nuclear accumulation of p53 protein (determined by immunohistochemical analysis), and increased risk of recurrence of bladder cancer with a decrease in overall survival [15–17]. In patients with TCC confined to the bladder, an accumulation of *p53* in the tumour-cell nuclei predicts a significantly increased risk of recurrence and death, independent of tumour grade, stage and lymph-node status. Nuclear *p53* reactivity or other measures of *p53* mutation should be considered for protocols of radical cystectomy and adjuvant treatment. Methodology for detecting the *p53* mutation is still evolving and overexpression of the protein may not always accompany mutations.

Other factors, such as tumour multicentricity, vascular invasion and continued exposure to carcinogens, may also present a risk, although this is not universally agreed upon.

Results of cystectomy for T1 tumour

It is clear that cystectomy is effective therapy for T1 tumours. Several studies indicate that 80–90% of patients survive 5 years with this modality, although up to 38% of specimens are tumour-free [18–20]. Early or immediate as opposed to delayed cystectomy appears to result in improved survival. Stöckle *et al.* [18] found that of 55 patients who underwent cystectomy at diagnosis, of mostly G3 tumours, 90% survived compared to 63% of those in whom surgery had been delayed. This observation is supported by Mohomed *et al.* [10].

Operative mortality has been dramatically reduced in recent cystectomy series to less than 1%. Additionally, concerns about surgery have been reduced due to improved quality of life after surgery, the use of nerve-sparing techniques for preservation of potency in males, and with the use of continent urostomies or orthotopic bladder substitutes. Continent urinary diversion and bladder neck sparing with orthotopic bladder substitutes with continence have also been described in women.

The objective of bladder-sparing treatment has taken on new meaning. It no longer just refers to treatment preserving the patient's own bladder but could include treatments that result in an acceptable bladder substitute. Overall, the burden of therapy is now much less and this should be carefully considered when the high progression and mortality rates are considered in high-risk patients. As recently noted by Lamm and colleagues, tumour progression cannot occur in the absence of persistent or recurrent tumour [21]. Finally, tumour markers may provide prognostic information in these patients that might permit prospective identification of poor prognosis patients [16].

Recommendations for management

All patients should undergo complete TUR of all visible bladder tumour with directed biopsy of suspicious areas. The role for random biopsy is controversial, but may alter treatment if sub-clinical Tis is detected, although there may be potential for implantation. Resection is followed by weekly intravesical BCG immunotherapy for 6 weeks, beginning 2–3 weeks after surgery, to allow wound healing. All patients should be cystoscoped at 3 months. If there is no tumour, maintenance BCG should be seriously considered. If there is persistent or recurrent G1–2 tumour or very localized G3, it may be appropriate to resect and begin BCG-induction therapy again [22]. A decision to proceed to cystectomy would also be very reasonable, particularly if the pathology is G3, multifocal and with Tis, or if the pathology indicates prostatic involvement.

The greatest gains will be achieved with those high-risk patients who present with localized disease, but are frequently destined to progress. With early appropriate therapy for those high-risk patients plus close follow-up, the mortality from the disease should be reduced. In fact, the potential impact on overall mortality could exceed that of doubling the complete-response rates of achieved with current chemotherapy. However, this does not seem probable in the immediate future. This statement bears examination.

If we accept that 20% of new patients with TCC have T1 and that up to 30% progress, 6 patients of 100 new bladder-tumour patients will progress, and potentially die from T1 tumour, if managed by TUR alone. If they are aggressively treated they might be cured. Furthermore, if we assume that half of new patients presenting with T2–4 disease, which comprise approximately 30% of new patients, have metastatic disease (up to 15% of the total) and that current complete-response rate with combination chemotherapy is 15%, chemotherapy will cure two patients of the T2–4 group. Doubling this will cure four patients which would be less than the six T1 patients potentially cured by cystectomy.

Therefore urologists have the potential to make the greatest impact on the overall survival of patients with bladder cancer simply by aggressively pursuing their current practice of careful cystoscopy, TUR and the use of initial BCG in T1 patients. Most importantly a crisp decision to aggressively treat patients that fail this initial management must be made.

Summary of indications for radical cystectomy in stage T1 disease

1. Selected initial tumours of high grade (G3) especially with Tis or prostatic involvement.
2. Patients who fail conservative therapy with TUR and intravesical immunotherapy.
3. Patients at apparent risk who overexpress *p53* as determined by immunochemistry.

References

1 Heney NM, Ahmed S, Flanagan MJ *et al.* Superficial bladder cancer: progression and recurrence. *J Urol* 1983; **130**: 1083–6.
2 Parmar MKB, Freedman LS, Hargreave TB, Tolley D. Prognostic factors for recurrence and followup policies in the treatment of superficial bladder cancer: report from the British Medical Research Council Subgroup on Superficial Bladder Cancer (Urological Cancer Working Party). *J Urol* 1989; **142**: 284–8.
3 Torti FM, Lum BM, Aston D, MacKenzie N *et al.* Superficial bladder cancer: the primacy of grade in the development of invasive disease. *J Clin Oncol* 1987; **5**: 125–30.

4 England HR, Paris AMI, Blandy JP. The correlation of T1 bladder tumour history with prognosis and follow-up requirements. *Br J Urol* 1981; **53**: 1981–6.

5 Jakse G, Loidl W, Seeber G, Hofstäder F. Stage T1 grade 3 transitional cell carcinoma of the bladder: an unfavourable tumour? *J Urol* 1987; **137**: 39–43.

6 Witjes JA, Keimeney LA, Schaafsma KL, Debruyne FMJ. The influence of review pathology on study outcome of a randomized multicentre superficial bladder cancer trial: members of the Dutch South East Cooperative Urological Group. *Br J Urol* 1994; **73**: 172–6.

7 Williams JL, Hammonds JL, Saunders N. T1 bladder tumours. *Br J Urol* 1977; **49**(7): 663–8.

8 Hellsten S, Glifberg I, Lindholme CE, Tehammar E. Therapy of bladder carcinoma: long-term results of a retrospective study of 214 cases. *Scand J Urol Nephrol* 1981; **15**: 115–20.

9 Smith G, Elton RA, Chisholm GD, Newsam JE, Hargreave TD. Superficial bladder cancer: intravenous chemotherapy and tumour progression or metastases. *Br J Urol* 1986; **58**(6): 659–63.

10 Mohamed SR, Mishriki SF, Persad RA *et al.* Urological audit: the role for an aggressive approach to high grade superficial bladder tumours. *Br J Urol* 1992; **70**: 156–60.

11 Bono AV, Benvenuti C, Damiano G, Lovisolo J. Results of transurethral resection and intravesical doxorubicin prophylaxis in patients with T1G3 bladder cancer. *Urology* 1994; **44**(3): 329–35.

12 Catalona WJ, Hudson MA, Gillen DP, Andriole GL, Ratliff TL. Risks and benefits of repeated courses of intravesical bacillus Calmette–Guérin therapy for superficial bladder cancer. *J Urol* 1987; **137**: 220–4.

13 Herr HW, Klein EA, Rogatko A. Local BCG failures in superficial bladder cancer. *Eur Urol* 1991; **19**: 97–100.

14 Soloway MS, Murphy W, Rao MK. Serial multiple site biopsies in patients with bladder cancer. *J Urol* 1978; **130**: 57–9.

15 Greenblatt MS, Bennett WP, Hollstein M. Mutation in the p53 tumor suppressor gene. *Cancer Res* 1994; **54**: 4855–78.

16 Esrig AS, Elmajian D, Groshen S *et al.* Accumulation of nuclear p53 and tumor progression in bladder cancer. *N Engl J Med* 1994; **331**: 1259–64.

17 Sarkis AS, Dalbagni G, Cordon-Cardo C *et al.* Association of p53 nuclear overexpression and tumor progression in carcinoma *in situ* of bladder. *J Urol* 1994; **152**: 388–92.

18 Stöckle M, Alken P, Engelmann U *et al.* Radical cystectomy — often too late? *Eur Urol* 1987; **13**: 361–7.

19 Bracken RB, McDonald MW, Johnson DE. Cystectomy for superficial bladder cancer. *Urology* 1981; **18**: 459–63.

20 Malkowicz SB, Nichols P, Lieskovsky G *et al.* The role of radical cystectomy in the management of high grade superficial bladder cancer (PA, P1, PIS, and P2). *J Urol* 1990; **144**: 641–5.

21 Lamm DL, Riggs DR, Traynelis CL, Nseyo UO. Apparent failure of current intravesical chemotherapy prophylaxis to influence the long-term course of superficial transitional cell carcinoma of the bladder. *J Urol* 1995; **153**: 1444–50.

22 Zhang GK, Uke ET, Sharer WC, Borkon WD, Bernstein SM. Reassessment of conservative management for stage T1N0M0 transitional cell carcinoma of the bladder. *J Urol* 1996; **155**: 1907–9.

CHAPTER 20

Carcinoma *in situ*

D.L. Lamm

Introduction

Transitional-cell carcinoma *in situ* of the bladder is a highly aggressive, life-threatening malignancy. The recognized lethality of carcinoma *in situ* (CIS) previously led to the use of radical cystectomy as the treatment of choice because treatment options available at the time, including transurethral fulguration, radiation therapy, and intravesical chemotherapy proved to be generally ineffective. In 1990, based on a Southwest Oncology Group comparison of Connaught bacillus Calmette–Guérin (BCG) and doxorubicin and six Tice-BCG studies, the United States Food and Drug Administration approved BCG for the treatment of CIS. No other treatment has received such approval. Continued experience confirms that BCG immunotherapy is now the initial treatment of choice for patients with CIS, and cystectomy can be safely reserved for the minority of patients who fail to respond completely to intravesical therapy. In this review I will summarize BCG immunotherapy for CIS and discuss treatment techniques, results, precautions, and alternative strategies.

Historical background

Carcinoma in situ

CIS of the bladder, first described in 1952 by Melicow [1], is a diffuse malignancy that can extend from the renal pelvis to penile urethra [2]. CIS may occur as primary disease, in association with papillary or solid tumours, or following tumour resection. Irritative symptoms are common [3] and patients often present with haematuria. Urinary cytology is positive in more than 90% of patients with CIS. Urinary cytology should be conducted in all patients suspected of having CIS because cystoscopic findings and even bladder biopsy may be falsely negative.

The clinical course of CIS is highly variable, but prior to the advent of BCG immunotherapy more than 50% of reported patients progressed to muscle-invasive disease [4]. Extensive, diffuse disease has a high risk for progression, but focal disease may exist for years and progress in as few as 8% of patients [5]. Focal CIS is the earliest stage in the evolution of invasive bladder cancer, and though the course is often protracted, regression of the disease is virtually unknown. These patients are optimal candidates for intravesical therapy. Diffuse, widespread disease is typically associated with irritative symptoms and as many as 34% of patients treated with cystectomy will be found to have unsuspected microinvasive carcinoma [6]. *In situ* disease extends to the distal ureter in as many as 57% of patients and to the prostatic urethra in as many as 62% [6]. Despite use of the most aggressive treatment — cystectomy — death from metastatic disease occurs in up to 6% of patients.

The results of radiation therapy for CIS are very disappointing. In a series of 11 patients treated with external beam radiation therapy 10 (91%) died at a mean follow-up of 3.5 years [5]. In a similar way, systemic chemotherapy may temporarily eradicate CIS, but local recurrence is virtually certain. The results of topical intravesical chemotherapy have been much more encouraging, and continue to have a role in the management of CIS. In a review of 448 patients treated with intravesical chemotherapy, the overall average complete response rate averages 48% (Table 20.1). Complete responses were reported in 38% of 89 patients treated with thiotepa, 48% of 212 patients treated with doxorubicin, and 53% of 147 patients treated with Mitomycin C [4]. In most series, fewer than 20% of patients treated with intravesical chemotherapy remain disease-free for 5 years or more, but some preliminary encouraging results have been reported with the combination of Mitomycin C and doxorubicin and the use of maintenance chemotherapy [7]. In the absence of a clear indication for intravesical chemotherapy, i.e. suspected or confirmed residual disease, unnecessary instillations should be avoided, because repeated instillation of thiotepa, doxorubicin, or Mitomycin C in normal rodent bladders is reported to induce atypia, CIS, and even invasive transitional-cell carcinoma [8].

BCG immunotherapy

BCG has been found to be highly successful in the treatment of CIS. A review of 34 series involving 1354 patients shows average complete-response rates to be 72% (Table 20.2). The lowest response rate in these series is 39% and every preparation studied thus far has been effective. Preparations do vary in viability, lipid composition, and antigenicity, but the differences in response rates listed in Table 20.2 relate primarily to differences in treatment schedules. The first Southwest Oncology Group (SWOG) study used once weekly for six weeks Connaught BCG instillations followed by single treatments at 3-month intervals. With 64 patients evaluable complete response was 70% and median duration of response was 39 months. In a second SWOG study the overall complete-response rate was increased to 87% when patients received an additional 3-week course of BCG at 3 months. Maintenance BCG therapy of three weekly treatments every 6 months for 3 years has yielded an estimated 4-year disease-free rate of 83%. BCG has supplanted the role of cystectomy in the initial treatment of CIS. It remains to be shown that initial cystectomy is superior to an initial trial of BCG, followed by cystectomy, for those who fail to have a complete response.

Table 20.1 Chemotherapy responses in CIS.

Study	Patients (*N*)	Complete response (%)
Thiotepa		
Koontz *et al.*	20	11 (55)
Prout	40	16 (40)
Stanisic *et al.*	24	6 (25)
Prout *et al.*	5	1 (20)
Subtotal	89	34 (38)
Doxorubicin		
Edsmyr and Anderson	8	7 (88)
Edsmyr *et al.*	30	20 (67)
Duchek and Pavone-Macaluso	9	4 (44)
Jakse *et al.*	15	10 (67)
Glashan	55	35 (64)
Ek *et al.*	22	2 (9)
Stanisic *et al.*	6	0
Lamm *et al.*	67	23 (34)
Subtotal	212	101 (48)
Mitomycin C		
Flüchter *et al.*	6	6 (100)
Harrison *et al.*	6	4 (67)
Issel *et al.*	14	4 (29)
Bouffioux	5	3 (60)
Powell	5	3 (60)
Soloway	12	5 (42)
Koontz *et al.*	20	9 (45)
Jauhiainen *et al.*	11	9 (82)
Cant *et al.*	12	5 (42)
Lucero and Wise	5	4 (80)
Hetherington *et al.*	4	4 (100)
Stricker *et al.*	19	15 (79)
Stanisic *et al.*	7	0
Soloway	21	7 (33)
Subtotal	147	78 (53)
Chemotherapy total response	**448**	**213 (48)**

Table source: Lamm DL. Carcinoma *in situ*. *Urol Clin North Am* 1992; **19**: 499–508.

Table 20.2 Comparison of bacillus Calmette–Guérin (BCG) strains in the treatment of CIS of the bladder.

Strain	Total number of patients	Number of series	Complete response rate (%)	Range of response rates (%)
Connaught	419	6	79%	70%–92%
Pasteur	218	6	74%	40%–80%
Tokyo	65	2	74%	63%–84%
Tice	277	6	71%	56%–82%
Evans	127	4	64%	53%–88%
A. Frappier	145	6	60%	39%–100%
S. African	13	1	69%	–
Danish	42	1	67%	–
Romanian	33	1	64%	–
RIVM	15	1	60%	–
Total	1,354	34	72%	39%–100%

Source: Lamm DL. BCG immunotherapy for transitional-cell carcinoma *in situ* of the bladder. *Oncology* 1995; **9**: 947–52.

Principles of BCG immunotherapy

Animal studies and extensive clinical experience have elucidated several factors of importance in optimizing the response to BCG immunotherapy. Animal studies demonstrate that the anti-tumour response is limited by tumour burden [9], so all visible tumour should be resected or fulgurated prior to initiation of treatment. Optimal response requires a sufficient number of viable organisms and direct juxtaposition of BCG and tumour cells. While a sufficient number of colony-forming units is required for response, the dose–response curve for BCG immunotherapy, like most biological response modifiers, is bell shaped [10]. In the murine model, optimal-antitumour response occurs with 10^7 colony forming units (CFU). In clinical trials of intravesical instillation effective doses appear to range from 1 to 10×10^9 CFU. The optimal dose has not been defined. A reduction in the dose of BCG could have major clinical relevance because Morales *et al.* [11] have shown that lower BCG doses significantly reduce the toxicity of intravesical BCG. Pagano and associates have data suggesting that 75 mg Pasteur BCG is not only less toxic but also more effective than the standard 150 mg dose [12].

Importantly, immune stimulation and antitumour response in patients receiving intravesical instillation appear to peak at the sixth weekly intravesical instillation. Continued administration after that time invokes suppressive-immune responses and serves only to increase the toxicity of treatment for most patients. As might be expected, subsequent weekly instillations in patients who have already received an initial course of BCG result in peak immune stimulation at 3 weeks [13]. This observation is of particular importance when considering optimal maintenance schedules, as discussed below.

Not all tumours are susceptible to immunotherapy. While we once considered tumour antigenicity to be required, the observation that BCG can stimulate natural killer cells, lymphocyte-activated killer cells, and distinctive BCG-activated killers, which can non-specifically kill malignant cells, suggests that tumour-specific antigenicity may not be required. Nevertheless, both in the murine bladder-tumour model and in patients, some transitional-cell carcinomas appear to be completely unresponsive to immunotherapy.

An intact immune system, and in particular a functional T-cell immune system and interleukin (IL)-2 induction, is required for response to BCG immunotherapy. Individual components of the immune system can be blocked in animal models, without eliminating the anti-tumour effect of BCG, as long as the function of cytotoxic T cells are preserved [14].

BCG treatment techniques

Experience with thousands of patients treated with BCG now confirms that the basic principles of BCG immunotherapy demonstrated in animal models apply to the clinic. Optimal response to BCG requires administration of sufficient numbers of viable organisms in direct juxtaposition to tumour cells. BCG immunotherapy is remarkably effective in transitional-cell carcinoma of the prostatic urethra, producing a complete response rate similar to that reported in the bladder, but as expected by the requirement for direct contact there appears to be no reduction in the occurrence of upper-tract tumours with intravesical instillation. Intravesical instillation results in contact of BCG with urethral tumours, but in the absence of reflux, no contact with upper-tract tumours.

Optimal response occurs when tumour volume is minimized. While the 100,000 cell limit seen in mice fortunately does not apply to man, I make every effort to resect all visible tumour and fulgurate areas of CIS prior to initiation of BCG immunotherapy. Early treatment protocols attempted to instill BCG as soon as possible after tumour resection, but subsequent experience has shown that early administration increases the risk of intravascular dissemination of BCG with the attendant complications. Therefore, BCG instillation is postponed for 1–2 weeks following transurethral bladder tumour resection.

Ratliff *et al.* [15] demonstrated that fibronectin is an important attachment mechanism for BCG. A retrospective review of the patients treated with BCG at Washington University, St. Louis, showed significant reduction of anti-tumour activity when BCG was given to patients taking clot inhibitors including aspirin, dipyridamole, and coumadin. A subsequent report by Rogerson confirmed these findings [16].

Optimal attachment of BCG occurs when BCG is diluted with preservative and bactericidal-free normal saline at pH 7.4. Attachment peaks 2 hours after instillation. As previously noted, with treatments repeated weekly, immune stimulation peaks at 6 weeks. It is remarkable that the initial treatment schedule found to be best resembles so closely that designed by Dr Morales as the original BCG treatment regimen [17].

Induction

Optimal BCG-induction therapy, in my opinion, is 6 weekly BCG instillations followed by a 6-week rest period and an additional 3 weekly instillations. In the SWOG study of 218 randomized patients with CIS, 6 weekly instillations resulted in the expected 73% complete-response rate [18]. With three additional treatments the complete response rates increased to 87% ($p < 0.04$). Importantly, as noted above, this '6 plus 3' schedule should not be converted to a '9' schedule, because continued instillation beyond 6 weeks suppresses immune response and has resulted in a disappointing recurrence rate.

Maintenance

Optimal maintenance therapy with BCG has now also been elucidated by studies from the SWOG [18]. In my previous experience, a single instillation of BCG at 3-month intervals was associated with a fourfold reduction in the rate (not incidence) of tumour recurrence [19]. Two subsequent controlled trials failed to demonstrate that monthly [20] or quarterly [21] BCG-maintenance therapy reduced the incidence of tumour recurrence. In patients with CIS who were disease-free at 3 months, continued 3 weekly maintenance-BCG treatments at 6 month intervals increased long-term disease-free status from the expected 65% to 83% ($p < 0.01$). In 270 patients with rapidly recurring, high-grade, or Stage-T1 superficial transitional-cell carcinoma, the results of maintenance BCG using 3 weekly instillations of 120 mg Connaught BCG was even more dramatic. In patients randomized to a single 6-week BCG course, an excellent long-term response was observed; 50% of patients remained disease-free for 4 or more years. In patients given maintenance therapy at 3 months, 6 months, and every 6 months to 3 years, long-term disease-free status was improved by 33%, to 83% tumour-free at 4 years ($p < 0.000001$).

Adjunctive chemoprevention

Epidemiological, *in vitro*, and animal-model studies have suggested that various vitamins, including vitamin A, B6, and C, may have a protective or even therapeutic effect in many cancers, including bladder cancer. Immunotherapy can markedly alter vitamin metabolism. In patients given IL-2 immunotherapy serum, vitamin C levels were depressed to undetectable levels in 12 of 15 patients [22] and 60% of patients were found to be hypovitaminemic for vitamin A, 80% for carotene, 90% for vitamin B6 and 45% for folate [23]. We evaluated long-term administration of recommended daily allowance versus RDA multivitamins plus megadoses of vitamins A, B6, C and E in 65 BCG-treated patients with superficial transitional-cell carcinoma, one-third of whom had CIS. In this randomized double-blind study, high-dose vitamin administration (Oncovite, Mission Pharmacal) was associated with a 40% long-term reduction in tumour recurrence ($p < 0.02$) [24]. While natural killer cell activity was not significantly elevated following BCG therapy in patients receiving RDA vitamins, significant increase was found in those receiving high-dose vitamins [25]. These remarkable results, which exceed the benefit currently reported with intravesical chemotherapy in superficial bladder cancer, need to be independently evaluated, but I currently recommend high-dose vitamin supplementation for all my bladder cancer patients.

Alternative immunotherapies

The remarkable success of BCG immunotherapy in superficial bladder cancer suggests that other immunotherapies may be equally effective. There is optimism that several new immunotherapies may be less toxic than BCG, or effective in patients who have failed BCG. While alpha-interferon, keyhole limpet haemocyanin, and bropirimine have demonstrated efficacy in superficial bladder cancer, to date no alternative treatment has achieved the level of success seen with current BCG-treatment schedules.

Interferons

Interferons are virtually non-toxic intravesically and have clear efficacy in the treatment of superficial bladder cancer. Using leukocyte gamma-interferon intramuscularly, three small studies found response rates ranging from 43% partial response to 75% complete response [26]. No response was seen when recombinant gamma-interferon was used, however [27].

The most encouraging results with interferon are reported using intravesical alpha-2b-interferon. In a dose–response study, Torti *et al.* reported a 25% complete response in papillary tumours and a 32% complete response in CIS using alpha-interferon in intravesical doses ranging from 50 to 1000 million units [28]. Remarkably, no significant toxicity was observed even at the highest dose. In a subsequent multi-centre randomized trial, reported by Glashan [29], 100 million units of alpha-interferon given weekly for 12 weeks and then monthly to 1 year was found to be significantly better than 10 million units given on the same schedule. Complete biopsy and cytological resolution of CIS occurred in 43% of patients randomized to 100 million units and only 5% of patients randomized to 10 million units. Importantly, complete response was observed in some patients who had failed a course of BCG immunotherapy and many of the responses were of long duration. While this study confirms the efficacy of interferon in the treatment of transitional-cell carcinoma, and demonstrates that 100 million units is superior to 10 million units, one should not conclude that the 100 million-unit dose or the schedule employed is optimal. The dose–response curve of biological response modifiers is typically bell shaped. We and others have observed excellent responses with 50–60 million-unit doses and we are currently using the 3 weekly, 6-month maintenance schedule found to significantly improve the results of BCG immunotherapy.

Continued research will be required to define the optimum interferon-treatment schedule and the ideal role of interferon in the management of superficial bladder cancer. Initial randomized comparison studies with BCG immunotherapy have confirmed that interferon is substantially less toxic, but also less effective than BCG. In a study reported by Kalble *et al.* [30], 5 of 32 patients (16%) treated with BCG had recurrence compared with 21 of 35 patients (60%) treated with alpha-interferon ($p = 0.003$).

Keyhole limpet haemocyanin (KLH)

Keyhole limpet haemocyanin is a highly antigenic, complex glycoprotein, with a molecular weight of 8 million that serves as the oxygen-carrying molecule for the mollusc *Megathura crenulata*. Since almost no one is exposed to this inedible mollusc, the highly antigenic protein was used as a monitor of immune competence as measured by delayed-type cutaneous hypersensitivity. Olsson *et al.* [31] originally used 5 mg intradermal inoculations of KLH to correlate immune competence with reduced risk for tumour recurrence in patients with superficial bladder cancer. Remarkably, patients who received intradermal KLH had a dramatic reduction in tumour recurrence. In a subsequent prospective trial of prophylactic KLH, one tumour occurred among nine immunized patients followed for 204 months, compared with seven recurrences in 10 non-immunized patients followed for 228 months. We investigated KLH in the animal model in the late 1970s, and while we confirmed an anti-tumour effect, we were unimpressed with the activity of KLH when compared with BCG. Fortunately, other investigators continued this pursuit and in 1988 Jurincic *et al.* [32] reported the results of a randomized comparison of 10 mg intravesical KLH and mitomycin. Tumour recurrence was reduced from 39% in the mitomycin group to 14% in the KLH group, and KLH was found to be essentially free of toxic reactions. In a subsequent randomized clinical trial, 30 mg of intravesical KLH was compared with ethoglucid [33]. Tumour recurrence was seen in 55% of patients treated with KLH and 61% of those treated with ethoglucid. Again, no toxicity of KLH was reported.

As with other biological-response modifiers, the optimal dose of KLH is unknown and the dose–response curve is expected to be bell shaped. Several animal model studies have confirmed that KLH has significant anti-tumour activity in bladder cancer, and an ongoing Phase I–II clinical trial has confirmed complete response in CIS with as little as 2 mg of intravesical KLH.

Bropirimine

Bropirimine is a pyrimidinone that has a wide variety of immune-stimulatory activities, including the induction of interferon and other lymphokines, enhancement of natural killer-cell activity and macrophage cytotoxicity, and heightened antibody production [34]. Bropirimine can be taken by mouth and is excreted in the urine in active form. Initial animal studies in transitional-cell carcinoma demonstrated marked inhibitory activity [35]. In a Phase 1 trial of oral bropirimine in 34 patients with papillary or *in situ* transitional-cell carcinoma of the bladder, 6 of 26 evaluable patients had complete response. In a subsequent multi-centre evaluation of bropirimine in 54 patients with CIS, 27 of whom had failed prior BCG therapy, complete response was seen in 50% of patients. These data suggest that bropirimine will have a future role in the management of transitional-cell carcinoma. An important future application for bropirimine may be the treatment or prophylaxis of transitional-cell carcinoma of the upper urinary tract. While BCG immunotherapy is effective when directly applied to upper tract tumours, the oral route of administration is far more convenient.

Conclusions

BCG in the treatment of CIS of the bladder represents perhaps the most successful application of immunotherapy to human malignancy. In contrast to historical series in which 50% of patients with CIS progressed to muscle-invasive disease, and complete response to surgical fulguration or intravesical chemotherapy occurred in a minority of patients, with current optimal BCG-induction treatments 87% of patients will have complete response, and with maintenance therapy using three weekly instillations every 6 months, 83% of complete responses are of 3 or more years duration. Patients remain at risk for extravesical recurrence of CIS, particularly in the distal ureters, and close surveillance is essential. With meticulous follow-up, however, most patients can be safely spared the trauma of radical cystectomy unless they fail to completely respond or become resistant to treatment. Patients with focal recurrence may also respond to intravesical chemotherapy or alternative immunotherapies, and these patients are important resources for the development of improved treatment alternatives for future patients.

References

1   Melicow MN. Histological study of vesical urothelium intervening between gross neoplasm in total cystectomy. *J Urol* 1952; **68**: 261–79.

2   Melicow MN, Hollowell JW. Intra-urothelial cancer: carcinoma *in situ*, Bowen's disease of the urinary system: discussion of 30 cases. *J Urol* 1952; **68**: 763–72.

3   Okaneya T, Ikado S, Ogawa A. The progress pattern of carcinoma *in situ* of the urinary bladder. *Nippon Hinyokika Gakkai Zasshi* 1991; **82**: 1227–32.

4   Lamm DL. Carcinoma *in situ*. In: Lamm DL (ed) *Superficial Bladder Cancer. Urol Clin N Am* 1992; Volume 19: 499–508.

5   Riddle PR, Chisholm GD, Trott PA *et al.* Flat carcinoma *in situ* of bladder. *Br J Urol* 1976; **47**: 829–33.

6   Utz DC, Farrow DM. Carcinoma *in situ* of the urinary tract. *Urol Clin North Am* 1984; **11**: 735.

7   Fukui I, Kihara K, Sekine H *et al.* Intravesical combination chemotherapy with Mitomycin C and doxorubicin for superficial bladder cancer: a randomized trial of maintenance versus no maintenance following a complete response. *Cancer Chemother Pharmacol* 1992; **30**: S37–40.

8   Friedman D, Mooppan UM, Rosen Y, Kim H. The effect of intravesical instillations of thiotepa, Mitomycin C and Adriamycin® on normal urothelium: an experimental study in rats. *J Urol* 1991; **145**: 1060–3.

9   Bast RC Jr, Zbar B, Borsos T *et al.* BCG and cancer. 1. *N Eng J Med* 1974; **290**: 1413.

10 Lamm DL, Reichert DF, Harris SC *et al.* Immunotherapy of murine transitional cell carcinoma. *J Urol* 1982; **128**: 1104–8.

11 Morales A, Nickel JC, Wilson JWL. Dose–response of bacillus Calmette–Guérin in the treatment of superficial bladder cancer. *J Urol* 1992; **147**: 1256–8.

12 Pagano F, Bassi P, Milani C *et al.* A low dose bacillus Calmette–Guérin regimen in superficial bladder cancer therapy: is it effective?. *J Urol* 1991; **146**: 32–5.

13 DeBoer E. Personal communication, 1994.

14 Ratliff TL, Gillen D, Catalona WJ. Requirement of a thymus dependent immune response for BCG-mediated antitumor activity. *J Urol* 1987; **137**: 155–8.

15 Ratliff TL, Kavoussi LR, Catalona WJ. Role of fibronectin in intravesical BCG therapy for superficial bladder cancer. *J Urol* 1988; **139**: 410–14.

16 Rogerson JW. Intravesical bacille Calmette–Guérin in the treatment of superficial transitional cell carcinoma of the bladder. *Br J Urol* 1994; **7**: 655–8.

17 Morales A, Eidinger D, Bruce AW. Intracavitary bacillus Calmette–Guérin in the treatment of superficial bladder tumors. *J Urol* 1976; **116**: 180–3.

18 Lamm DL, Crawford ED, Blumenstein B *et al.* Maintenance BCG immunotherapy of superficial bladder cancer: a randomized prospective Southwest Oncology Group Study. *J Urol* 1992; **147**: 274A (242).

19 Lamm DL. Bacillus Calmette–Guérin immunotherapy for bladder cancer. *J Urol* 1985; **134**: 40–7.

20 Badalament RA, Herr HW, Wong GY *et al.* A prospective randomized trial of maintenance versus nonmaintenance intravesical bacillus Calmette–Guérin therapy of superficial bladder cancer. *J Clin Oncol* 1987; **5**: 441–9.

21 Hudson MA, Ratliff TL, Gillen DP *et al.* Single course versus maintenance bacillus Calmette–Guérin therapy for superficial bladder tumors: a prospective, randomized trial. *J Urol* 1987; **138**: 295–8.

22 Marcus SL, Petrylak DP, Dutcher JP *et al.* Hypovitaminosis C in patients treated with high-dose interleukin 2 and lymphokine-activated killer cells. *Am J Clin Nutr* 1991; **54**: S1292–7.

23 Baker H, Marcus SL, Petrylak DP *et al.* Effect of interleukin-2 on some micronutrients during adoptive immunotherapy for various cancers. *J Amer Col Nutr* 1992; **11**: 482–6.

24 Lamm DL, Riggs DR, Shriver JS *et al.* Megadose vitamins in bladder cancer: a double blind clinical trial. *J Urol* 1994; **151**: 21–6.

25 Lamm DL, Riggs DR, DeHaven JI. Enhanced natural killer (NK) cell activity with BCG and vitamin treatment. *J Urol* 1994; **151**(Abstr 991): 475A.

26 Sargent ER, Williams RD. Immunotherapeutic alternatives in superficial bladder cancer. *Urol Clin N Amer* 1992; **19**: 581–9.

27 Grups J, Frohmuller H, Ackermann R. Can recombinant human gamma-2 interferon prevent recurrence of high-grade superficial bladder tumors? *Cancer Detect Prev* 1987; **10**: 405–9.

28 Torti F, Shortliffe L, Williams R *et al.* Alpha-interferon in superficial bladder cancer: a Northern California Oncology Group study. *J Clin Oncol* 1988; **6**: 476–83.

29 Glashan R. A randomized controlled study of intravesical alpha-2b-interferon in carcinoma *in situ* of the bladder. *J Urol* 1990; **144**: 658–61.

30 Kalble T, Beer M, Staehler G. Intravesical prophylaxis with BCG versus interferon A for superficial bladder cancer. *J Urol* 1994; **151**(Abstr 22): 233A.

31 Olsson CA, Chute R, Rao CN. Immunologic reduction of bladder cancer recurrence rate. *J Urol* 1974; **111**: 173–6.

32 Jurincic C, Engelmann U, Gasch J. Immunotherapy in bladder cancer with keyhole-limpet hemocyanin: a randomized study. *J Urol* 1988; **139**: 723–6.

33 Flamm J, Bucher A, Holtl W. Recurrent superficial transitional cell carcinoma of the bladder: Adjuvant topical chemotherapy versus immunotherapy: A prospective randomized trial. *J Urol* 1990; **144**: 260–3.

34 Rios A, Stringfellow DA, Fitzpatrick FA *et al.* Phase I study of 2-amino-5-bromo-6-phenyl-4(3H)-pyrimidinone (ABPP), an oral interferon inducer in cancer patients. *J Biol Resp Modifiers* 1986; **5**: 330–8.

35 Simmons WB, Reichert DF, Lucio RM, Lamm DL. Pyrimidinone interferon inducers in the treatment of murine transitional cell carcinoma. *78th annual AUA* 1983; **169**(Abstr 309): 330A.

CHAPTER 21

Follow-up of patients with superficial transitional-cell carcinoma of the bladder

P.D. Abel

Introduction

Is post-diagnostic management of superficial (pTa and PT1) [1] transitional-cell carcinoma of the bladder (TCCB) tailored to suit individual cases according to the currently available data on the natural history of the disease? Although bladder cancer is a heterogeneous disease, it is follow-up (FU) of the so called superficial TCCB that makes up the larger part of the workload of urologists involved in the treatment and management of bladder cancer. Yet FU, consisting of regular life-long check cystoscopies (CC) and intravenous urograms (IVU), is by convention mandatory in all cases and is often conducted according to rigid protocols without giving due consideration to the individuality of the patient or the characteristics of the tumour.

The anticipation of disease progression with sufficient accuracy to justify radical therapy while a lesion is still amenable to local treatment is the rationale underlying follow-up in the pTa/pT1 category of TCCB [2]. Smith [3] suggested that of all medical interventions only about 15% are supported by solid scientific evidence. Is there any evidence to indicate that the natural history of superficial TCCB is altered by conventional follow-up policies?

Endoscopic follow-up: present practice

Following complete resection of newly diagnosed TCCB, traditionally used follow-up protocols (as well as those of major research bodies including the EORTC and MRC) normally involve CC being conducted every 3 months for 1 year following surgery after which they are conducted at 6-monthly intervals for the second year and then once per year for the remainder of the patient's life assuming no new TCCB develop [4]. During the first 3 years this usually involves seven cystoscopies, although up to 10 cystoscopies are advocated by some urologists [5]. In the event of new superficial tumours developing a return to 3-monthly examinations, in line with the traditional follow-up schedule after the first diagnosis, is recommended.

In England and Wales around 9500 new cases of bladder cancer are diagnosed annually [6]; 70–80% of these are superficial [7,8], suggesting that a minimum of 50 000 CC are conducted in the initial 3 years following newly diagnosed superficial TCCB. Most newly diagnosed patients are aged over 70 years and a high proportion have co-morbid conditions. These factors should be taken into account in spite of the lower morbidity rates and reduced discomfort of FU made possible with newer technologies such as flexible cystoscopy with local anaesthesia.

Natural history of superficial TCCB: is it influenced by diagnostic or check cystoscopies and their timing?

The assumption that all bladder cancers are initially non-invasive, but undergo an ordered sequence of steps to invade lamina propria, detrusor muscle, perivesical fat and then metastasize, appears to be the basis of the rationale for follow-up check cystoscopies. If this were correct, the identification and destruction of new tumours before they are able to progress would be very important. However, the majority of new occurrences of superficial TCCB are of the same grade and pT category as the initial tumour and do not progress. This is particularly the case following pTa disease [9–12]. In actual fact, the vast majority of patients suffering from muscle-infiltrating TCCB (80–90%) present initially with invasive tumours; of the remainder only 10–20% have had a history of previous superficial disease [11, 13–15]. Brawn [13] reported that of the patients presenting with infiltrating disease at first diagnosis, up to 25% had undergone cystoscopy at some point previously. For all of these patients the cystoscopy notes revealed that no tumour had been detected.

According to Mommsen *et al.* [16], the influence of early diagnosis on prognosis has not been convincingly demonstrated. From a survey of data relating to both haematuria-screening clinics and the utilization of urine cytology in groups at risk, Bishop [17] concluded that the influence of early diagnosis on survival times was only marginal. There was minimal evidence to suggest that differences in patient management, including delay of treatment (median 48 days from referral), contributed to outcome, according to a study by Gulliford *et al.* [18], who identified the most important prognostic factors to be age, haemoglobin at presentation and pT category. Surprisingly, those patients treated after the shortest delay had the shortest survival times, probably due to recognition of the fact that they had advanced disease and as a result prompted the earliest intervention. This observation carries the implication that clinicians recognize and target the resources available in accordance to the greatest need.

An influential study involving 100 consecutive grade-1 TCCB patients was published by Greene *et al.* in 1973 [19]. Depth of tumour infiltration was not reported in the study. Of the 100 patients, 73 developed new tumours. Of these, 15% and 8% developed their first new occurrence after 5 and 10 years, respectively. Of the new tumours reported, 10 infiltrated the bladder wall and were identified between 3 months and 13 years following diagnosis (mean 8 years). The authors' widely quoted conclusions suggested that the original tumours should 'all be considered carcinomas' and that these patients should 'undergo periodic urological examination, at least every 2 years, for the rest of their lives'. No data were presented, however, to prove that such policies would be predictive of those TCCB destined to become invasive or cause death.

In subsequent studies aspects of the work of Greene *et al.* were supported, specifically patterns of new tumour occurrence, but prognostic groups have recently been further classified. Of those patients with superficial TCCB between 50% and 70% develop new superficial disease after first diagnosis. Of these, only approximately 10% go on to develop progression to a deeper pT category and/or worse grade [20,21].

Up to the year 1978, pT1 was the only histopathological category allowed by the UICC TNM staging system. This sole category included all TCCB infiltrating up to but no deeper than lamina propria (excluding carcinoma *in situ* [CIS]). After this date, pTa, a new UICC histopathological category, was defined which specifically included those tumours that had not invaded and penetrated the basement membrane. Lamina propria, but not bladder muscle, invasion is category pT1 TCCB. A similar classification had originally been proposed by Jewett and Strong in 1946 [20]. There is now much evidence in support of the subdivision of superficial TCCB into pTa and pT1, as an important prognostic factor. Of all superficial TCCB 20–30% are pT1 and up to 80% are pTa.

In 1980, Anderstrom *et al.* [21] reported 5-year mortality rates of 24% in 99 patients with pT1 disease compared to rates of less than 1% in 77 patients with pTa tumours. Prospective studies, reported by Heney *et al.* [8], revealed that 30% of pT1 TCCB patients progressed to muscle infiltration within a median follow-up of 39 months compared to only 4% of pTa TCCB patients progressing within the same median follow-up period.

The studies of Cutler *et al.* [7] revealed that only 3% of pTa patients, compared to 24% of pT1 patients, went on to infiltrate muscle. The muscle infiltrating new-occurrence developed within 12 months of diagnosis in two-thirds of the pT1 patient group. Abel *et al.* [22] reported that, within a 3-year follow-up period, none of the patients with pTa disease developed a new muscle-infiltrating tumour, but 46% of patients presenting with pT1 TCCB did develop such a tumour.

That pTa tumours followed-up for long periods rarely progress has been confirmed in other studies. In a review of 414 cases of grade-1 and -2 pTa TCCB Fitzpatrick *et al.* [23] indicated that, in individual patients, it proved impossible to predict the duration of tumour-free intervals or the development of new tumours, but important prognostic factors were identified. In the first 10 years of follow-up approximately half (45%) of the patients had no new tumour occurrences. Additionally, if the first CC was tumour-free, 79% of patients remained clear over this time period. Conversely, approximately 90% of patients with new occurrences at first CC went on to develop new tumours; these patients had a 35% risk of new occurrence at each future check cystoscopy. It is clear that the detection of a new tumour at the initial CC is of considerable prognostic importance, but a proportion of tumours detected at the first CC may have been missed and remained behind at initial diagnosis. In the 84% of cases where patients had single tumours there was an 80% chance of remaining tumour-free. Only 19 patients (4.5%) developed muscle-infiltrating disease. Regular CC had failed to identify any of these patients before muscle infiltration had already occurred. Of those patients who eventually progressed in pT category, half had never been free of new tumour occurrence at CC. However, 2 had been completely tumour-free for 3 and 8 years, respectively. Detection of new tumours at first CC is also reported by Palmar *et al.* [24] to be a poor prognostic indicator for future tumour development, although, in their studies it was apparently independent of pT category.

In a study of 170 patients followed-up for 1–15 years, describing the rate of new tumour occurrence in pTa disease (excluding dysplasia or CIS) [25], only 3% of participants developed muscle-infiltrating disease. Sixty-two (49%) of 125 patients with solitary tumours at diagnosis stayed tumour-free. Conversely, the prognostic importance of multiple-tumour formation was emphasized by the fact that only 5 of 45 patients (11%) with multiple tumours remained tumour-free. It is worth recording that of the 5 patients who developed muscle-invasive cancer, 3 did so in spite of the fact that they had been followed-up with regular CC. This indicates that regular follow-up only appeared to have been of benefit in two (1%) of the patients in this series (if it is assumed that these 2 patients did not present with interval-symptoms between hospital visits). A zero progression rate for G1pTa TCCB (3% for all pTa TCCB) was reported by Kiemeney et al. [26]. All things considered, however, the aim of accurately defining the risk of progression in individual patients continues to elude us.

The striking difference between the behaviour of grade-3 pT1 and pTa TCCB lesions is revealed in a review by Birch and Harland [27]. In about 40% of cases followed-up between 24 and 106 months, muscle-infiltrating progression occurred [27].

The rate of superficial new occurrence may approach 80% if managed with transurethral resection (TUR) alone [28]. Tumour-free interval was only modestly affected by intravesical agents or radiotherapy and neither had an effect on tumour progression. Independent indicators of a poor prognosis again included multiplicity. In this group of patients the use of cystectomy continues to be controversial [29]. Taking into account whether lamina propria invasion is confined to the stalk (pT1a) or descends beneath it (pT1b) may provide a beneficial subclassification of pT1 TCCB. Using this system a significantly higher rate of progression for pT1b TCCB (53%) compared to pT1a (7%) has been reported by Hasui et al. [30].

From the above data it should be clear that the poor prognosis TCCB of superficial disease emanates almost entirely from patients with pT1 disease.

Technical factors in incorrect TMN classification of superficial bladder cancer

Inadequate surgery that goes unrecognized may be far more common than realized and may explain in part the poorer prognosis of pT1 compared to pTa disease. In a series of 46 patients with pT1 disease [31], surgeons believed, according to the operative report, that they had achieved complete removal of tumour in 40 of the patients. The site of original tumour was re-resected at a second operation, in all patients, 8–14 days later at which time only 13 patients were clinically suspected to have residual disease. However, residual TCCB was detected in 20 (43.5%) of the histological specimens. The extent of the lesions was misjudged even by experienced surgeons. According to Kolozsy [32], improved biopsy techniques that assess adequacy of surgery and reduce such errors are warranted. In some cases of multiple TCCB it is possible that tumours are left behind after initial TUR, resulting in seemingly 'new' occurrences at subsequent CC, another source of error.

Inter- and intra-individual variation in the interpretation of tumour grade by histopathologists in frank TCCB has been reported [33]. Such variation also occurs in the interpretation of pT category [34]. Clearly, even where experienced urologists are concerned, similar variations in the interpretation of clinical T category occur at TUR [31]. However, there is evidence to suggest that this may not be especially important [35]. In a study of the influence of local and review pathology on outcome, Witjes *et al.* [35] conducted a randomized multi-centre study of superficial bladder cancer. Their conclusion was that although review pathology caused substantial changes in the pathology results, the results of treatment remained unchanged and the results of prognostic-factor analysis hardly altered at all.

When interpreting data gathered from routine surgical and pathological practice all of these factors should be taken into account, otherwise they are likely to lead to distortion of the results of clinical as well as academic studies. It seems unlikely that misinterpretation of tumour biopsy results will ever be entirely eliminated, but improvements in training and a systematic approach to tumour biopsy should at least lead to a reduction in such misinterpretation.

Other prognostic indices in superficial bladder cancer

In order that the available resources can be concentrated on the management of those patients at greatest risk, the challenge is to isolate predictors for those superficial tumours that are most likely to progress to muscle infiltration.

Tumours with the best prognosis are solitary at diagnosis. Multifocal urothelial abnormality and an increased rate of new occurrences are indicated by even one additional tumour [23,24]. One of the most useful prognostic indicators for new tumour occurrence and progression is thought to be dysplastic and/or neoplastic changes within seemingly normal-looking urothelium. It is from these sites that new frank tumours may evolve; hence these tumours are not recurrences, but new occurrences. In order to identify cellular dysplasia (field change), random biopsy of macroscopically normal urothelium in all cases of TCCB has been encouraged, particularly where solitary tumours are concerned. Recently, however, this course of management has been challenged. Richards *et al.* [36] detected 'wide variations between different pathologists in the reported incidence of dysplastic change' and 'on second review of the same sections at least 6 months later, pathologists reproduced their own assessment on only 62% of occasions'. The authors concluded that due to the difficulties in defining abnormalities, with both consistency and accuracy, biopsies of cystoscopically normal urothelium may be of no use in influencing therapy.

There is a need to identify other prognostic indicators that are possibly less subjective, for instance failed response to intravesical BCG therapy (such as the detection of persistent pT1 disease within 6 months of initiating treatment [37]) or the presence of new occurrence at first CC [23,24]. In patients failing to respond to intravesical epodyl a 75% risk of the development of muscle-invasive tumours has been reported [38], compared to a 14% risk in complete responders. According to Mulders *et al.* [39], the location of a tumour appears to have a significant influence on new occurrence-free interval with high risk being associated with the presence of at least one TCCB at the prostatic urethra, posterior wall and trigone. Another important prognostic indicator of progression, reported by Crawford [40], is the presence of tumours exceeding 5 cm in size.

Does regular check cystoscopy influence clinical management?

Check cystoscopy allows accurate classification of grade and category of new occurrences and permits their treatment. However, management is often not changed even when adverse prognostic features, that suggest high risk of progression, are detected. For example, for patients with newly diagnosed or new multiple G2/G3 pT1 TCCB, which are high risk and reported to have progression rates greater than 50% [27], further CC may be the only follow-up proposed. Unless management is influenced by the findings, recording the natural history of TCCB in individual patients is valueless.

Perhaps Thompson *et al.* [41] best illustrated this point when they 'identified late invasive recurrence *despite* long-term surveillance for superficial bladder cancer'. The fact that 7 of 20 patients who were tumour-free for 5 years subsequently developed muscle-infiltrating disease was used in support of regular CC despite the clear lack of benefit these regular examinations had brought.

Intravenous urography (IVU): follow-up protocol

The exclusion of both obstructive uropathy and upper-tract TCCB is the underlying rationale for the performance of intravenous urography (IVU) at diagnosis. However, in a retrospective review of a study of routine follow-up IVU, involving 337 patients over 9 years, it was concluded that if the reason for undertaking the study was to exclude upper-tract urothelial tumours it was neither necessary nor cost-effective in patients with bladder tumours [42]. Not one case of unsuspected upper-tract tumour was found in this series. In 250 patients followed up for a median period of 8.7 years [43] only 3 cases of upper-tract TCCB were detected. These authors reported that the IVU findings did not affect prognosis in patients with invasive ureteric disease. Obstruction of the upper-urinary tract was identified in 18 of the 250 participating patients. In a study involving 180 patients who had undergone cystectomy and ileal conduit, it was revealed that of the 10 upper-tract TCCB, developing between 1 and 9 years of follow-up, none was identified using routine urography. In these patients, a diagnosis had been made when they returned for the investigation of new symptoms [44].

The routine use of excretory urography for screening for new upper-tract tumours is not supported by the data from the above studies. Other techniques, including radionuclide renography, have been advocated for detecting upper-urinary tract obstruction [43].

Rationale for present follow-up policies : a summary

The present follow-up policies for superficial TCCB evolved in order to identify and destroy all new tumours as soon as they are detected. They were based on the reasoning that frequent check examinations enabled earlier detection (and that this was important), that pTa and pT1 TCCB behaved in a similar way biologically and that management could (and would) be changed according to the new tumour's characteristics. Whether present FU policies have a significant influence on the natural history of bladder cancer is, however, doubtful and disease progression is not anticipated with sufficient accuracy following regular CC to justify radical therapy when a lesion is still responsive to local treatment.

In the region of 50% of all TCCB (up to 80% of superficial TCCB) are non-invasive (pTa). Those remaining, including pT1, all penetrate the basement membrane. pT1 TCCB comprise about 10% of all TCCB and about 20% of superficial TCCB and are therefore relatively rare. pT1 category disease (particularly those that are G3) are almost entirely responsible for the 10–20% progression rate of superficial tumours. In less than 5% of cases do pTa tumours develop new muscle-infiltrating tumours. Of the patients with muscle-infiltrating TCCB the vast majority (80–90%) have never had tumours passing through a superficial stage in the sense that they were identifiable clinically before invasion occurred. Patients who have low-grade solitary pTa TCCB at diagnosis with no new occurrence at first CC have the best prognosis.

Proposal and rationale for suggested new follow-up protocols

It is proposed that follow-up protocols be rationalized in accordance with the behavioural, histopathological and clinical characteristics of superficial TCCB in individual patients, as discussed above, taking into account co-morbidity and the age of the patient. Further refinements of these follow-up policies should be encouraged by new prognostic indices.

Diagnostic cystoscopy
The most important investigation a patient will undergo is diagnostic TUR and as a result this should only be conducted or supervised by experienced urologists.

The aims are to:
- distinguish solitary or count multiple tumours
- remove tumour(s) completely, including muscle, for assessment of depth of infiltration and for histological diagnosis by resecting:
  exophytic tumour,
  tumour base (to define muscle invasion) and
  resection base (to define tumour clearance)
- biopsy randomly from seemingly normal mucosa
- record sites of tumour and adequacy of resection to aid distinction, at subsequent CC, between inadequate resection, new local occurrences at the site of original tumour(s), and new tumours at new sites (new tumour development should be confirmed only after complete removal of all initially presenting tumours, even if multiple procedures are required) and,
- review histology sections with pathologists and reach a concensus on pT grade and category.

A 'p' category must be assigned since depth of invasion cannot be based on clinical assessment alone [45].

Check cystoscopy: general

Appropriately trained or supervised clinicians should perform this procedure. To confirm the presence of carcinoma or dysplasia, its grade and the pT category, adequate biopsy is required. Adequate biopsy implies taking representative resection samples of new frank tumours with detrusor muscle, as well as additional random biopsies. It is inadequate to perform cystodiathermy alone. Both for prognostic purposes and to ensure that the original tumour is completely removed the initial post-diagnostic cystoscopy is particularly important [23]. Other than this the procedure followed for diagnostic cystoscopy should be used.

pTa tumour(s): follow-up

To confirm adequate resection of the initial TCCB, and/or to identify new occurrences of TCCB, patients should undergo first CC as day-cases at 3–4 months.

Of the patients tumour-free at first check:
1. those who presented with a solitary TCCB should have a CC 12 months later and, if still clear, be considered for discharge. It is extremely unlikely that these patients will have any significant new occurrence.
2. patients who presented with multiple TCCB should undergo subsequent cystoscopy at 12-monthly intervals; because of the greater risk of new tumours this should be continued until 3 tumour-free years have passed at which time discharge is considered.

Genuine new occurrences at first check
These patients require local re-staging as described above. They have a further check at 3–4 months, unless there is progression, when more radical therapy may need to

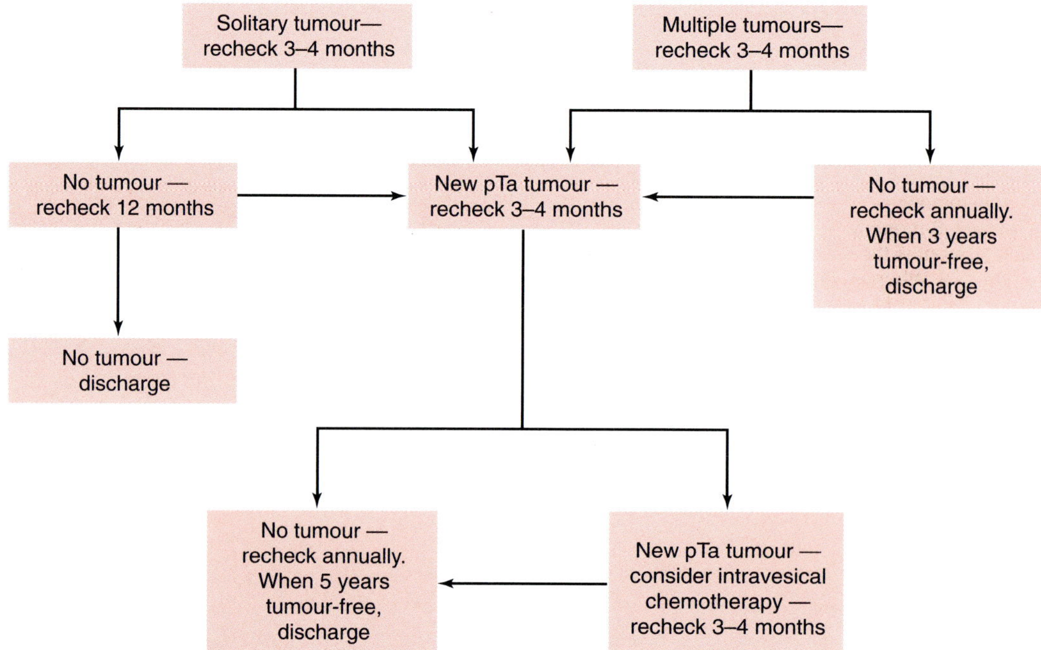

Figure 21.1. Suggested protocol for management of newly diagnosed pTa tumour.

be considered. Then, if tumour-free, patients re-enter a cycle of yearly checks due to the higher risk of new tumours and progression. After 5 tumour-free years discharge may be considered. Although progression will not develop in 95% of these patients, the greatest risk of progression is carried by those patients who are never tumour-free [23].

Additional treatment, such as intravesical chemo- or immunotherapy, is required in cases of multiple new occurrences that are uncontrollable by resection alone. However, there is no definitive evidence that progression is effectively prevented by any of the existing intravesical agents [46].

When discharged, patients need to be advised to return (and their general practitioner informed accordingly) if irritative lower-urinary tract symptoms or haematuria develop; these may indicate further tumour formation.

pT1 tumour(s): follow-up

By definition, these tumours have breached the basement membrane and are thus invasive. If basement-membrane penetration is indicated by histology, but the biopsy contains no muscle or complete resection is believed unlikely, it is important to re-resect within 2–4 weeks. The data from Klan [31] suggest that early re-resection may, in the near future, become routine in all cases of pT1 TCCB. Otherwise, first CC should be performed at 3–4 months if the tumour is moderately or well differentiated.

If the bladder remains clear and random mucosal biopsies are normal, further CC should be performed 6 monthly for the first year and then annually until 5 tumour-free years have passed. Re-staging is mandatory if there are new tumours. Although new pTa tumours are managed as described above, a need for more frequent (3–4 monthly) checks, and the probability that radical therapy may be required, is suggested by persistent pT1 disease.

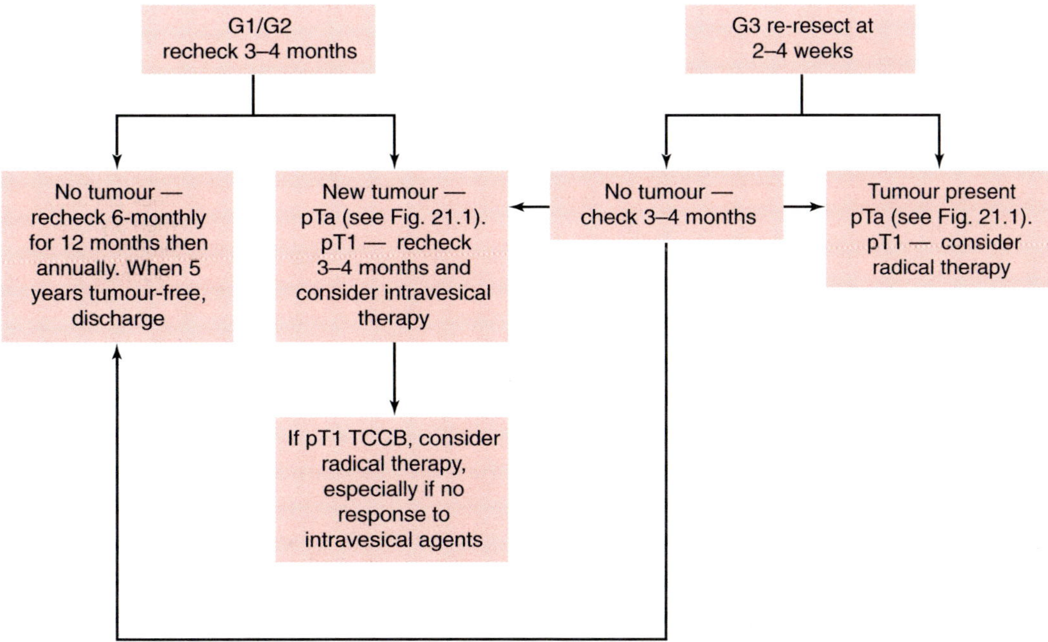

Figure 21.2. Suggested protocol for management of newly diagnosed pT1 tumour.

The superficial TCCB carrying the worst prognosis is that of G3 pT1 TCCB [27]. If the primary tumour is not removed completely and with certainty at first resection or if there is new G3pT1 occurrence or CIS early radical treatment is probably indicated [27]. Initial CC should be conducted within 2–4 weeks and re-resection of previously resected areas should be performed, even if no tumour is apparent [31]. If the patient is clear, CC should be conducted again within 4 months and then at intervals of 6 months for a year followed by examinations once a year until 5 tumour-free years have elapsed.

Consequences of new suggested policies

If these policies are followed, the number of CC in patients with no new occurrences could be reduced by over 50% in the first 2 years after diagnosis and about 40% of patients could be discharged within 3 years of diagnosis. Patients with high risk for progression will remain easily identifiable, due to new occurrences, and monitored accordingly. Resources will be directed more appropriately to those patients most likely to benefit from them. There are likely to be considerable potential savings in costs.

The following illustrates the potential for saving on costs relating to pTa tumours: the pTa category accounts for approximately 50% of bladder TCCB (about 5000 cases in the UK annually) [6] and of these approximately half (2500) never have another new tumour. Using conventional protocols seven CCs in the first 3 years following diagnosis would be required (35 000 cystoscopies); a further 7 CC would be required in the subsequent 7 years (a total of 14 per patient, or a total of 70 000 CC for all pTa cases). If, in at least half of these cases, CC are only performed 3 times in 10 years (that is 7500 CC) then a saving of 27 500 CC in the pTa group will be made. Based on an estimate of cost of £500 per cystoscopy, a projected potential saving of over £13 million over a 10-year period for each year's cohort of patients could potentially be made. Additionally, reduced patient morbidity would represent a corresponding unquantifiable gain. It is, however, unlikely that cash savings of this magnitude would be achieved as the vast majority of hospital costs are fixed [47]. More importantly, urologists would have more time to treat other clinical problems.

Other follow-up strategies

The data of Gulliford *et al.* [48] relating to 240 men (< 75 years) with superficial bladder cancer first diagnosed in 1982, and followed-up for a median period of 6.1 years, support a policy in which efficiency of follow-up for patients with superficial bladder cancer is improved. They suggested dividing patients with different follow-up requirements into groups according to their relative risks of new occurrence and progression. Taking this concept a step further, and basing their suggestions on Medical Research Council studies [24], Hall *et al.* [49] proposed three major prognostic groups, namely good-risk, medium-risk and poor-risk. The first group, comprising 60% of cases, encompasses those patients with solitary TCCB at presentation and no new occurrence at first CC. The medium-risk group, comprising 30% of cases, encompasses those patients who have either multiple TCCB at diagnosis, and who are tumour-free at first CC, or have solitary TCCB with new occurrence at the first CC.

The final group, comprising 10% of cases, includes those patients having multiple TCCB at presentation and new occurrence at first CC. The prognostic group determines the intensity and duration of follow-up and this varies between groups. That all patients receive intravesical agents after diagnostic resection, as this decreases the new occurrence rate, was an additional recommendation made by the authors. However, although up to one-half of patients may benefit from intravesical agents, the risks to the remaining half, who do not require further therapy, need to be considered as well, however small the morbidity may be. These criteria proved straightforward when subsequently applied to routine clinical practice using retrospective data [50]. However, the necessity for caution was emphasized by the fact that of the 127 group-1 patients studied 46% did develop new occurrence within 3 years. Morris *et al.*'s [51] key finding was that of patients with superficial bladder cancer who had been tumour-free for a period of more than 2 years, none developed invasive new occurrence. However, despite such evidence the authors' conclude that 'some form of follow-up' and perhaps 'alternative methods of assessment' are 'desirable'. This is presumably for an indefinite period of time but without giving any evidence of benefit. Conclusions such as this can only cause confusion; TCCB of clinical importance were not identified by these authors and it is not at all clear why in the face of the evidence of their own data, clinicians continue to advocate follow-up policies that appear to have been based on flimsy evidence.

Summary of data and recommendations

- None of the currently used follow-up policies, for patients with superficial TCCB, can be said to be superior to the other on the basis of the scientific evidence available. However, that frequency and period of follow-up may safely be reduced is suggested by studying the literature. Rationalization and review of follow-up policies is needed, but without new policies gaining general and widespread support consideration will need to be given to the medico-legal implications.
- pTa and pT1 TCCB have to be distinguished and clearly differentiated. The blanket term 'superficial' must be abandoned. For clarity, it would be best if only the pT category were used. However, if other descriptions must be used, suitable terms might be 'superficially invasive' for pT1 cases and 'noninvasive' for pTa TCCB.
- In order for classification to be accurate, adequate biopsy, including muscle, is needed at every stage of diagnosis and follow-up. Recognition of the limitations of histopathologists in interpreting grade/pT category, and the limitations of clinicians performing inadequate resections and under-staging, is essential. It may become mandatory to perform early resection (at 2–3 weeks) in patients with pT1 disease and review tumour sections, in joint histology meetings, before the most appropriate management is decided upon. Histopathologists and urologists with the appropriate training are required.
- The term 'recurrences' refers to the development of either a new tumour at the same location as a previously completely resected tumour or residual disease at the site of the original tumour(s) (this suggests incomplete resection). The term recurrence is misleading when misapplied and another term such as 'new occurrences' [52] should be coined to indicate areas of new disease.

- A more important end-point than new pTa occurrence is progression and this is the case for both the management and prognosis of the individual patient (although as a prognostic indicator for developing progression new occurrence may be useful). Progression should be taken to mean:

    new tumours at a deeper pT category and/or

    de-differentiation to a poorer grade and/or

    metastases.

- In order to stop traditional practices prevailing, well organized, prospective, controlled studies of superficial TCCB are required to address the above points.

Finally, much of this chapter is concerned with the measures of outcome that are disease-based (new tumour occurrence/progression) rather than patient based (e.g. quality and duration of survival). Some patients, such as those who have had many CC but no new tumours, may believe that their treatment was worse than the disease. Studies of patient based outcome measures are warranted.

References

1 U.I.C.C.. *TMN classification of malignant tumours.* 3rd ed. Geneva: Union Internationale Contre le Cancer, 1978.

2 Whitmore WF. Toward the rationale management of bladder cancer: an overview. *Urology* 1988; **31**(Suppl.): 5–8.

3 Smith R. Where is the wisdom? *BMJ* 1991; **303**: 798–9.

4 Tolley DA, Hargreave TB, Smith PH *et al.* Effect of intravesical mitomycin C on recurrence of newly diagnosed superficial bladder cancer. *BMJ* 1988; **296**: 1759–61.

5 Flamm J. The value of tumour-associated tissue inflammatory reaction in primary superficial bladder cancer. *Urol Res* 1990; **18**: 113–17.

6 Office of Population Censuses and Surveys, Cancer Statistics Registration. *Cases of diagnosed cancer registered in England and Wales, 1985.* Series MBI, No 18. London: H.M.S.O., 1990.

7 Cutler SJ, Heney NM and Friedell GH. Longitudinal study of patients with bladder cancer: factors associated with disease recurrence and progression. In: *Bladder Cancer,* A.U.A. Monographs Vol 1. Eds. Bonney WW and Prout GR. Baltimore: Williams and Wilkins, 1982.

8 Heney NM, Ahmed S, Flanagan MJ *et al.* Superficial bladder cancer: progression and recurrence. *J Urol* 1983; **130**: 1083–6.

9 Friedell GH, Jacobs JB, Nagy GK. The pathogenesis of bladder cancer. *Am J Path* 1977; **89**: 431–42.

10 Skinner DG. Current state of classification and staging of bladder cancer. *Cancer Res* 1977; **37**: 2838–42.

11 Prout GR, Griffin PP and Shipley WU. Bladder carcinoma as a systemic disease. *Cancer* 1979; **43**: 2532–9.

12 Droller MJ. Transitional cell cancer: upper tracts and bladder. In: *Campbell's Urology.* Eds. P.C. Walsh RF, Gittes AD, Perlmutter and T.A. Stamey. New York: W.B. Saunders, 1986.

13 Brawn PN. The origin of invasive carcinoma of the bladder. *Cancer* 1982; **50**: 515–19.

14 Kaye KW and Lange PH. Mode of presentation of invasive bladder cancer: reassessment of the problem. *J Urol* 1982; **128**: 31–3.

15 Newman LH, Tannenbaum M and Droller MJ. Muscle-invasive bladder cancer: does it arise de novo or from pre-existing superficial disease? *Urology* 1988; **32**: 58–62.

16 Mommsen S, Aagaard J, Sell A. Presenting symptoms, treatment delay and survival in bladder cancer. *Scand J Urol Nephrol* 1983; **17**: 163–7.

17 Bishop MC. The dangers of a long urological waiting list. *Br J Urol* 1990; **65**: 433–40.

18 Gulliford M, Petruckevitch A and Burney P. Survival with bladder cancer: associations of treatment delay, type of surgeon and modality of treatment. *BMJ* 1991; **303**: 437–40.

19 Greene LF, Hanash KA, Farrow GM. Benign papilloma or papillary carcinoma of the bladder? *J Urol* 1973; **110**: 205–7.

20 Jewett HJ and Strong GH. Infiltrating carcinoma of the bladder: relation of depth of penetration of the bladder wall to incidence of local extension and metastasis. *J Urol* 1946; **55**: 366–72.

21 Anderstrom C, Johansson S, Nilsson S. The significance of lamina propria invasion on the prognosis of patients with bladder tumours. *J Urol* 1980; **124**: 23–6.

22 Abel PD, Hall RR, Williams G. Should pT1 transitional cell cancers of the bladder still be classified as superficial? *Br J Urol* 1988; **62**: 235 9.

23 Fitzpatrick JM, West AB, Butler MR *et al.* Superficial bladder tumours (stage pTa, grades 1 and 2): the importance of recurrence pattern following initial resection. *J Urol* 1986; **135**: 920–2.

24 Parmar MKB, Freedman LS, Hargreave TB *et al.* Prognostic factors for recurrence and follow-up policies in the treatment of superficial bladder cancer. *J Urol* 1989; **142**: 284–8.

25 Morgan JDT, Bowsher W, Griffiths DFR *et al.* Rationalisation of follow-up in patients with non-invasive bladder tumours. *Br J Urol* 1991; **67**: 158–61.

26 Kiemeney LALM, Witjes JA, Heijbroek RP *et al.* Predictability of recurrent and progressive disease in individual patients with primary superficial bladder cancer. *J Urol* 1993; **150**: 60–4.

27 Birch BRP, Harland SJ. The pT1 G3 bladder tumour. *Br J Urol* 1989; **64**: 109–16.

28 Mulders PFA, Hoekstra WJ, Heybroek RPM *et al.* Prognosis and treatment of T1G3 bladder tumours. A prognostic factor analysis of 121 patients. *Eur J Cancer* 1994; **30A**: 914–17.

29 Harland SJ. Aggressive superficial bladder cancer. *Eur J Cancer* 1994; **30A**: 899–900.

30 Hasui Y, Osada Y, Kitada S *et al.* Significance of invasion to the muscularis mucosae on the progression of bladder cancer. *Urology* 1994; **43**: 782–6.

31 Klan R, Loy V and Huland H. Residual tumour discovered in routine second transurethral resection in patients with stage T1 transitional cell carcinoma of the bladder. *J Urol* 1991; **46**: 316–18.

32 Kolozsy Z. Histopathological "self control" in transurethral resection of bladder tumours. *Br J Urol* 1991; **67**: 162–4.

33 Ooms ECM, Anderson WAD, Alons CL *et al.* Analysis of the performance of pathologists in the grading of bladder tumours. *Hum Path* 1983; **14**: 140–3.

34 Abel PD, Henderson D, Bennett MK *et al.* Differing interpretations by pathologists of the pT category and grade of transitional cell cancer of the bladder. *Br J Urol* 1988; **62**: 339–42.

35 Witjes JA, Kiemeney LALM, Schaafsma HE *et al.* The influence of review pathology on study outcome of a randomised multicentre superficial bladder cancer trial. *Br J Urol* 1994; **73**: 172–6.

36 Richards B, Parmar MKB, Anderson CK *et al.* Interpretation of biopsies of "normal" urothelium in patients with superficial bladder cancer. *Br J Urol* 1991; **67**: 369–75.

37 Herr HW, Badalament RA, Amato DA *et al.* Superficial bladder cancer treated with bacillus Calmette-Guerin: a multivariate analysis of factors affecting tumour progression. *J Urol* 1989; **141**: 22–9.

38 Mufti GR, Virdi JS, and Hall MH. Long-term follow-up of intravesical epodyl therapy for superficial bladder cancer. *Br J Urol* 1990; **65**: 32–25.

39 Mulders PFA, v.d.Meyden APM, Doesburg WH *et al.* Prognostic factors in pTa-pT1 superficial bladder tumours treated with intravesical installations. *Br J Urol* 1994; **73**: 403–8.

40 Crawford ED. Recent advances in treatment of superficial bladder cancer. *Urology* 1992; **40** (Suppl.): 2–7.

41 Thompson RA, Campbell EW, Kramer HC *et al.* Late invasive recurrence despite long-term surveillance for superficial bladder cancer. *J Urol* 1993; **149**: 1010–11.

42 Walzer Y and Soloway MS. Should the follow-up of patients with bladder cancer include routine excretory urography? *J Urol* 1983; **130**: 672–3.

43 Booth CM, Kellett MJ. Intravenous urography in the follow-up of carcinoma of the bladder. *Br J Urol* 1981; **53**: 246–9.

44 Hastie KJ, Hamdy FC, Collins MC *et al.* Upper tract tumours following cystectomy for bladder cancer. Is routine intravenous urography worthwhile? *Br J Urol* 1991; **67**: 29–31

45 Chisholm GD, Hindmarsh JR, Howatson AG *et al.* TMN (1978) in bladder cancer: use and abuse. *Br J Urol* 1980; **52**: 500–5.

46 Newling D. Intravesical therapy in the management of superficial transitional cell carcinoma of the bladder: the experience of the EORTC GU group. *Br J Cancer* 1990; **61**: 497–9.

47 Beech R, Larkinson J. Estimating the financial savings from maintaining the level of acute services with fewer hospital beds. *Int J Health Planning Management* 1990; **5** :89–103.

48 Gulliford M, Petruckevitch A and Berney P. Can efficiency of follow-up for superficial bladder cancer be increased? *Annals RCS Eng* 1993; **75**: 57–61.

49 Hall RR, Parmar MKB, Richards AB *et al.* Proposal for changes in cystoscopic follow-up of patients with bladder cancer and adjuvant intravesical chemotherapy. *BMJ* 1994; **308**: 257–60.

50 Reading J, Hall RR, Parmar MKB. The application of prognostic factor analysis for Ta,T1 bladder cancer in routine urological practice. *Br J Urol* 1995; **75**: 604–7.

51 Morris SB, Gordon EM, Shearer RJ *et al.* Superficial bladder cancer: for how long should a tumour-free patient have check cystoscopies? *Br J Urol* 1995; **75**: 193–6.

52 Soloway MS. Rationale for intensive intravesical chemotherapy for superficial bladder cancer. *J Urol* 1980; **123**: 461–6.

CHAPTER 22

Satisfaction with life during BCG therapy

A. Böhle, F. Balck, J. von Wietersheim
and D. Jocham

Introduction

Intravesical therapy of recurrent superficial bladder carcinoma with bacillus Calmette–Guérin (BCG) is clinically established and is considered to be highly effective [1,2,3]. However, this treatment is associated with a high rate of side-effects, such as dysuria, burning and bladder spasms [4]. Severe systemic complications are rare [5].

Traditionally, the objectives for successful cancer therapy are 'hard' data, such as freedom from recurrence and progression rate or survival. 'Soft' data, such as the subjective wellbeing of the patient or his or her 'quality of life' have only recently been recognized in oncological therapy [6,7] However, most of these data relate to advanced carcinomas. Today, quality of life is defined operationally and includes several domains of daily life, such as functional status, psychological strain, social interaction, sexuality and body image, symptoms of disease, side-effects and satisfaction with medical therapy [8]. Therefore, the evaluation of such a construct as 'quality of life' is complex. However, the assessment of the general quality of life is usually of minor value to the physician if, by specific questions, it does not also deal with the very special situation of the patient with regard to disease, surgery or chemotherapy. Therefore, a modular approach has been suggested [9,10] in which a general assessment of the quality of life is combined with questions on the particular disease or therapy. A specific instrument for this purpose needs to be constructed for each disease and therapeutic entity.

In order to clarify whether the distressing local symptoms of intravesical BCG immunotherapy influence the patient's quality of life, this aspect was prospectively examined, together with the side-effects in patients receiving BCG. This survey provides insight into the specific wellbeing of patients receiving intravesical therapy for superficial bladder carcinoma.

Methods

During this pilot study 30 patients with superficial urethelial bladder carcinoma at stages pTa–pT1, G1–G3 were examined. The average age of patients was 67 ± 11.4 years; 5 women and 25 men were treated. Informed consent was obtained from the patients for every treatment procedure. Intravesical therapy with BCG was commenced 14–21 days after the last transurethral resection (TUR) of the bladder tumour. BCG (8.1 mg), strain Connaught (Immucyst®, Cytochemia, Germany), was dissolved in 50 ml saline and instilled intravesically with a 12 French catheter. Instillations were performed regularly between 8.00–9.00 a.m. in the hospital. Patients were asked to drink large quantities of fluid and to avoid physical activity on the day of the instillation. Six instillations were given at weekly intervals; no maintenance therapy was performed in these patients.

Examination of the quality of life

The quality of life in patients was documented with a clinically valid and standardized [10] questionnaire, derived from the Münchner Lebensqualitäts Dimensionen Liste (MLDL) [11]. A comparable method was also used by the European Organization for Research and Treatment of Cancer (EORTC) in the assessment of the quality of life in patients with bronchial carcinoma [9]. Previous studies on the MLDL had shown a satisfactory discriminant and convergent validity, together with a rather high internal consistency of this instrument [10,11]. Our quality-of-life questionnaire consisted of two parts. In the first part, the satisfaction with different aspects of life was assessed. These aspects were general wellbeing (including physical and mental state, energy, and health in general), work (including business or domestic work, financial situation, leisure activities, independence in everyday life, and everyday life in general), illness (including coping with disease, abilities, self-esteem, and person in general), family (including everyday life with partner, sexual activity, family, and position in family), friends and social contacts (including contact and number of friends and acquaintances, contact with other people, and medical treatment). The answers were graded on a 5-point scale as 'very satisfied' to 'very dissatisfied'. From these 21 items a total score was reached by transforming the sum of the scores into a scale ranging from 0 (highest dissatisfaction) to 100 (highest satisfaction with life).

The second part of the quality-of-life questionnaire consisted of six additional items, which were analysed separately. In these, the degree to which patients were affected by their complaints, the impairment of mood by the health situation, the degree of dissatisfaction with life because of the health situation, a general rating of the physical situation and a general rating of the quality of life were assessed. The quality-of-life questionnaire was given to the patients three times: Questionnaire-1 recorded the 2-week time period *prior* to onset of BCG therapy and was issued to the patient on the day of discharge from hospital subsequent to TUR. In the quality-of-life questionnaire-2, the 6-week period *during* intravesical BCG treatment was evaluated, with patients receiving the questionnaire subsequent to the six intravesical instillations. Quality-of-life questionnaire-3 analysed the 6-week period following therapy and was issued to the patient at the 3-monthly follow-up examination (6 weeks after the last BCG instillation, i.e. approximately 3 months subsequent to TUR). The patients were asked to complete the questionnaires themselves. The quality-of-life questionnaires were usually completed within 5–10 minutes.

Analysis of side-effects

Side-effects of intravesical therapy were assessed by a questionnaire, which had been used previously in another clinical study, on BCG-related symptoms in patients with vesico-ureteral reflux [12]. This questionnaire contains eight items. Patients were requested to indicate their frequency of micturition during the day and night, and to indicate the occurrence of further typical symptoms (i.e. dysuria, haematuria, secretion of mucus, nausea, fatigue, chills, joint pain, fever) during the 6-weekly course of instillation. Furthermore, the patients were asked to give a subjective assessment of the severity of these side-effects on a 4-point scale, ranging from: mild, moderate to severe and extremely severe. In an open question the patients were able to report on special symptoms which had not been mentioned in the questionnaire. The time necessary for completion of the side-effects questionnaire was 2–3 minutes. With each instillation the patients received seven side-effects questionnaire, i.e. a total of 42 for the whole course of treatment. The questionnaires were completed daily. Thus, 1260 side-effects questionnaires were in circulation.

In order to establish a synoptic presentation, all side-effects were summarized in an index. For this purpose, data were summarized into three values per week, day 1 (instillation) and day 2, days 3–4 and days 5–7 were summarized, respectively.

Statistics

Analysis of the data on the quality-of-life items showed no significant difference from the normal distribution, so parametric statistical evaluations were suitable. For the comparison of the quality-of-life scores at different periods the analysis of variance with repeated measurement design (MANOVA) was used. Data of the side-effects questionnaire were not normally distributed, therefore, non-parametric statistics were used. Different periods were analysed using the Friedman test. Correlations between items of the quality-of-life questionnaires and the side-effects questionnaires were calculated by means of the Spearman rank-correlation coefficient. The calculations were performed on a personal computer utilizing the SPSS®/Windows program.

Results

All patients returned their quality-of-life questionnaires and the response rate was calculated at 100%. The evaluation for the side-effects questionnaires after termination of the study showed that 36 questionnaires had not been received or were returned blank. The returned fraction of side-effects questionnaires was calculated at 97% (Table 22.1).

Table 22.1 Return quota of the quality of life and side-effects questionnaires.

	LEZU-questionnaire	NW-questionnaire
Expected (n)	90	1,260
Received (n)	90	1,224
Return quota	100%	97%

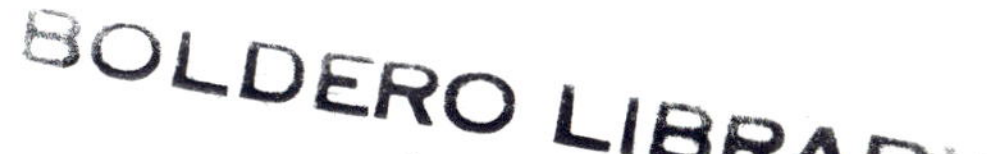

General satisfaction with life

In the patients examined, a relatively high total score of satisfaction with life at a median of 84 points could be demonstrated; this is comparable to satisfaction with life in the normal population [13]. Statistical analysis did not show any difference between the three periods — before, during and after BCG therapy (Fig. 22.1). Thus, intravesical BCG therapy was not found to have a significant influence on general satisfaction with life.

The subjective assessment of state of health was rated by the patients; the mean rating was 4.8 points (Fig. 22.2). On a further 7-point scale, asking for the subjective

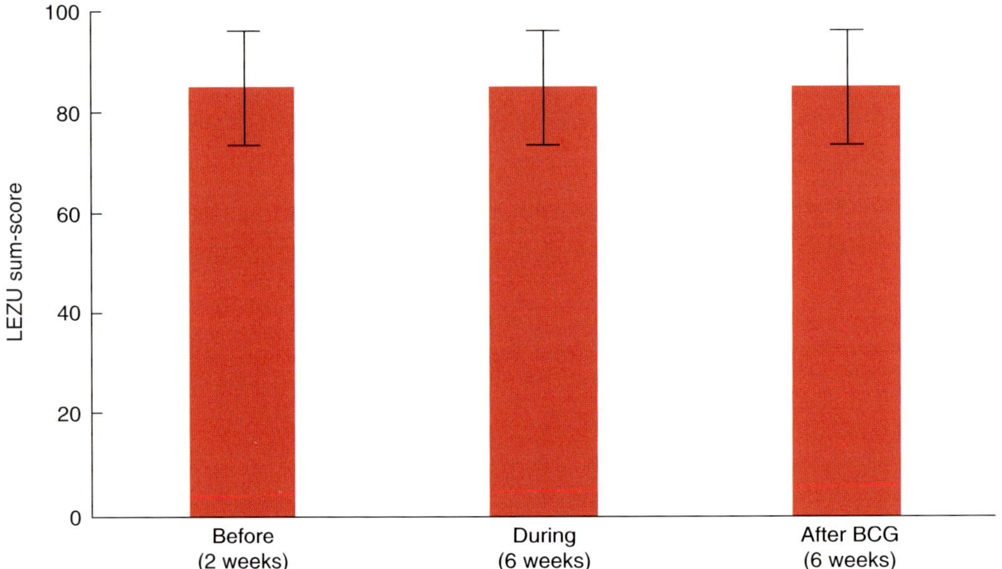

Figure 22.1. 'General Satisfaction with Life' calculated from 21 questions in the LEZU-questionnaires on three periods of interest, prior to, during and after intravesical BCG therapy.

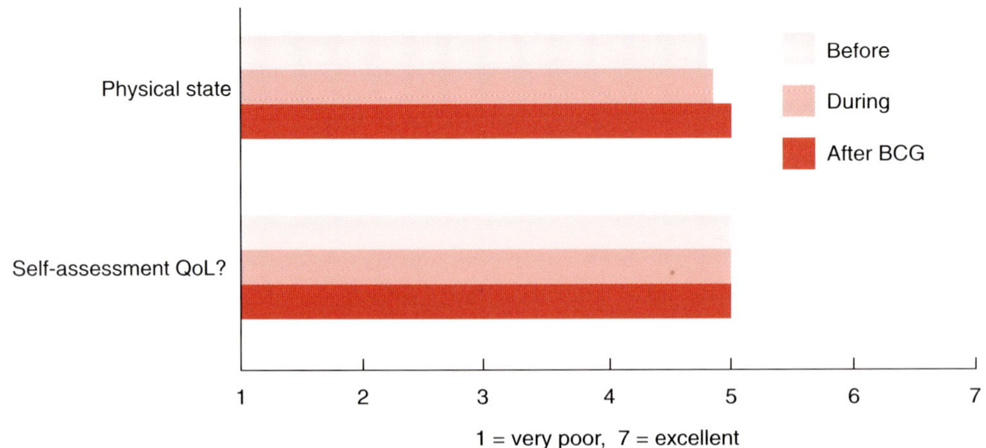

Figure 22.2. Results of supplementary questions on the performance and on the quality of life on the LEZU-questionnaire prior to, during and after BCG therapy. (How would you assess your general physical state during the last 6 weeks? In all, how would you assess the quality of life during the last 6 weeks?).

assessment on the patient's quality of life, patients rated themselves at a median of 5. Neither of the questionnaires revealed a significant difference between the three periods of interest.

Assessment of side-effects

By means of the daily assessment of side-effects, the course of the clinically known symptoms of intravesical BCG therapy could very well be observed and documented. After the first instillation only a small number of patients indicated dysuric symptoms. This ratio, however, increased to approximately 60% of patients during the course of the following instillations. The frequency of micturition during the day and night also decreased (Figs. 22.3 and 22.4); on the day of treatment, micturition showed the

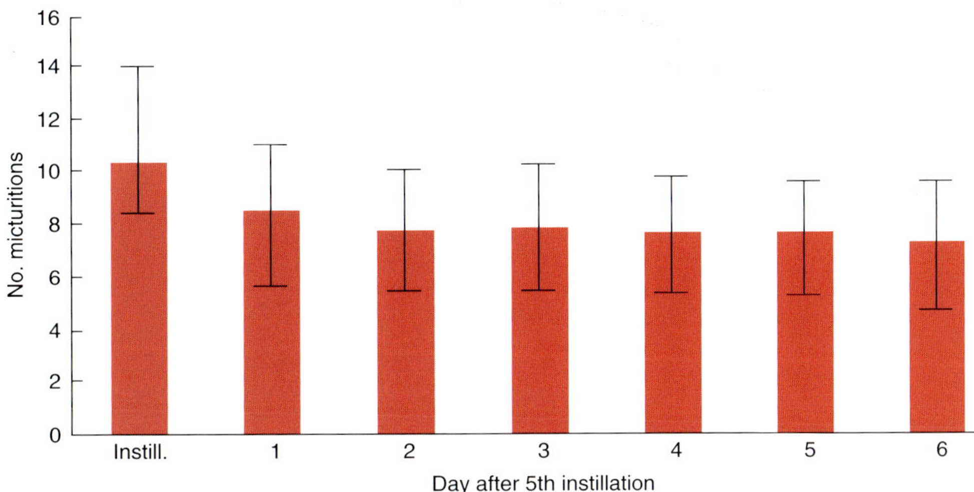

Figure 22.3. Daily frequency of micturition in the 5th week of instillation. The highest frequency of micturition is seen on the day of instillation.

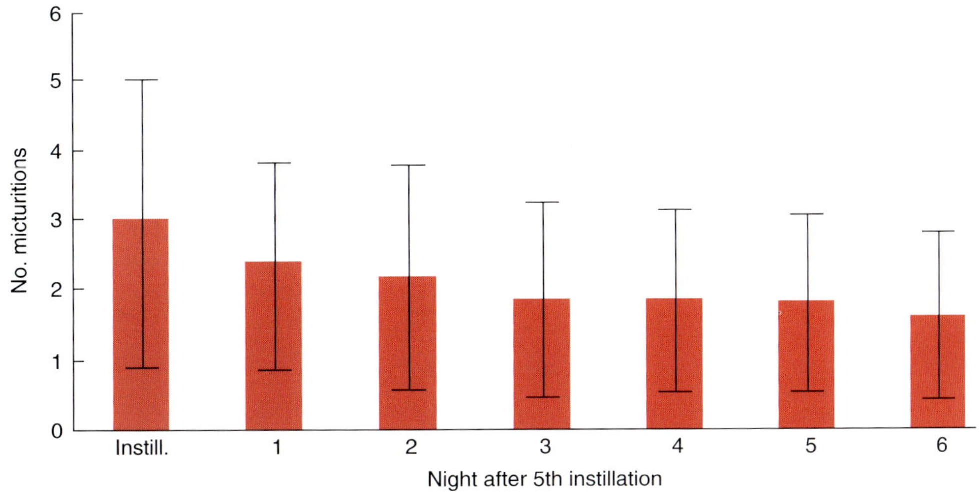

Figure 22.4. Nocturnal frequency of micturition in the 5th instillation week. Similar course of symptoms as in Figure 22.3. Highest frequency of micturition immediately after the instillation.

highest frequency (mean during day = 10 times, during the night = 3 times), whereas, on the following days, the frequency of micturition significantly decreased. The mean frequency of micturition increased steadily during the 6-week course of instillation (Fig. 22.5).

The mean rating of the subjective evaluation of the side-effects during the course of instillation was 'moderate'. The evaluation 'too severe' was never indicated by a patient during the treatment course (Fig. 22.6).

By reducing the side-effects rating to three measurements per week, the typical course of the symptoms after instillation could be quantitatively assessed, showing increased side-effects on the first 2 days with a decrease in symptoms thereafter.

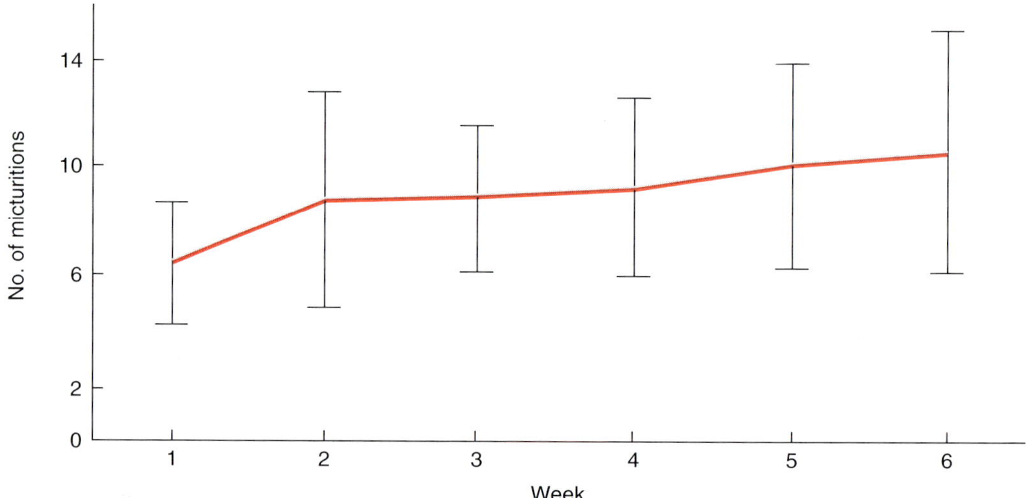

Figure 22.5. Mean daily frequency of micturition during the 6-week instillation course.

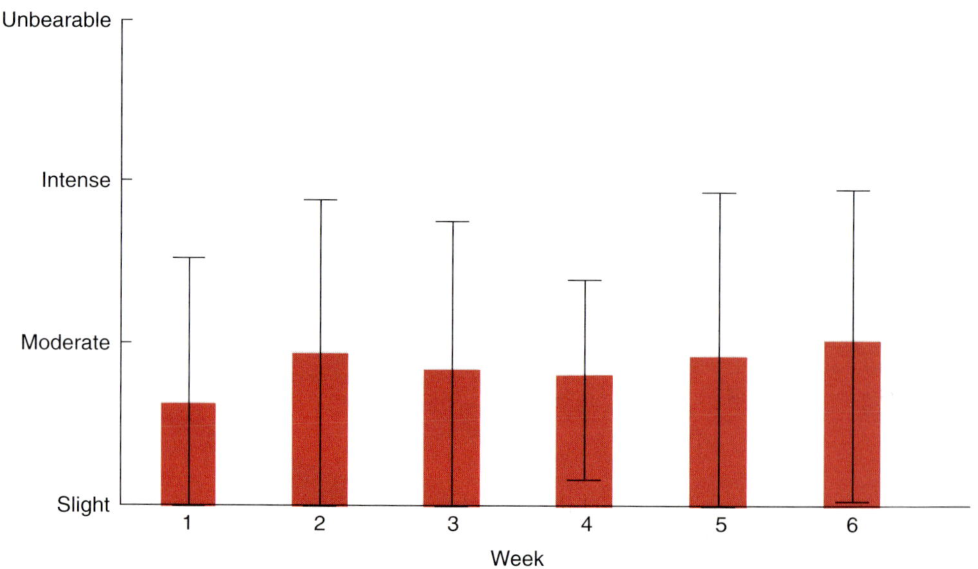

Figure 22.6. Mean values per week of daily subjective assessment of symptoms on the side-effects questionnaire (the complaints were classified from poor to too intense).

During the final week of treatment, again, the total score of side-effects was increased without a tendency to regress.

Discussion

The principles of assessment of quality of life by a modular approach, consisting of a 'general' and a 'special' part, were adhered to in our pilot study. The domains of the 'General Satisfaction with Life' were assessed psychometrically before, during and after therapy [14]. The specific situation of 'local intravesical therapy', on the other hand, was taken into account by the frequent use of the side-effects questionnaire. The results argue in favour of the applicability of this concept in studies on superficial carcinoma of the bladder.

A good acceptance of the survey by the patients could be observed, as demonstrated by the high response rate to the quality-of-life questionnaire as well as to the side-effects questionnaires. During intravesical treatment with repeated instillations and a resultant increase in side-effects, daily questioning seems necessary. The possibility of establishing a side-effects index, in which these daily-assessed data are reduced to summarized scores of longer periods, offers the opportunity of comparing different therapy regimes and therapeutic schedules [15,16]. Therefore, this approach is suggested for further multicentric comparative trials of superficial bladder cancer.

In general, the assessment of the quality of life in the form presented was well suited to the situation of patients with superficial bladder carcinoma. Obviously, the therapy-induced side-effects were not so pronounced, as to impair satisfaction with life. In this pilot study, a rather low incidence of side-effects as compared to more extensive Phase III studies was detectable [17–19]. A reason for the high degree of satisfaction with life in the patient group analysed, may be the good prognosis of the disease and the prospects of contributing to therapy by co-operation. Therefore, assessment of satisfaction with life can be expected to increase the compliance of patients in further trials [20].

In conclusion, in this survey on intravesical BCG therapy against superficial bladder carcinoma recurrences, it could be shown that a prospective assessment of the quality of life and of the local symptoms of intravesical therapy is a satisfactory approach to gain knowledge on the well-being of this special patient group. Such knowledge could contribute to the development of further clinical studies and to the improvement of intravesical therapy.

References

1   Lamm DL, Crawford ED, Blumenstein BA *et al.* SWOG 8795: a randomized comparison of bacillus Calmette–Guérin and Mitomycin C prophylaxis in stage Ta and T1 transitional cell carcinoma of the bladder. *J Urol* 1993; **149**: 282A.

2   Lamm DL. Carcinoma *in situ. Urol Clin N Am* 1992; **19**: 499–508.

3   Lamm DL. Long-term results of intravesical therapy for superficial bladder cancer. *Urol Clin N Am* 1992; **19**: 573–80.

4   Lamm DL. Complications of bacillus Calmette–Guérin immunotherapy. *Urol Clin N Am* 1992; **19**: 565–72.

5   Lamm DL, Stogdill VD, Stogdill BJ, Crispen RG. Complications of bacillus Calmette–Guérin immunotherapy in 1278 patients with bladder cancer. *J Urol* 1986; **135**: 1352–4.

6   Fossa SD, Aaronson NK, Calais da Silva F *et al*. Quality of life in patients with muscle-infiltrating bladder cancer and hormone-resistant prostatic cancer. *Eur Urol* 1989; **16**: 335–9.

7   Aaronson NK, Bullinger M, Ahmedzai S. A modular approach to quality of life assessment in cancer clinical trials. *Rec Results Cancer Res* 1988; **111**: 231–49.

8   Aaronson NK, Calais da Silva F, Yoshida O *et al*. Quality of life assessment in bladder cancer clinical trials: conceptual, methodological and practical issues. *Prog Clin Biol Res* 1986; **221**: 149–70.

9   Aaronson NK, Bullinger M, Ahmedzai S. A modular approach to quality-of-life assessment in cancer clinical trials. In: Scheurlen H, Kay R, Baum M (eds) *Cancer clinical trials: a critical appraisal*. Berlin: Springer-Verlag, 1988; 231–49.

10   Heinisch M, Ludwig M, Bullinger M. Psychometrische Testung der Münchner Lebensqualitäts Dimensionen Liste (MLDL). In: Bullinger M, Ludwig M, v. Steinbüchel N (eds) *Lebensqualität bei kardiovaskulären Erkrankungen*. Göttingen: Hogrefe, 1991; 73–90.

11   Bullinger M. Forschungsinstrumente zur Erfassung der Lebensqualität bei Krebs — ein Überblick. In: Verres R, Hasenbring M (eds) *Jahrbuch der Medizinischen Psychologie III. Psychosoziale Onkologie*. Berlin: Springer-Verlag, 1989; 45–57.

12   Böhle A, Schüller J, Knipper A, Hofstetter AG. Bacillus Calmette–Guérin treatment and vesicorenal reflux. *Eur Urol* 1990; **17**: 125–8.

13   Glatzer W, Zapf W (eds) *Lebensqualität in der BRD*. 'Objektive Lebensbedingungen und subjektives Wohlbefinden'. Frankfurt/Main: Campus Verlag, 1984.

14   Moinpour CM, Feigl P, Metch B *et al*. Quality of life end points in cancer clinical trials: review and recommendations. *J Natl Cancer Inst* 1989; **81**: 485–95.

15   Nordstroem G, Nyman CR, Theorell T. Psychosocial adjustment and general state of health in patients with ileal conduit urinary diversion. *Scand J Urol Nephrol* 1992; **26**: 139–47.

16   Raghavan D, Grundy R, Lancaster L. Assessment of quality of life in long-term survivors treated by first-line intravenous cisplatin for invasive bladder cancer. *Prog Clin Biol Res* 1988; **260**: 625–31.

17   Mansson A, Johnson G, Mansson W. Quality of life after cystectomy. Comparison between patients with conduit and those with continent caecal reservoir urinary diversion. *Br J Urol* 1988; **62**: 240–5.

18   Witjes JA, v.d. Meijden APM, Witjes WPJ *et al*. A randomised prospective study comparing intravesical instillations of Mitomycin-C, BCG-Tice, and BCG-RIVM in pTa–pT1 tumours and primary carcinoma *in situ* of the urinary bladder. *Eur J Cancer* 1993; **29A**: 1672–6.

19   Richardson JL, Marks G, Levine A. The influence of symptoms of disease and side effects of treatment on compliance with cancer therapy. *J Clin Oncol* 1988; **6**: 1746–52.

20   Yancik R, Edwards BK, Yates JW. Assessing the quality of life of cancer patients: practical issues in study implementation. *J Psychosoc Oncol* 1989; **7**: 59–74.